Cryotherapy in Sport Injury Management

Kenneth L. Knight, PhD, ATC
Indiana State University

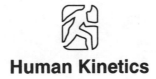

Human Kinetics

To John H.P. Maley of the Chattanooga Corporation,
for his many contributions to physical medicine.

Library of Congress Cataloging-In-Publication Data

Knight, Kenneth L.
    Cryotherapy in sport injury management / Kenneth L. Knight.
        p.   cm.
    Includes bibliographical references and index.
    ISBN 0-87322-771-9 (paper). -- ISBN 0-87322-894-4 (book & VHS
video). -- ISBN 0-87322-895-2 (book & PAL video)
    1. Sports injuries--Cryotherapy.   I. Title.
    [DNLM: 1. Cryotherapy. 2. Athletic Injuries--therapy.   QT 261
K69c   1995]
RD97.K65   1995
617.1'06329--dc20
DNLM/DLC
for Library of Congress   95-18201
                                                                        CIP

ISBN: 0-87322-771-9 (book); 0-87322-894-4 (book and video VHS package);
0-87322-895-2 (book and video PAL package)

Copyright © 1995 by Kenneth L. Knight

Permission notices for material printed in this book from other sources can be found on pages 300-301.

Developmental Editor: Christine Drews; **Assistant Editors:** Dawn Roselund and John Wentworth; **Editorial Assistants:** Jennifer Hemphill and Alecia Mapes Walk; **Copyeditor:** Jay Thomas; **Proofreader:** Dawn Barker; **Typesetting and Text Layout:** Angela K. Snyder; **Text Designer:** Judy Henderson; **Paste-Up:** Denise Lowry and Tara Welsch; **Cover Designer:** Jack Davis; **Photographer (cover):** Chris Brown; **Photographer (interior):** Paul Hightower, PhD; **Medical Illustrator:** Beth Young; **Mac Illustrator:** Studio 2D; **Printer:** United Graphics

Printed in the United States of America

10   9   8   7   6   5   4   3   2   1

Human Kinetics
P.O. Box 5076, Champaign, IL 61825-5076
1-800-747-4457

Canada: Human Kinetics, Box 24040,
Windsor, ON N8Y 4Y9
1-800-465-7301 (in Canada only)

Europe: Human Kinetics,
P.O. Box IW14, Leeds LS16 6TR, United Kingdom
(44) 1132 781708

Australia: Human Kinetics,
2 Ingrid Street, Clapham 5062, South Australia
(08) 371 3755

New Zealand: Human Kinetics, P.O. Box 105-231, Auckland 1
(09) 523 3462

Contents

Preface

Cryotherapy—the use of cold—is one of the most inexpensive and widely used therapeutic modalities for treating and rehabilitating acute sport injuries. Even so, its use is hindered because of confusion concerning why, when, and how to apply its various techniques.

Ever since I was introduced in 1967 to cryokinetics for injury rehabilitation, I have had a fascination, bordering on obsession at times, with trying to understand cryotherapy and improve my ability to use this modality. For over 20 years I used various cryotherapeutic techniques almost daily in working with athletic teams at four colleges and universities. Most of my scholarly work during the past 20-plus years has been devoted to researching and writing about cryotherapy.

In *Cryotherapy*, the precursor to this book, I attempted to summarize the vast research and literature on the topic. In this book, I have updated the science, expanded the book from 15 to 21 chapters, and extensively reorganized the content. The additional chapters on inflammation, wound repair, and rehabilitation will provide readers with a more solid basis for understanding cryotherapy and using cryo techniques with other therapy.

I am convinced that technique needs theory, and theory needs technique—whether in the training room, library, or research laboratory. For example, to understand the influence of cryotherapy as a first-aid measure, you must understand the inflammatory process. And to fully appreciate the effects cryotherapy has during rehabilitation, you must understand the entire rehabilitative process. Theory and practice cannot be separated, and the organization of this book reflects their interrelationship.

Part I gives a brief overview of cryotherapy: what, when, where, how, and why. Part II reviews in depth the pathological and physiological responses of bodily tissues to injury and cryotherapy and provides a theoretical basis for the cryotherapy techniques used in dealing with acute musculoskeletal conditions. Clinical techniques are presented, with abundant illustrations, in Part III. The extensive references (organized for scholars), Subject Index, and Author Index will be extremely useful to many readers. References are cited in a letter-number format (e.g., B64, H13) explained on page 255.

Students and clinicians will appreciate the clear explanations and illustrations of techniques. The physiological and theoretical basis will help clinicians understand *why* as well as how and when to use the techniques.

Scientists and scholars will also benefit from this volume. The more than 600 references and the comprehensiveness of the information presented makes this the most extensive and up-to-date resource on cryotherapy.

My favorite word is "Why?" Most progress comes after asking this one-word question. Remember though, questions are much easier to come by than answers.

My guide in preparing this book has been the words of Sir Francis Bacon, who said:

Read not to
   Contradict and refute,
Nor to accept
   And take for granted,
But to
   Weigh and consider.

We are fortunate that many clinicians, scholars, and scientists have provided written information to weigh and consider. Although I have not agreed with the conclusions some have reached, their research findings and writings have been useful. No doubt some of the ideas in this book will ultimately prove to be less than adequate. That is all right—if it stimulates people to prove them to be so.

   I trust that you will find this book useful and that it will lead to greater understanding of the theory and clinical application of cryotherapy, thereby resulting in better athletic health care and further research.

Acknowledgments

Many, many people have contributed to this work: John Maley, Rainer Martens, Chris Drews and her crew, Jay Thomas, Dr. Paul Hightower, The Interlibrary loan staff at Cunningham Memorial Library at Indiana State University, Coaches John Bensen, Sark Arslanian, and Ralph Hunter, Dr. John Roberts, Dr. Ben Londeree, Dr. Bob Behnke, Dr. Chris Ingersoll, former students, colleagues, and Shari Knight. Your assistance in many and varied ways is greatly appreciated. Although my name is on the cover, the work was truly a team effort.

My first book on cryotherapy was the brainchild of John Maley. His vision and moral and financial support were responsible for its delivery. Rainer Martens envisioned a very different approach to the material and encouraged me to develop this version. Chris Drews and her staff have been super to work with; her encouragement, understanding, and flexibility kept a very busy professional working weekends and evenings at a part time job. Jay Thomas helped me craft the words to express my ideas more clearly. And Paul Hightower, a busy academic himself, was most accommodating in reshooting many of the photographs because I wanted something a little different. Thank you all.

Well over 500 of the articles referenced in this work (and numerous others that turned out to be unsuitable) were obtained for me by the interlibrary loan staff of Indiana State University's Cunningham Memorial Library. Without their support this work would have been much more difficult, if not impossible.

Coach Bensen introduced me to the athletic training field; Coach Arslanian taught me to love it, encouraged me to excel, and gave me my first two professional positions. Coach Hunter gave me the opportunity and trusted me to try some unorthodox cryotherapy in the 1960s. Dr. Roberts and Dr. Londeree of the University of Missouri-Columbia guided my early cold research, and an encouraging comment on the first paper I wrote for Dr. Roberts helped sustain me through a most difficult period. Dr. Londeree was a hard taskmaster, for which I'm grateful. Bob Behnke and Chris Ingersoll, my colleagues at ISU, have contributed to this work in numerous ways. Bob's writings helped stimulate much of my early work, and Chris is doing some great work on the effects of cold on pain and proprioception.

The praise and encouragement, criticism and challenges of my research, and opinions by students and professional colleagues have stimulated me to continue to dig and to develop and refine these ideas. Thank you all.

And what can be said about the contribution of a loving and supportive eternal companion? Thank you, Shari.

Technique Tips

Introduction to Cryotherapy

In the two chapters of this part, I attempt to give an overview of cryotherapy as it is used in the management of acute musculoskeletal injuries. Chapter 1 defines *cryotherapy*, introduces numerous cryotherapeutic techniques, outlines physiological responses, touches upon some of the confusion concerning cryotherapy, and briefly presents the rationale for its use in treating various types of injuries. Each of these topics is covered in more depth in later chapters of the book.

In chapter 2, I present a historical perspective of the use of cryotherapy. Heat vs. cold, cold and immediate care, the use of cold for rehabilitation, the history of cryokinetics, cold and muscle spasm, pain, and postsurgical cryotherapy are the major topics.

1

The What and Why of Cryotherapy

Few professional, college, or high school sporting events in North America take place without ice or cold packs on the sidelines. Almost without exception cold is used immediately after an injury to limit pain and swelling (B3, B10, H9, H59). This helps the injury seem less serious, and the athlete usually proceeds through rehabilitation more quickly.

Cryotherapy is not limited to immediate care. Its use extends to physical therapy departments, rehabilitation clinics, operating rooms, pain centers, and elsewhere. Rehabilitation is quicker with cryotherapy because therapeutic exercises can begin earlier and become more effective when they are alternated with cold. With this modality spasticity is lessened, surgical complications are reduced, organs are preserved for transplantation, and the list of benefits goes on. One nurse has claimed that cold is the most effective and underused physical modality for pain (E67).

But confusion over cryotherapy is almost as widespread as its popularity.

WHY THE CONFUSION?

There are numerous definitions of *cryotherapy* and many opinions about why and how certain cryotherapeutic techniques should be used, when to apply them, and how the cold affects, or what happens within, the tissue. This confusion limits and even prevents effective use of the techniques.

With sport injuries, part of the confusion stems from the fact that cold is applied as part of both immediate-care (see Figure 1.1) and later rehabilitative procedures. Cold can be effective during both phases of injury management, even though the objectives differ.

The major cause of confusion, however, is that medical and allied health clinicians practice an art. Using cryotherapy—or any therapeutic modality—for sport injury management is an art. The modality's effectiveness depends largely on the skill and technique of the clinician who administers it. Both experience and science guide the art (and are influenced by the art), but the art and technique almost always precede the science (see Figure 1.2).

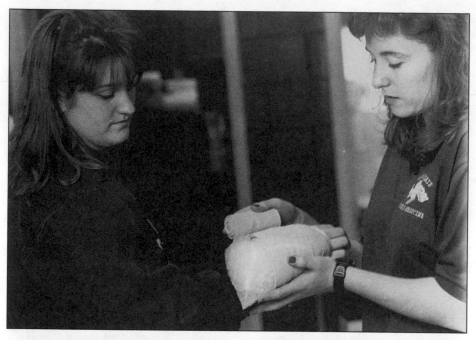

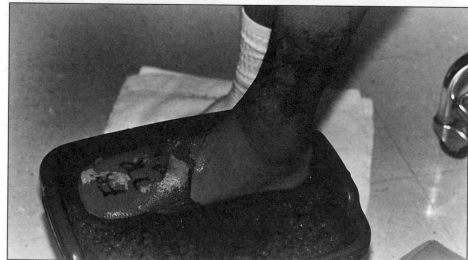

Figure 1.1   Even though cryotherapy is used for both immediate care (top) and rehabilitation of sport injuries (bottom), the rationale and application protocol are different. Failure to recognize these differences is one of the sources of great confusion concerning cryotherapy.

Figure 1.2   Medical or clinical practice is an art influenced by both experience and tradition and science and theory. Clinical practice in turn influences both; additional experience may alter tradition and can stimulate experimental investigation, which may solidify or alter accepted theories.

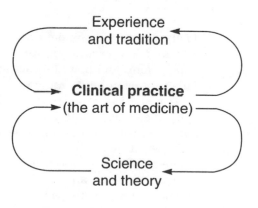

Experience
and tradition

Clinical practice
(the art of medicine)

Science
and theory

Unfortunately, the physiological bases of cryotherapy are not nearly as well understood as are the clinical responses to it. Attempts to explain the clinical successes of cold have led to overly simplistic explanations that sometimes do not stand up under close scrutiny (A18, C42, F19). Some explanations contradict others, and some are even self-contradictory.

We must continue to expand the theoretical basis for our work with good science. Chapman's (E17) advice should be followed: After critically analyzing the published research about the effects of five groups of physical modalities on the management of pain, she concluded that most researchers had compared various modalities with one another but had not included a control group. She concluded:

> Do the results of these studies indicate that all modalities are equally effective, or equally ineffective? . . . Further research is necessary to justify the continued use of physical modalities in clinical practice and to define their short- and long-term therapeutic value. This research should be designed with randomized controlled trials including a control group not receiving any other physical modality. And, since most physical modalities are used in physical rehabilitation to prepare the patient for subsequent exercise therapy, such studies should also include trials with the exercise component.

Despite confusion and a need for further research, however, some powerful cryotherapeutic techniques exist, and great healing art is being practiced with these techniques. Learn them, perfect them, and adjust them as good science tweaks their theoretical basis, and use them to improve or restore health and vitality to the injured.

WHAT IS CRYOTHERAPY?

Cryotherapy means different things to different people. To some people it is putting an ice pack on a sprained ankle, while to others it is massaging a sore muscle with a large ice cube before stretching the muscle. Still others see it as spraying −60°C liquid nitrogen on a tumor to freeze and destroy it. Who is right? They all are.

Cryotherapy means, quite literally, "cold therapy." So any use of ice or cold applications for therapeutic purposes is cryotherapy (see Figure 1.3). Stated another way, cryotherapy is the therapeutic application of any substance to the body that results in the withdrawal of heat from the body, thereby lowering tissue temperature. Each of the following techniques is cryotherapy:

- Ice or cold-pack application for immediate care of acute injuries
- Ice massage
- Running cold water over a burn
- Cryokinetics (alternating cold applications with active exercise)
- Cryostretch (alternating cold applications with muscle stretching)
- Cold-water baths (cold whirlpool or immersion in a "slush bucket")
- Cryosurgery
- Ice or cold-pack application following orthopedic surgery
- Whole-body hypothermia prior to abdominal or organ transplant surgery
- Treating trigger points with ice

Because the techniques are used for a wide range of therapeutic objectives, to refer to a specific technique as cryotherapy leads to confusion and ambiguity. Refer to individual techniques by their specific names to avoid the confusion. Think of the term *cryotherapy* only in the broad sense, as an umbrella term covering all the specific techniques.

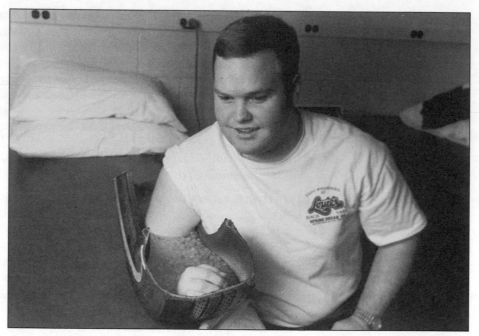

a

Figure 1.3 These photos illustrate three of the many types of cryotherapy, which is the use of cold for any therapeutic purpose: (a) ice slush immersion of a baseball pitcher's elbow following a ball game helps minimize delayed onset muscle soreness; (b) ice massage to the quadriceps as part of rehabilitation for a pulled muscle; and (c) cryosurgery with liquid nitrogen to remove a wart on the hand. *(continued)*

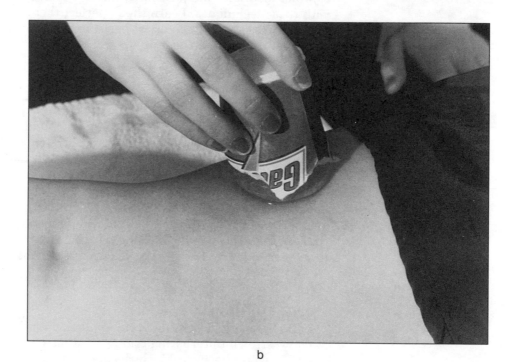

b

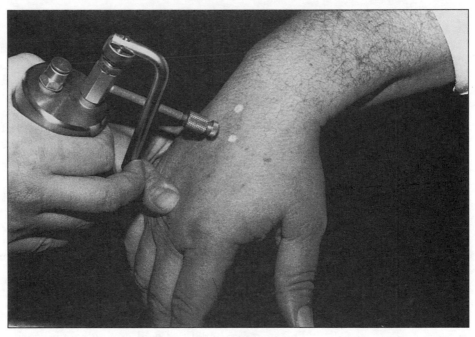

c

Figure 1.3
(continued)

Uses of Cryotherapy

- Decreasing pain, swelling, and secondary hypoxic injury in an acute injury
- Allowing active exercise earlier when rehabilitating an acute joint sprain
- Decreasing pain and spasm in an acute pulled muscle (strain)
- Decreasing pain, swelling, and secondary hypoxic injury resulting from orthopedic surgery
- Destroying tissue during cryo-surgery

- Assisting in stretching connective tissue
- Reducing pain and cramps during menstruation
- Eliminating or minimizing cold-sore development
- Preventing hair loss during chemotherapy
- Minimizing pain when medications are injected

CRYOTHERAPEUTIC TECHNIQUES

Cryotherapeutic techniques can be grouped into five major categories, based on the objectives for using them.

Immediate care—cooling acutely injured musculoskeletal tissue immediately after an injury, as part of first aid

Rehabilitation—cooling tissue during rehabilitation of various musculo-skeletal pathologies as an adjunct to other therapy

Surgical adjunct—cooling tissue prior to, during, or after surgical procedures

Cryosurgery—freezing tissue for surgical purposes

Miscellaneous—techniques that don't fit into one of the previous four categories

Immediate Care

The primary objectives during immediate care are (a) to prevent further injury and (b) to minimize adverse sequelae (sequelae are events that follow and are a result of the injury). For most acute musculoskeletal injuries you prevent injury by removing the injured person from the environment in which he or she was hurt. For athletes this usually means taking them out of practice or the game.

Adverse sequelae to injury include secondary injury, pain, swelling, and muscle spasm. (Contrary to popular belief, however, inflammation is not an adverse sequela. When a hematoma is involved, the inflammatory process is needed for healing to take place [J44].) If they are applied quickly enough following the injury, cold applications are beneficial because they diminish all these adverse sequelae. And although cold also decreases the inflammatory response, the decrease in metabolism and secondary hypoxic injury more than compensates for the diminished inflammation. Chapters 4, 5, and 6 expand on the theoretical basis, and chapters 15 and 16 present the application.

Rehabilitation

The primary benefit of cold during rehabilitation is that it decreases pain and muscle spasm and thereby allows earlier mobilization. Not only does the proper use of exercise speed the healing process (J34, 35), but lack of exercise during the early stages of rehabilitation may result in permanent disability (J15). Caution must be observed, though; exercise that is too vigorous may result in permanent disability. The optimum conditions for healing depend on the very fine balance between returning to full normal function at the earliest possible time and protecting injured body parts from overstressing the injury and from reinjury (J15). Chapters 3, 4, and 9 through 13 expand on the theoretical basis, and chapters 15 and 17 through 19 present the application.

Surgical Adjuncts

Cryotherapy is often used before, during, and after surgical procedures. The objective is the same as during immediate care of acute injuries: to decrease metabolism so as to diminish secondary hypoxic injury. Chapters 6, 7, and 17 will expand on this point.

Cryosurgery

Cryosurgery is a surgical technique that uses ultralow-temperature (-20° to -70°C) probes to freeze tissue and thereby destroy it (G19, G58). A detailed discussion of cryosurgery is beyond the scope of this book; readers who desire more information on cryosurgery should consult the references just given and those found in chapter 11.

Miscellaneous

Such techniques as limiting menstrual cramps and pain, limiting cold sores, and numbing painful injections are grouped together in the miscellaneous category. These techniques are discussed in chapters 20 and 21.

WHAT HAPPENS WHEN COLD IS APPLIED?

The pathophysiological effects of cold have been reviewed by many (A1-A47). These effects may be grouped into seven primary categories:

- Decreased temperature
- Decreased metabolism
- Inflammatory effects (decreased or increased)
- Circulatory effects (decreased or increased)
- Decreased pain
- Decreased muscle spasm
- Increased tissue stiffness

The immediate response to cold applications is tissue cooling. If the cooling is severe enough (-20 to $-70°C$ or -4 to $-94°F$), the tissue is destroyed (as in cryosurgery). During sports medicine applications the tissue is usually cooled to a surface temperature of $1°$ to $10°C$ (33 to $50°F$). Cooling to this temperature causes the tissue reactions just noted.

The physiological effects of cold application are not as straightforward as clinicians of the past have thought. Such effects as decreased pain, muscle spasm, metabolism, and inflammation appear to be universally accepted, although the mechanisms by which they occur have not been fully explained (A20, A38). Interestingly, it appears that some types of inflammation and muscle spasm are stimulated rather than decreased by cold. There is great confusion in the literature concerning the circulatory effects of cold applications, with reports that cold applications result in increased blood flow and reports that they result in decreased blood flow, although those who have proposed increased blood flow have had either nonexistent or arbitrary explanations for when blood flow increases and decreases. In Part II we'll look at these issues in more detail.

Not all of the effects of cold are beneficial during sport injury management, so if cryotherapy is not used properly it could be detrimental rather than beneficial.

HEAT VS. COLD: WHEN AND WHY

Table 1.1 lists the physiological responses of local tissue to therapeutic applications of heat and cold, along with the efficacy or desirability of each of these effects during various phases of sport injury management.

Acute Injuries: Immediate Care

Decreased metabolism is the most important effect of cold during immediate care because it limits secondary hypoxic injury (G50, J44). Decreased metabolism is partially, but not completely, counteracted by another effect—decreased circulation—which lowers oxygen delivery and therefore contributes to secondary hypoxic injury (see chapters 7 and 16 for a more complete discussion). Cold also is beneficial during these procedures because it decreases muscle spasm and pain.

Heat application is contraindicated during immediate care because increased metabolism would promote secondary hypoxic injury and thus aggravate the injury.

Acute Injuries: Rehabilitation

Decreased circulation, metabolism, and inflammation and increased tissue stiffness are detrimental to rehabilitation following acute injury (G1, G55);

Table 1.1   Use of Cryo- and Thermotherapy During Acute and Chronic Sports Injury Management

Physiological effects	Efficacy during immediate care of acute/chronic injuries		Efficacy during rehabilitation of acute/chronic injuries	
Of cold:				
Decreased circulation	0	0	–	–
Decreased metabolism	+ + +[1]	0	–	–
Decreased inflammation	–	+	–	+
Decreased pain (anesthesia)	+	+	+ + +[3]	+
Decreased muscle spasm	+	0	+	0
Increased tissue stiffness	0	0	–	–
Overall	+	[5]	+	?
Of heat:				
Increased circulation	0	0	+	+
Increased metabolism	– – –[2]	0	+	+
Increased inflammation	+	–	+	–
Decreased pain (analgesia)	+	+	0[4]	+
Decreased muscle spasm	+	0	+	0
Decreased tissue stiffness	0	0	0	+
Overall	–	[5]	–	+

[1]Inhibits secondary hypoxic injury; [2]Promotes secondary hypoxic injury; [3]Allows/requires active exercise; [4]Often does not facilitate active exercise; [5]There is no immediate care of chronic injuries.

the need at this time is for increased circulation and metabolism. Decreased pain and decreased spasm are desirable. A mathematician would probably conclude from these contrasting considerations that there is no benefit to using cryotherapy during rehabilitation. For many cryo techniques this is true.

However, the exercise component of cryokinetics provides benefits that more than compensate for the cold-induced decreases in circulation and metabolism (B14, C47, E49). Exercise-induced vasodilatation during cryokinetics is much greater than that which results from heat applications. In addition, exercise retards the development of adhesions, reverses neural inhibitions (B20, H36, J15), and activates the lymph system (G20). Much of the tissue debris from the injury is removed from the area via the lymphatic system (H30). Since lymphatic flow requires muscular action to "pump" its fluid, active exercise is essential. Since pain prevents active exercise for many days after even minor joint sprains (E49, J15), cold-induced pain relief allows active exercise much earlier than would be possible otherwise (B14, E49, H36, H70). Increased tissue stiffness hinders active exercise, and so is listed as a negative effect during rehabilitation.

Cryokinetics can also begin much earlier than thermal therapy (B14, H11, J45). Thermotherapy cannot be applied until the vascular system is repaired; to do so would cause additional secondary hypoxic injury. This repair is usually not complete until 48 to 72 hours following injury. Cryokinetics can begin 1 to 24 hours following injury (B3).

Heat applications are not as effective as cold applications as an adjunct to exercise during acute injury rehabilitation. Although both decrease pain, active exercise is not facilitated by heat as it is by cold (A24). Exercise following heat applications often invokes a return of the pain and muscle spasm that were present prior to the heat application, although this does not seem to be true with chronic injuries.

Post-Acute Injuries

Post-acute refers to an acute injury after 10 to 15 days have elapsed. Dull soreness is more often a problem than is sharp pain; soreness responds better to heat than to cold applications. Decreased range of motion at this time can be the result of either muscle spasm or contracted connective tissue. Treat muscle spasm with cold, but treat connective tissue with a combination of heat, stretching, and cold.

Chronic and Overuse Injuries

There is no immediate care for overuse injuries. Since the onset of these injuries is gradual, there is little vascular collapse and therefore little fear of secondary hypoxic injury.

Rehabilitation of chronic injuries is also confused (B15, B30, B33, B51, J70). Usually there is little or no muscle spasm, and pain occurs only during extended activity. An overactive inflammatory response would seem to call for cold applications to decrease the inflammatory process. There is no evidence, however, that cold is beneficial.

A popular therapy for tendinitis is to apply hot packs before, and cold packs after, practice. Like other chronic-injury therapy, however, there is no evidence to support or refute this regimen. My clinical impression is that ultrasound applications applied twice daily for 10 days is as effective as any other therapy (but I have no research data to support this method).

SUMMARY

- *Cryotherapy* is an umbrella term that refers to many techniques involving cold applications.
- To obtain the maximum benefit from any therapeutic modality, you must understand the specific needs of the patient and the physiological response to specific modalities.
- The local physiological responses to cold applications include decreased temperature, metabolism, inflammation, circulation, pain, and spasm and increased tissue stiffness. Some of these responses are beneficial, others detrimental, during various phases of sport injury management.
- Decreased metabolism is the major benefit during immediate care of acute injuries because it limits development of secondary hypoxic injury.
- Heat applications are usually preferred for post-acute injury management to reduce soreness and as an adjunct to stretching connective tissue contractures.
- During rehabilitation, cold applications are used as an adjunct to active exercise.
- There is no evidence for or against cryotherapy for chronic injuries.

2

Historical Perspective

Cryotherapy is a relatively new, complex, and misunderstood concept. Only since the early 1950s has cold been a regular part of sport injury management, and the bounds within which it is used, explanations for why it is used, and what occurs when it is used continue to be debated. As a result, cold is often used improperly. Figure 2.1 provides an overview of the use of cold treatments through history.

As noted previously, part of the confusion with cryotherapy stems from its use in both immediate-care and rehabilitation procedures. Laboratory and clinical research during the 1970s, 1980s, and 1990s has helped refine the theoretical rationale for and application of cryotherapy, thus resolving some of the confusion.

HEAT VS. COLD

One of the dominant theories of physical medicine (treatment with such physical modalities as heat, light, and electricity) during this century is that the rate of tissue healing can be increased by increasing blood flow to the tissue. Since heat applications increase metabolism and blood flow, clinicians have assumed that heat applications increase the rate of healing. Much of the research during the 1950s and 1960s was devoted to changes in blood flow resulting from various heat modalities.

Early in the century heat applications dominated. However, toward the middle of the century cold began to be recognized as beneficial during the immediate-care phase of treating acute injuries. By the late 1960s the philosophy of athletic trainers was to treat acute injuries with cold for the first 24 to 72 hours and then follow with heat, "Once the bleeding stopped." Other health professionals lagged behind. In the mid-1980s one of our out-of-season athletes at Indiana State University went to the student health center on a Sunday for a metatarsal sprain. The nurse advised him to go home and soak the injured area in a hot bath. He questioned her, suggesting that

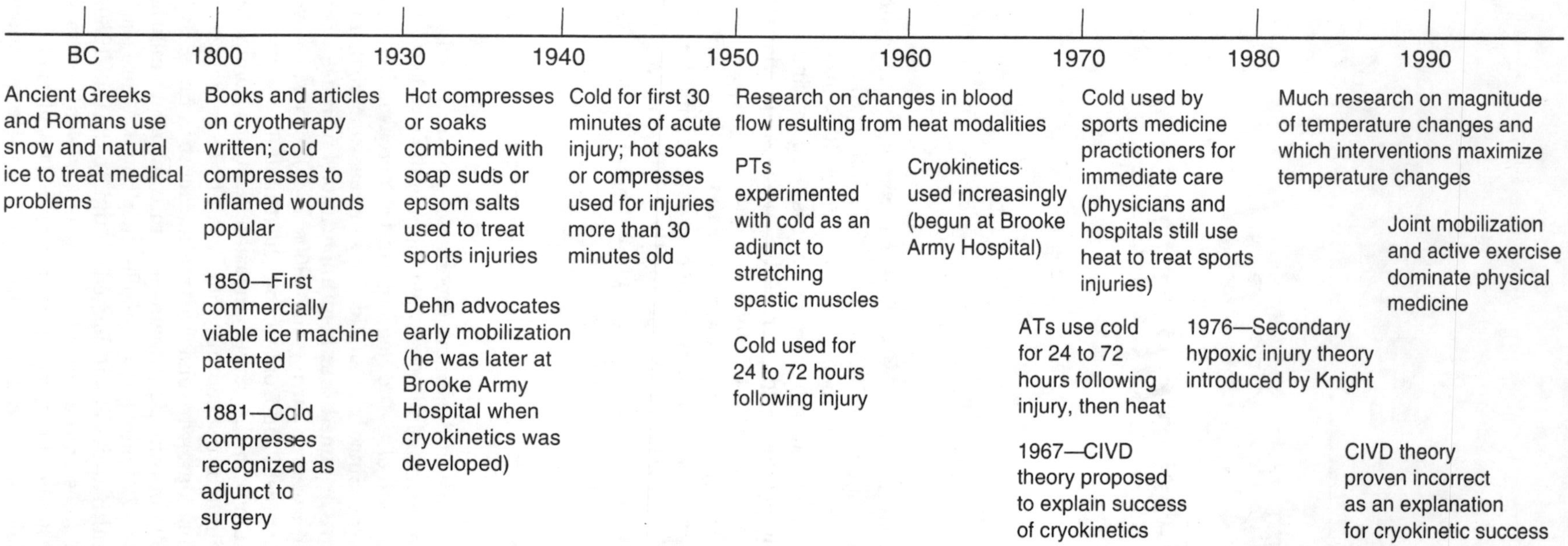

BC	1800	1930	1940	1950	1960	1970	1980	1990
Ancient Greeks and Romans use snow and natural ice to treat medical problems	Books and articles on cryotherapy written; cold compresses to inflamed wounds popular	Hot compresses or soaks combined with soap suds or epsom salts used to treat sports injuries	Cold for first 30 minutes of acute injury; hot soaks or compresses used for injuries more than 30 minutes old	Research on changes in blood flow resulting from heat modalities	Cryokinetics used increasingly (begun at Brooke Army Hospital)	Cold used by sports medicine practictioners for immediate care (physicians and hospitals still use heat to treat sports injuries)		Much research on magnitude of temperature changes and which interventions maximize temperature changes
	1850—First commercially viable ice machine patented	Dehn advocates early mobilization (he was later at Brooke Army Hospital when cryokinetics was developed)		PTs experimented with cold as an adjunct to stretching spastic muscles				Joint mobilization and active exercise dominate physical medicine
	1881—Cold compresses recognized as adjunct to surgery			Cold used for 24 to 72 hours following injury		ATs use cold for 24 to 72 hours following injury, then heat	1976—Secondary hypoxic injury theory introduced by Knight	
						1967—CIVD theory proposed to explain success of cryokinetics		CIVD theory proven incorrect as an explanation for cryokinetic success

Figure 2.1 An historical overview of cryotherapy.

perhaps an elastic wrap and ice pack would be better. "Oh," she replied, "elastic wraps and ice packs are only for sprained ankles."

During the 1950s physical therapists began experimenting with cold applications as an adjunct to stretching spastic muscles (F17, F18, F28, F30, F31), and in the following decade physical therapists and athletic trainers began treating acute joint sprains by alternating cold and active exercise in a treatment called cryokinetics (B10, B16, B20, B29). The popularity of cold applications during rehabilitation grew. The question of when is it safe to begin rehabilitation—that is, to begin heat applications—no longer needed an answer because cold has replaced heat as the preferred modality during rehabilitation.

Joint mobilization and active exercise are beginning to dominate physical medicine in the 1990s. This, along with an increased understanding of the physiological responses to heat and cold, has lead to a more balanced use of heat and cold as adjuncts to active exercise during rehabilitation.

EARLY MEDICAL USES OF COLD

Cold applications of snow and natural ice were used by the ancient Greeks and Romans to treat a variety of medical problems (see reference A26 for numerous references to the early use of heat and cold). Many books and articles were written about cryotherapy in the early 19th century, and by 1835 the application of cold compresses to inflamed wounds was quite popular (A26). Patented in 1850 by a Florida physician, the first commercially viable ice machine made ice and air-conditioned rooms for the doctor's malaria patients (A26).

COLD AND IMMEDIATE CARE

Cold compresses were a recognized adjunct to surgery as early as 1881 (A4). But in the 1930s the common treatment for acute sport injuries was hot compresses or soaks combined with soap suds or epsom salts (J53). Sports medicine textbooks of the 1940s advocated cold treatments for acute injuries, but only for 30 to 60 minutes and only if applied within the first 30 minutes after injury (J8, J9). For injuries more than 30 minutes old, hot soaks or compresses were prescribed whether or not ice had been used initially. During the 1950s the time period for using cold was extended to the first 24 to 72 hours following injury (B4, J13, H83). In 1961, athletic trainers were arguing the merits of heat vs. cold applications for initial treatment of athletic injuries (B4).

By the early 1970s cold was used almost universally by sports medicine practitioners for immediate care (H4, H59) but not by the medical community as a whole (H4, B44). Many physicians and hospitals continue to use or recommend hot packs for all phases of sport injuries management.

During the 1970s and 1980s efforts were made to expand the theoretical basis for the use of cold applications in immediate care—to understand why cold applications were beneficial and how and when they should be applied. The common rationale for using cold was that it decreased blood flow, thus decreasing hemorrhaging, and thereby decreased swelling (A17, A22, A25, A41, B21, B24, B31, B45, B47, H34, H69, H72, H76, H83). In 1976, however, I introduced the secondary hypoxic (oxygen-deficient) injury theory (G50), which asserts that the beneficial effect of treating acute musculoskeletal injuries with ice is that the cold decreases metabolism in the tissues in the vicinity of the injury that has escaped damage by the trauma. This then allows many cells to survive the period of decreased oxygen delivery that results from compromised circulation attributable to injury to blood vessels and the inflammatory process. Swelling, according to the theory, is due less to hemorrhaging and more to edema that results from increased free protein and oncotic pressure (a force that attracts water) in the injured tissue.

Part of the basis of the secondary hypoxic injury theory was recognizing that swelling often occurs for hours following an injury, while direct hemorrhaging into the tissue is most often stopped by clotting, which occurs within minutes after the injury. Since cold applications are rarely applied sooner than 5 to 10 minutes after the injury (during which time the injury is evaluated and the athlete is removed from the playing area) and since it takes time for a superficially applied cold pack to affect deep tissues, the decreased-hemorrhaging theory did not seem a viable explanation for the dramatic effects of immediate cold applications. Most authors of athletic training textbooks now accept the secondary hypoxic injury theory (A42, H34), although those in other fields still cling to the decreased-hemorrhaging theory (I7).

During the 1980s and 1990s much research was conducted to determine the magnitude of temperature decreases during cryotherapy and which types of therapeutic intervention maximized temperature decrease. For instance, crushed-ice packs result in greater temperature decreases than commercial cold packs (C49), and crushed ice applied to the ankle for 30 minutes decreases temperature more than 20-minute applications do (H48, H56) but not significantly less than 45- or 60-minute applications (H48). Elastic wraps applied under the cold pack insulate the tissue from the cold (H73), while ice packs applied over the cold pack provide equal pressure to the underlying tissue (H74) and maximize the cooling effects. Rewarming (heat conduction from warmer surrounding tissue) following cold application is much slower than cooling, except in the fingers (C45, H40, H56). Exercise prior to application of the cold pack has no effect on the rate of cooling and subsequent rewarming; the elevated tissue temperature prior to application is maintained during and following application (H40). Minimal activity, such as showering and walking on crutches, accelerates rewarming following cold application; thus, the first reapplication of the cold pack should occur more quickly than subsequent reapplications. Too-frequent reapplication may cause too much tissue cooling (H56).

The dominant question to be answered now is, How cold is cold enough? Future research must determine the optimal temperature for treating acute injuries.

USE OF ICE FOR REHABILITATION: THE HISTORY OF CRYOKINETICS

Using cold applications during rehabilitation of acute sprains, strains, and contusions appears to have begun at Brooke Army Hospital in the early 1960s, although Mead, Knott and their co-workers (F17, F18, F28, F30, F31) had been using cold applications for treating spastic disorders during the 1950s. The first reports from the Brooke group appeared in 1964: Grant (B10) and Hayden (B16), a physician–physical therapist team, described their treatment of soldiers who had assorted musculoskeletal injuries suffered during basic training with a new method that they termed *cryokinetics*, referring to a combination of cold and exercise (Figure 2.2).

Dehn (J15) must also be credited as a force behind cryotherapy. He was chief of orthopedic surgery at Brooke Army Hospital and a colleague of Grant and Hayden's (personal communication with Keith Markley, MD, San Antonio, who trained under Dehn, 1985). Dehn began advocating early mobilization in the 1930s. According to Markley, Dehn was sometimes fanatical with nurses, driving them to get patients up and moving after surgery as soon as they came out of anesthesia. Since Grant and Hayden were responsible for rehabilitation of Dehn's patients, his philosophy of early mobilization no doubt influenced them.

Grant and Hayden's procedure began with either ice massage or ice immersion (depending on the area of the body being treated) to anesthetize the injured body part (B16). This took from 3 to 20 minutes and was ceased when the patient reported numbness. Once numbed, the body part was exercised with active (voluntary) movement. If discomfort recurred, the ice was reapplied. Each treatment consisted of five to six exercise bouts alternated with ice applications. Hayden (B16) reported that all but 3 of 1,000 patients returned to duty within 2 days of beginning treatment with cryokinetics, but she did not give any theory or rationale for her success. Grant (B10) reported that over 80% of 7,000 patients were discharged from health services with less than three formal treatments. He postulated that early motion and restoration of normal function in the involved area was the key to symptomatic improvement and that the use of ice is simply an adjunct measure used to relieve pain and allow such early motion.

Since the reports of Grant and Hayden, hospital physical therapists (D14, E57, F6, F16, F25, F42) and athletic trainers (B20, B21, B29, B42, B47, C6, H70) have reported apparent dramatic success with cryokinetics. Juvenal (B20) wrote in 1966 about a football player with a sprained ankle who would normally have been sidelined for two to three weeks. After x-rays and consultation with a team physician, cryokinetics was started. In less than 72 hours the student was able to return to full contact with no limitation of movement and a minimum of pain. Reports such as this caused many to begin using the new technique (A15, A46, B2, B3, B29, C16, C22), and clinical success stimulated discussion as to the reason for its success (A3, A15, A37, B29, C16, C22). The most prevalent speculation was that cold-induced vasodilatation increased blood flow to the tissue, a contradiction to the prevalent theory at the time that cold was beneficial during immediate care because it caused vasoconstriction.

In 1967, Moore et al. (B29) presented case studies involving athletic rehabilitation with cryokinetics and discussed possible mechanisms to account for the quicker rehabilitation that they felt they had achieved with this technique. They stated that cold prepares the area for exercise and that exercise was of "paramount importance" to the success of cryokinetics. But they also introduced the idea that cold-induced vasodilation (CIVD) might be involved, even though they felt that the response was not fully understood and had "been unable to find applicable evidence to give an adequate physiological rationale" for cryokinetics. Subsequent writers discussed CIVD as if it were an established fact (B21, C1, C6, C16, C22). None of these authors presented original data to support CIVD; their writings were based on the research and opinions of others.

We (C47) attempted to substantiate the occurrence of CIVD during cryokinetics by using strain gauge plethysmography to measure blood flow to the ankle during six combinations of heat, cold, and exercise. There was no CIVD; in fact, just the opposite occurred: blood flow decreased during a 25-minute cold-pack application and remained depressed for 20 minutes following application. Our conclusions were that the success of cryokinetics

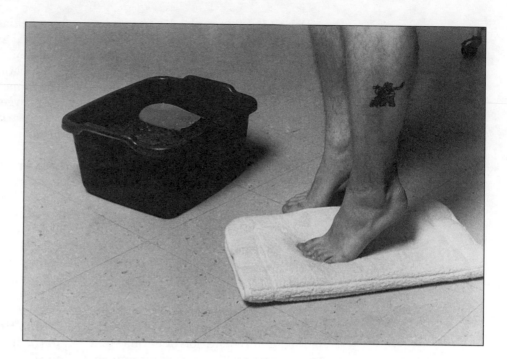

Figure 2.2 Cryokinetics, developed in the mid-1960s, led the way to aggressive rehabilitation of sport and orthopedic injuries that became common in the 1980s.

was due to the early exercise and that the role of cold was only to decrease pain and thereby allow earlier and more intense normal active exercise. Subsequent research substantiated our initial findings (see chapter 9).

Although cryokinetics is just being discovered by some professionals and is being touted as a "new" treatment (B19), it is a tried and true technique in the arsenal of many athletic trainers.

SUMMARY

Although there is little doubt in practitioners' minds about the efficacy of cold during both immediate care and rehabilitation, there has been little direct research to substantiate its use or to explain the mechanisms by which it works. Consequently, we cannot yet give a definitive explanation of the effects of cold on sport-induced inflammation. But peripheral research provides a basis for working hypotheses, which future research must examine and refine.

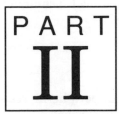

PART
II

The Scientific Basis of Cryotherapy

Part II presents the theoretical rationale for the use of various cryotherapeutic techniques and research concerning the efficacy of these techniques.

THEORY VS. TECHNIQUE

When used properly, cryotherapy techniques are powerful tools for managing musculoskeletal pathology, both during the initial-care phase of acute trauma and during rehabilitation of assorted musculoskeletal pathologies. Improper applications, however, can impede both phases of injury management by delaying or preventing the application of more beneficial therapy.

To gain the greatest benefit from cryotherapy, the needs of the patient must be matched with a technique that will meet those needs. This requires a theoretical basis: an understanding of the body's pathophysiological responses to the specific injury or disease and the body's physiological responses to the therapy. Some clinicians might reject the need for a theoretical basis for cryotherapy, claiming that the important thing is knowing how to apply cryotherapy, not how or why it works. Their underlying—and faulty—assumption is that there is no room for improving current technique.

Application must be based on theory. The closer to truth or reality theory is, the more refined and beneficial technique will be. Conversely, faulty theory can lead to improper and incomplete clinical applications. For instance, the idea that cold-induced vasodilatation (CIVD) results from cryotherapy gave rise to the false notion that blood flow could be increased more as a result of cold applications than heat applications. This in turn led to the use of cold whirlpools and cold water soaks without other therapy. Thus, proper treatment was delayed because the patient and therapist mistakenly believed that blood flow to the injury was being increased when in fact it was being decreased. But knowing that cold decreases blood flow leads to the conclusion that during rehabilitation cold applications must be followed by therapeutic exercise (C43, C46) and that the exercise stimulates the repair processes.

The search for substantiated pathophysiological explanations for the various cryotherapy techniques must go on. As it does, clinical techniques will improve and patients will receive better health care.

CENTRAL AND LOCAL RESPONSES

There is both a central, or core, response and a local, or peripheral, response to cold applications. The central response has been reviewed elsewhere (A2, A6, A20, C66, H21) and will not be dealt with here; this book is concerned only with the local response.

PATHOPHYSIOLOGY

The scientific basis for cryotherapy involves both pathology and physiology, sometimes called pathophysiology. Pathology is the study of diseases. Physiology is the study of the functions of cells, tissues, and organs of the living body. The pathophysiological basis of cryotherapy thus involves an investigation of how cold applications affect the functioning of normal and injured cells, tissues, and organs of the body.

Chapter 3 is a review of the normal inflammatory response, including the pathology of injury, the physiology of edema formation, and wound healing. Principles of rehabilitation follow in chapter 4. These two chapters form the foundation for investigating the use of cold in both immediate care and rehabilitation. Since all pathophysiological effects of cryotherapy are a result of decreased temperature, we devote chapter 5 to temperature changes.

The subsequent chapters are organized around immediate care and rehabilitation. Topics most important to immediate care are presented first. Chapter 6, on the effects of cryotherapy on metabolism and inflammation, explains the theoretical basis for using ice as part of the immediate care of injuries. This is followed by a discussion in chapter 7 of rest, ice, compression, elevation, and stabilization for managing acute sport injuries. And since the basis for using ice following surgery is similar to the rationale for immediate care of injuries, discussion of the presurgical and postsurgical uses of ice are next, in chapter 8.

Rehabilitation is covered in chapters on circulation (chapter 9), neurological effects (chapter 10), pain (chapter 11), muscle spasm (chapter 12), and tissue stiffness (chapter 13). The last chapter (chapter 14) of Part II concerns problems, precautions, and contraindications.

Throughout these chapters I have included "technique tips" that point to specific applications of the principles being discussed. Use these chapters to understand why cold is used in the various techniques. Use this science to influence and improve your art of sport injury care.

3

Inflammation and Wound Repair

In order to understand the effects of cold during sport injury management, you must understand inflammation—the body's pathological response to injury—and how injured tissues heal. In this chapter I will explain what inflammation and wound repair are, why inflammation is a necessary part of acute-injury care, and why cold applications are necessary in treating acute injuries. I will also touch briefly on how cold applications help decrease swelling and pain.

THE INFLAMMATORY RESPONSE

Inflammation, or the *inflammatory response*, is the local, tissue-level response of the body to an irritant. Inflammation has a threefold purpose (J24):

- To defend the body against alien substances
- To dispose of dead and dying tissue so that repair can take place
- To promote regeneration of normal tissue

There are five cardinal signs of inflammation:

- Pain
- Swelling, or edema
- Redness
- Heat
- Loss of function

These are *signs* of inflammation—indicators that the inflammatory process is taking place—not the inflammatory response itself. They may be caused by processes other than inflammation.

A common misconception is that one of the primary advantages of treating acute injuries with ice is that ice diminishes the inflammatory response. Ice does do this. The preceding list of purposes of the inflammatory response, however, indicates just how important inflammation is; diminishing the

21

inflammatory response only delays the healing process (J44). This misconception may be the result of confusing the inflammatory response with the signs of inflammation—specifically, confusing "swelling" with "inflammation." Using ice to control pain and swelling is helpful; limiting inflammation is not, even if there are some negative side effects of inflammation.

Inflammation consists of eight overlapping phases. They occur in the order listed here, but may happen to be occurring simultaneously at different places around an injury site because the response progresses at different rates in different parts of the tissue.

Phases of Inflammation

1. Injury
2. Ultrastructural changes
3. Metabolic (hypoxic) changes
4. Activation of chemical mediators
5. Hemodynamic changes
6. Permeability changes
7. Leukocyte migration
8. Phagocytosis

Injury

Any event that impairs tissue structure or function and thereby alters the cells' ability to carry out their normal homeostatic mechanisms will cause the inflammatory response. An injury may be so minor that the injured person is unaware of it; still, the inflammatory response occurs. Most sport injuries are caused by trauma, either (a) *macrotrauma*, also called "impact" or "contact," or (b) *microtrauma*, also known as "overuse," "cyclic loading," or "friction" (J44). Although trauma is the main cause of injury in athletics, there are many other causes of injury that result in the same basic inflammatory response. These include the following:

- Physical agents (e.g., burns and radiation)
- Metabolic factors (hypoxia)
- Biological agents (e.g., bacteria, viruses, and parasites)
- Chemical agents (e.g., acids, gases, organic solvents, and chemicals within the body)
- Normal secretions, either in abnormal locations (such as gout), or in increased quantity in a normal location (such as stomach ulcers)
- Iatrogenic agents (e.g., side effects from chemotherapy)

The magnitude of specific reactions may vary according to the causative agent.

Ultrastructural Changes

Ultrastructural changes involve the breakdown and eventual disruption of the cell membrane so that the cell's contents spill out into the extracellular spaces (J24, J26). With sports injuries, ultrastructural changes occur primarily as a result of trauma and secondarily as a result of hypoxia (oxygen deficiency) or enzymes (chemicals), explained next. Often, secondary hypoxic injury occurs in cells adjacent to cells that have undergone primary traumatic injury.

Metabolic (Hypoxic) Changes

The normal functioning of a cell requires energy, which is usually supplied by aerobic metabolism (J29). When a cell is deprived of oxygen (a state known as *hypoxia*), it switches to anaerobic metabolism (glycolysis) to produce energy. Glycolysis alone cannot continue for long, however, and continued hypoxia leads to a steady decrease in energy production. Membrane functions slow down as the energy necessary to maintain them decreases (I8). Of particular importance is the decreased activity of the sodium pump, which is responsible for maintaining the concentration of intracellular sodium at a very low level (Figure 3.1). As the sodium pump's activity slows or stops, the sodium concentration within the cell and its organelles rises, causing increased amounts of water to pass into the cell, which then begins to swell. Excessive swelling causes the cell to burst. Prolonged anaerobic metabolism also leads to intracellular acidosis. The buildup of acid within the cell further impairs membrane integrity.

One cellular organelle is the lysosome, whose function is to supply enzymes that digest foreign material entrapped within the cell. If the membranes of the lysosome accidentally rupture, as a result of acidosis or failure of the sodium pump, its contents begin digesting other cellular components, including the cell membrane.

Activation of Chemical Mediators

Histamine, bradykinin, and other chemicals whose job is to notify the rest of the body that cells have been damaged and to mobilize the body's resources to handle the situation (Figure 3.2) are activated by ultrastructural changes. These chemicals modify and regulate the rest of the inflammatory response, to attempt to neutralize the cause of the injury and begin removing the cellular debris so that repair can take place.

Hemodynamic Changes

Hemodynamic changes result in the mobilization and transport of defense components of the blood to the injury site and the securing of their passage through the vessel wall into the tissue. These changes occur in vessels within the injured area that were not disrupted by the trauma and in vessels on the periphery of the injury. Specifically, arteries dilate, enhancing blood flow (Figure 3.3). At the same time, many previously inactive capillaries and venules open. Thus, total blood flow to the area increases, but the rate

Figure 3.1 The sodium pump is an active process (i.e., requires energy to function) that maintains a sodium gradient across the cell membrane by actively moving sodium that passively diffuses into the cell, back out of the cell. As sodium is pumped out of the cell, potassium is pumped into it. Reprinted from Guyton (J29).

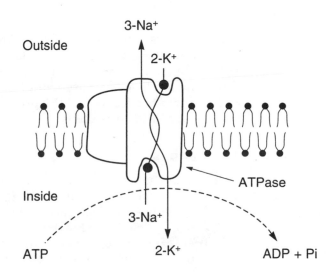

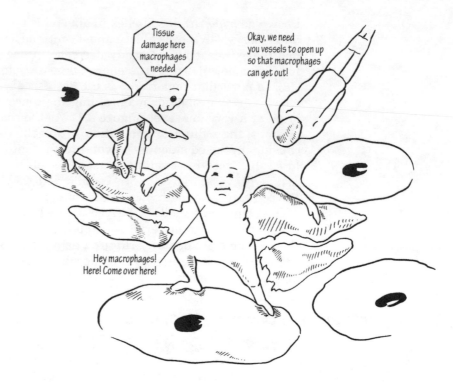

Figure 3.2 Chemical mediators act as "traffic cops" after being released by injured tissue. They activate numerous processes necessary for mobilizing and attracting white cells to the injury site.

Figure 3.3 Inactive vessels (a) open following injury (b) so as to flood the area with blood and decrease the rate of blood flow in individual vessels. These steps allow white cells to move from the center of the vessel to the walls and to slow down.

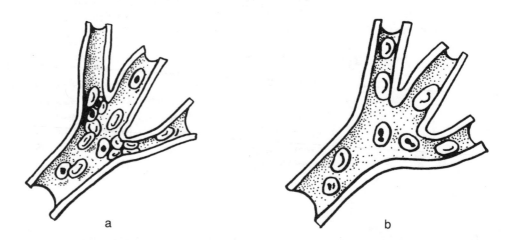

of flow through individual vessels slows. Sometimes complete stagnation occurs. The slowing of blood flow allows leukocytes (white blood cells) to fall out of the stream line, or middle of the vessel, and move to the margins. They tumble along the margin until they adhere to the endothelium (vessel wall) or to other leukocytes (Figure 3.4). Eventually, the endothelium becomes paved with these cells.

Permeability Changes

Both histamine and bradykinin increase the permeability of small blood vessels. The endothelial cells of the vessels seem to contract, or round up, thereby pulling away from each other (Figure 3.5) and leaving sizable gaps through which gathered leukocytes can move out of the vessel and to the injury site (Figure 3.6). Even though the gap is sizable in comparison with its normal state, the leukocytes have to work to escape.

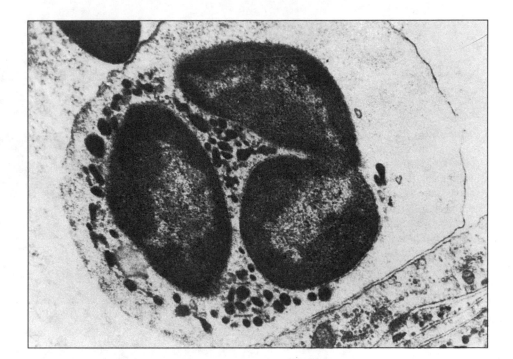

Figure 3.4 Electron micrograph of a white cell (polymorph) adhering to the vessel wall. Soon it will crawl along until it finds a gap in the vessel wall through which it can escape.
Photo courtesy of the Upjohn Corporation (G77).

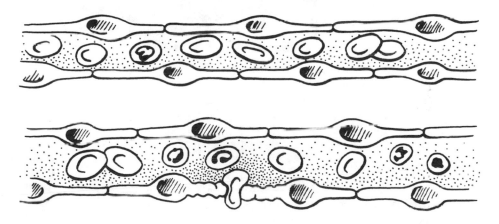

Figure 3.5 Endothelial cells of the vessel wall contract so that the gap between them enlarges, thus making it easier for white cells to move out of the vessel.

Although increased permeability occurs primarily to allow leukocytes to move toward the injury, it also allows great amounts of protein-rich fluid to escape. This results in increased viscosity of the blood, sometimes even to the point that cells become so packed in the vessel that they cannot move, blocking circulation.

Leukocyte Migration

Once outside the vascular wall, leukocytes begin migrating to the injury site in a concentration-limited fashion (Figure 3.7); that is, the number of leukocytes becomes greatest at those sites where the greatest tissue damage has occurred and is least in those areas of little or no tissue damage. This occurs in response to the concentration of chemical mediator in the area, which is greatest at the sites of greatest tissue damage.

The two types of leukocytes that play the primary role in sport injury–induced inflammation are the neutrophils and macrophages (Figure 3.8). Neutrophils travel faster than macrophages and so arrive at the injury site

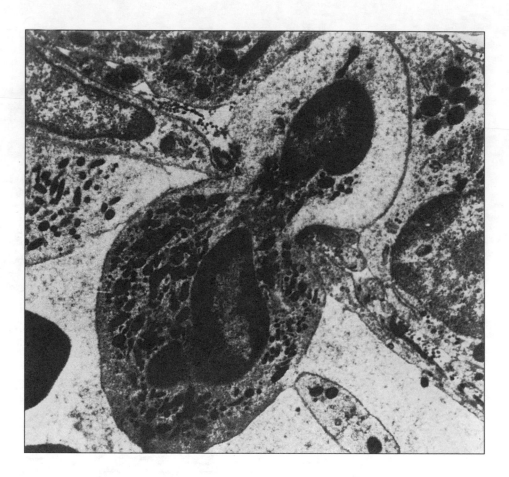

Figure 3.6 Electron micrograph of a neutrophil squeezing through an endothelial gap from the vessel into the tissue. Note the platelet (lower right) and portion of another neutrophil (upper left) adhering to the neutrophil.
Photo courtesy of the Upjohn Corporation (G77).

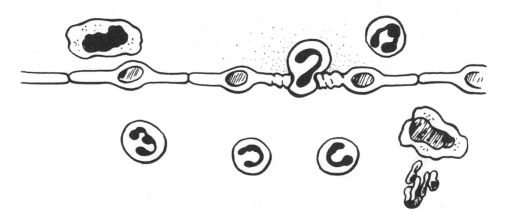

Figure 3.7 White cells migrate to the injury site in a concentration-limited fashion (i.e., the white cells congregate in proportion to the degree of injury).

first. They provide only a temporary first line of defense, though, since they are short-lived (about 7 hours) and incapable of reproduction. When they die they release chemical mediators that attract macrophages, adding to the concentration of chemical mediator released by the cells.

Macrophages live for months and can reproduce, thus providing a long-lasting second line of defense. In addition to phagocytosis, macrophages release potent enzymes that may destroy connective tissue, thus adding to the injury; release chemical mediators that may prolong inflammation; release substances responsible for fever; release factors that aid in healing; and secrete proteins that are important in defense mechanisms.

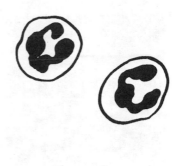

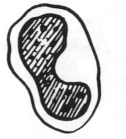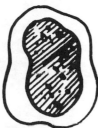

Figure 3.8 Neutrophils (also known as polymorphs; on top) and macrophages (bottom) are the most common white cells. Because neutrophils are smaller, they migrate out of the vessel first. But they soon die and add to the cellular debris that must be cleaned up by the macrophages.

Phagocytosis

Phagocytosis is the process of digesting cellular debris and other foreign material into pieces small enough to be removed from the injury site via the lymph vessels. As leukocytes arrive at the injury site, they begin removing tissue debris and any foreign material, such as bacteria, that is present. The leukocyte engulfs a bacterium or cell particle by invaginating its own membrane, which then closes around the particle and forms a sac (Figure 3.9). This sac, or phagosome, moves into the interior of the cell, where it unites with one or more lysosomes to become a phagolysosome. The contents of the lysosome spill into the phagosome and begin digesting its contents. This way, the cell can use powerful enzymes to digest foreign material without causing its own destruction.

Once the contents of the phagosome are broken down into very small units of protein (free protein), the contents are discharged into the intracellular space. This increased free protein increases tissue oncotic pressure (discussed later in this chapter) and thus increases edema and swelling.

CHRONIC INFLAMMATION

When the inflammatory response is unable to eliminate the cause of the injury (such as repeated overuse) and restore normal function to the injured tissue, *chronic inflammation* ensues (J24). Macrophages proliferate and release chemical mediators that attract additional macrophages. The more macrophages accumulate, the less stress or overuse it takes to keep the process going. Thus activity that is normally nontraumatic becomes an inflammatory stimulus. Words ending in *-itis*, such as *bursitis* and *tendinitis*, are used to designate conditions thought to involve chronic inflammation. However, although these conditions result from microtrauma, not all involve an inflammatory reaction. Clinically diagnosed Achilles tendinitis (G22) and patellar tendinitis sometimes show no evidence of an inflammatory reaction. One explanation for the lack of inflammation is that microtrauma can cause significant structural disruption and microvascular damage can occur, causing pain and other clinical symptoms, before the classic inflammatory process is set into action (J44).

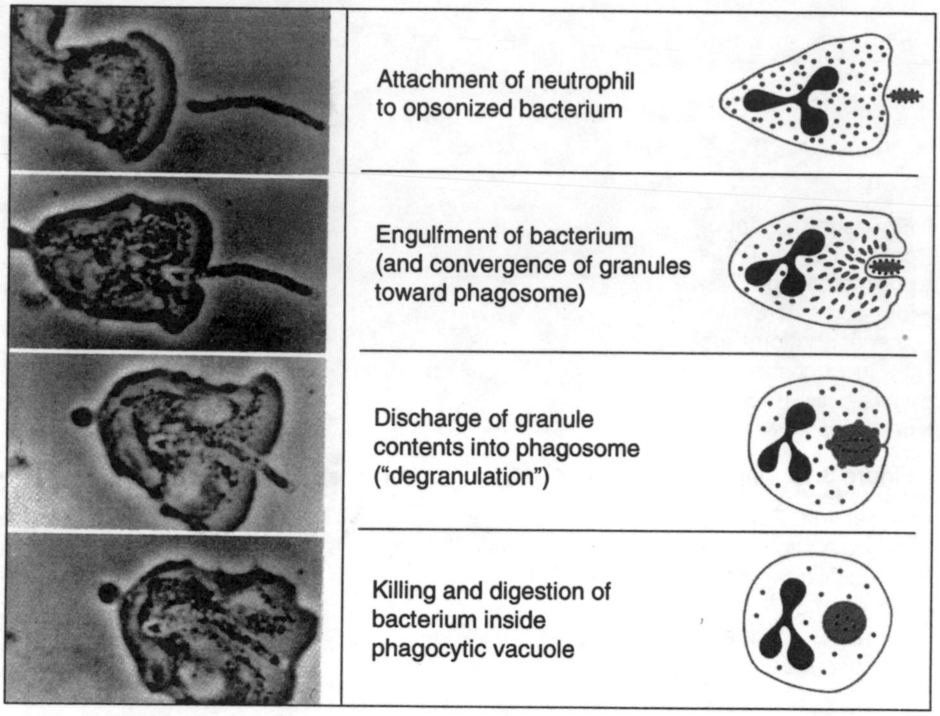

Attachment of neutrophil to opsonized bacterium

Engulfment of bacterium (and convergence of granules toward phagosome)

Discharge of granule contents into phagosome ("degranulation")

Killing and digestion of bacterium inside phagocytic vacuole

Figure 3.9   Schema illustrating phagocytosis of a strand of bacteria by a neutrophil. Actual photomicrographs on left, artist's rendition on right.
Courtesy of the Upjohn Corporation (G77).

THE SPORT INJURY MODEL

What happens when a muscle is pulled or an ankle sprained? Although every injury is somewhat different, the following model should help you understand the processes that occur following acute trauma. We begin with an "ideal" area of tissue composed of a number of cells; several blood vessels, with branches, to supply these cells with oxygen and nutrients; and two pain neurons (Figure 3.10).

When an injury occurs, whether a contusion caused by direct compression or a sprain or strain caused by a stretching force, immediate ultrastructural changes take place in muscle, connective tissue, or both (Figure 3.11); nerves and blood vessels may also be broken. All this damage is called primary traumatic damage, because it was caused directly by the trauma. The damaged tissue becomes debris that will have to be removed from the area before new cells can replace the damaged ones. The cellular debris releases chemical mediators to signal the body that an injury has taken place. The torn nerves send impulses to the brain that are interpreted as pain.

Blood hemorrhages from the broken vessels (Figure 3.12) into the extravascular spaces, causing swelling. The bleeding is usually short-lived, however, due to the clotting mechanism, in which fibrin and blood platelets close the damaged vessel (H32, H49, H64, H77). Fibrin, a protein in the blood, forms strands that grow into a network somewhat like a fish net. The fibrin net captures circulating platelets and forms a plug that seals the damaged vessel (Figure 3.13), sometimes completely plugging it so that circulation through it is stopped. The area is left with a mass of whole blood and cellular debris, which together are known as a hematoma (Figure 3.14).

As the hematoma forms, pressure is exerted on undamaged pain neurons in the area, resulting in additional pain. Besides such outward responses to pain as the awareness of hurting and nausea, the body responds with muscle spasm and inhibition of muscular strength and range of motion (B43). These responses are efforts by the body to protect itself by splinting the area and thus preventing aggravation of the injury.

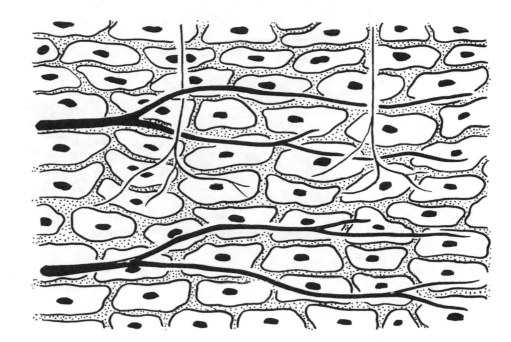

Figure 3.10 Injury model—normal: a hypothetical drawing of normal (uninjured) tissue cells, blood vessels, and nerves.

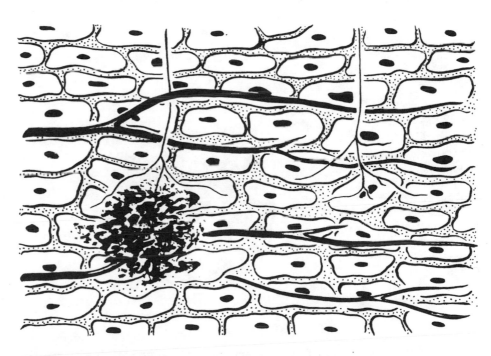

Figure 3.11 Injury model—primary injury; trauma, such as a contusion, causes ultrastructural changes to tissue cells, blood vessels, and nerves. All tissues damaged by the trauma have suffered primary injury. Damage to nerves causes pain.

The body's response to the hematoma is to remove it. It does so through the last four phases of the inflammatory response: hemodynamic changes, permeability changes, leukocyte migration, and phagocytosis. These events take place in the circulatory vessels on the periphery of the injury. Leukocytes are released into the tissue so that they can break down the tissue debris of the hematoma. The debris, as small pieces of free protein, can then be removed from the area by the lymphatic system. Once the hematoma is removed, wound healing or repair can take place.

The inflammatory response is not all positive, however. Slower blood flow in the vessels on the periphery of the injury and decreased blood flow from the damaged vasculature mean less oxygen is delivered to cells in the vicinity

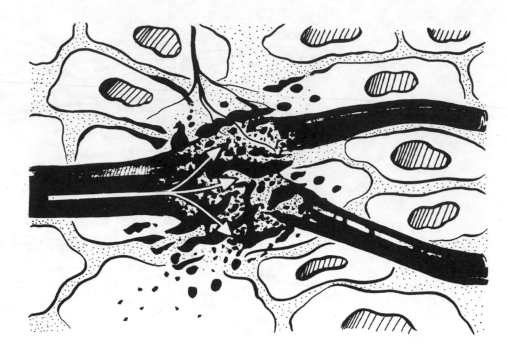

Figure 3.12 Injury model—hemorrhaging from a ruptured blood vessel into the tissue.

Figure 3.13 Injury model—clot; strands of fibrin begin forming immediately after injury. The fibrin strands crisscross in a fishnet fashion and begin entrapping platelets (left). Within minutes, a solid plug, or clot, is formed (right).

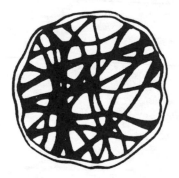

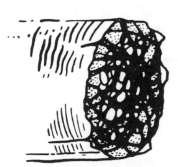

of the primary traumatic injury. If this hypoxic state is prolonged, metabolic changes occur in these cells, and they undergo secondary hypoxic injury. Thus, the total amount of damaged tissue is increased, and more debris is added to the hematoma.

SECONDARY INJURY

The body's response to primary traumatic damage leads to further tissue damage, known as secondary injury. This occurs in cells on the periphery of the primary traumatic injury (G31, G61, G76). Two separate mechanisms result in secondary injury: enzymatic action and hypoxia.

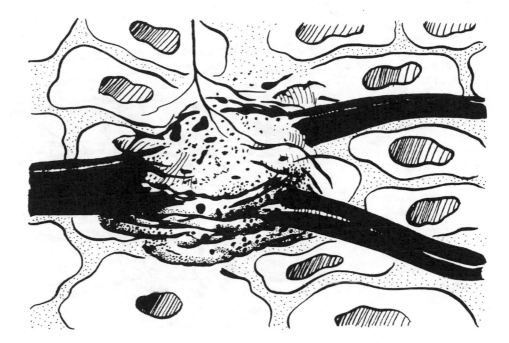

Figure 3.14 Injury model—hematoma; primary injury debris (damaged tissue, blood vessels, and nerve cells) and the hemorrhaged blood (both solid and liquid portions) are trapped in the tissue and are called a hematoma.

Secondary Enzymatic Injury

Enzymes designed to digest cellular debris are activated and released from the lysosomes of dead cells (G76, G77). If these enzymes come into contact with nearby live cells, they will begin breaking down the cellular membrane of the live cells, leading to additional cellular death.

Secondary Hypoxic Injury

The term *secondary hypoxic injury* was coined in 1976 to describe the tissue damage resulting from a metabolic imbalance secondary to acute traumatic sports injuries (G50). Secondary hypoxic injury results from inadequate oxygen delivery to tissues on the periphery of the primary traumatic injury. Blood flow ceases in injured vessels distal to the site of injury and is decreased in other vessels in the area because of inflammatory stasis and sludging (G62, G78, G86). The resultant lack of oxygen ultimately brings about cellular edema and bursting, acidosis, and lysosymal digestion, as described previously. Both the breakdown of the cellular membrane and the intracellular release of lysosomal enzymes lead to cell death (Figure 3.15). The resulting debris is added to the hematoma (Figure 3.16). Thus the total amount of damaged tissue is increased.

The inflammatory process is summarized in Figure 3.17.

SWELLING: HEMORRHAGING AND EDEMA

Swelling results from two processes already described: direct hemorrhaging into traumatized tissues and edema. Hemorrhaging results in initial swelling, whereas swelling that occurs hours after the injury is due to edema.

Figure 3.15 Injury model—secondary hypoxic injury; viable cells in the immediate area of the injury, but which escaped damage by the trauma, undergo metabolic changes because of oxygen deficiency which results from injured blood vessels and circulatory slow-down induced by the inflammatory response. In areas where the oxygen deficiency is severe enough and long enough, the cells die.

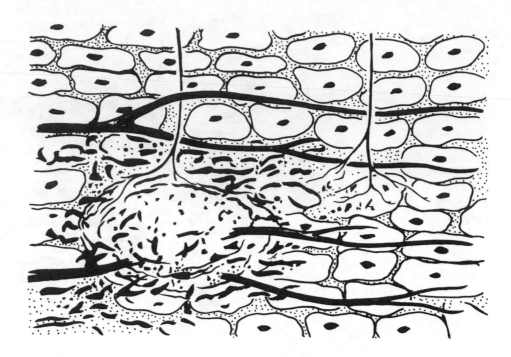

Figure 3.16 Injury model—growing hematoma; the hematoma expands as cellular debris from secondary injury is added to the debris of primary injury and hemorrhaging. As the inflammatory process breaks down the cellular debris into free protein, edema occurs. Additional secondary injury occurs (see cells at far left).

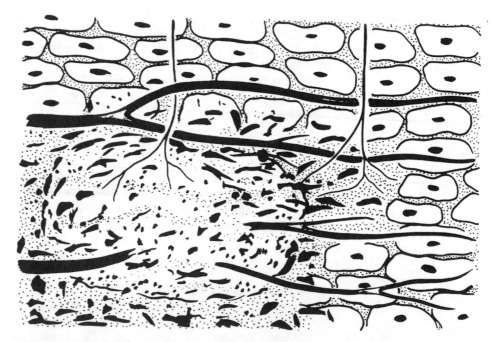

Whenever blood vessel walls are damaged as part of an injury, hemorrhaging occurs and continues as long as the vessel wall remains open. Under normal conditions, clotting occurs within a few minutes following injury (H28, H44), thus sealing the vessel walls and stopping the hemorrhaging.

Edema Formation

If the normal back-and-forth movement of fluid between capillaries and uninjured tissue is upset so that more fluid flows into the tissue than flows out of it, the result is edema, the accumulation in the tissues of the fluid

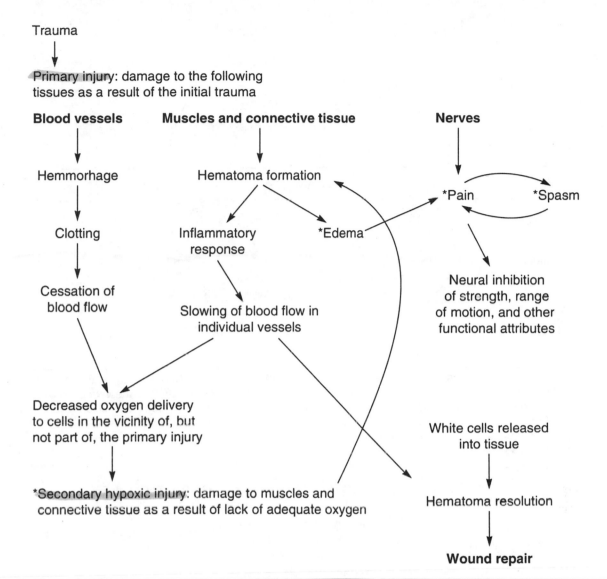

Figure 3.17 Summary of the response of the inflammatory system to acute trauma. Those phases of the response that are benefited by cold application to the injury site are labeled (*) and explained in the text.

portion of the blood. The longer the fluid dynamics are out of balance, the greater the edema accumulation and the greater the swelling.

Normal Fluid Exchange

In normal tissue, fluid constantly passes between the vascular system and the extracellular spaces (Figure 3.18). Normally, about two thirds of the fluid that passes into the tissues is reabsorbed directly into the vascular system. The other third is returned to the blood via the lymphatic system (H30). Two factors make the free movement of fluid possible. First, water molecules diffuse through the capillary walls several thousand times more rapidly than blood flows along the capillary (H21). Second, there is a difference in pressure between the inside and outside of the vessels. This pressure, called *capillary filtration pressure* or *transcapillary pressure*, is the sum of five pressures, resulting from Starling Forces (H54). Five components influence filtration pressure, according to the following formula:

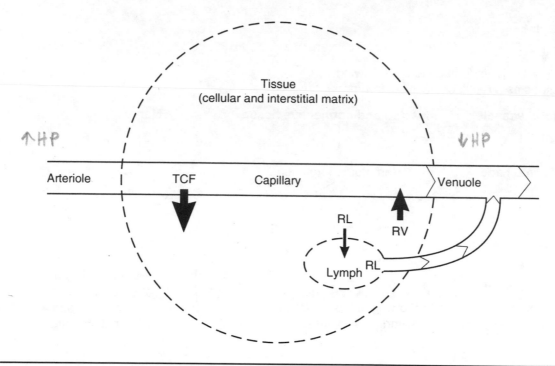

Figure 3.18   Fluid moves constantly between the circulatory system and tissue. Under steady state conditions, the amount of fluid that moves out of the capillary (TCF) is reabsorbed; two-thirds directly into the venous end of the capillary (RV) and one-third into lymph vessels (RL) which empty into the venous system. This fluid movement is caused by differences in fluid presure (hydrostatic and oncotic) in the capillary and tissue as explained in the text. Edema results when the pressures are upset so that more fluid moves out of the capillary than what is reabsorbed. Modified from Hargers (J82).

$$CFP = (CHP + TOP) - (COP + THP + EFP),$$

where

CFP = capillary filtration pressure,
CHP = capillary hydrostatic pressure,
TOP = tissue oncotic pressure,
COP = capillary oncotic pressure,
THP = tissue hydrostatic pressure, and
EFP = external force pressures.

Hydrostatic pressure is pressure exerted by a column of water. The higher the column of water, the greater the pressure. Anyone who has swum has experienced hydrostatic pressure. The deeper you go, the higher is the column of water above you and the greater the pressure. Similarly, hydrostatic pressure is exerted by the water portion of the blood and tissues: Capillary hydrostatic pressure forces fluid out of the capillary, and tissue hydrostatic pressure forces fluid back into the capillary. *Oncotic pressure* (also called colloid osmotic pressure) is the pressure resulting from the attraction of fluid by free protein. Tissue oncotic pressure tends to pull fluid out of the capillary, while capillary oncotic pressure tends to pull fluid back into the capillary.

External force pressure results from tissue elasticity and bandages. Since these are not factors in normal fluid filtration, and are not a part of the Starling Equation, they only come into play if the area is swollen. More about this later.

It is the sum of these pressures that determines which way the fluid passes. At the arterial end of capillaries, capillary hydrostatic pressure dominates; capillary filtration pressure is thus positive, so fluid moves out of the capillary and into the tissues (H3, H21, J29). Toward the venous end of the capillary, capillary hydrostatic pressure decreases and pressures that cause reabsorption increase, causing fluid to move back into the capillary. If all the pressures along the length of the capillary are summed and averaged, the average net capillary filtration pressure is slightly positive. This accounts for the fluid that is not reabsorbed but removed from the area via the lymphatic system (Table 3.1).

Fluid Exchange in Injured Tissue

With injury the average capillary filtration pressure increases as a result of an increase in tissue oncotic pressure (C38; Table 3.2). Tissue oncotic pressure rises because of the increased amount of free protein in the area that has come about as a result of the breakdown by macrophages of tissue debris from primary injury and secondary hypoxic injury and of hemorrhaged whole blood. Also, some free protein escapes from the circulatory system during the period of hemorrhaging (if a vessel was damaged) or as a result of the increased permeability. The result is that more fluid passes out of the capillaries in the vicinity of the injury and less is reabsorbed, resulting in edema and swelling. The greater the injury, the more free protein and eventually more edema.

This process accounts for the delayed nature of most swelling. Both second- ary hypoxic injury and the breakdown of tissue debris by macrophages occur over an extended period of time. Edema, therefore, begins minutes to hours

---

Table 3.1   Capillary Filtration Pressure Components and Their Effect on Fluid Exchange Between Capillaries and Tissue

Capillary filtration pressure component	Tendency to move fluid into tissue	Average normal pressure (mmHg)*
Capillary hydrostatic	+	23
Tissue oncotic (osmotic)	+	10
Tissue hydrostatic	–	1 to 4
Capillary oncotic		25
External	–	0
Net (overall)	**	4 to 7

*Estimates of these values differ from text to text. These values came from Ryan and Majno, 1977 (G77).
**If sum is +, fluid moves into tissue; if –, out of tissue.

Table 3.2   Changes in Capillary Filtration Pressure Components Following Injury

Capillary filtration pressure component	Tendency to move fluid into tissue	Average normal pressure (mmHg)	Change due to injury
Capillary hydrostatic	+	23	~
Tissue oncotic (osmotic)	+	10	↑ ↑ ↑ ↑ ↑
Tissue hydrostatic	–	1 to 4	↑
Capillary oncotic	–	25	~
External	–	0	~
Net (overall)	*	+4 to 7	↑ ↑ ↑ ↑ ↑

*If sum is +, fluid moves into tissue; if –, out of tissue.

after injury and continues to develop for many hours. The swelling that occurs immediately after the injury is due to direct hemorrhaging.

Not only does secondary hypoxic injury result in increased edema, but increased edema can contribute to increased secondary hypoxic injury. Two mechanisms are involved (H21). First, as edema develops, the distance between the blood vessel and tissue cells increases. This makes it more difficult for oxygen and nutrients to diffuse from the circulatory system to the tissue. Second, edema fluid can compress the blood vessel, decreasing circulation to the area.

If swelling is due to edema, why does the area turn black and blue? Wouldn't this be due to oxidized blood? Some of it is, but much of the discoloration in muscle may be the result of oxidized myoglobin from damaged musculature.

How Does Cold Decrease Swelling?

Cold applications are usually applied after clotting has occurred and so have no effect on hemorrhaging. Moreover, once edema has developed, cold applications cannot reverse it. But cold can prevent edema from occurring if applied soon enough after the injury. Cold diminishes secondary hypoxic injury, so there is less free protein in the tissues. Thus, there is less tissue oncotic pressure, the major cause of edema. The details of this process are discussed in chapter 8.

■ DON'T DELAY IN APPLYING COLD PACKS

Apply ice packs as quickly as possible following injury. The quicker you apply the ice, the quicker you slow metabolism. Thus, you protect more tissue from secondary hypoxic injury and have less total tissue damage.

Do not, however, forgo a thorough evaluation of the injury just to apply ice packs more quickly. This is the "golden period" for evaluation—the time when you will be able to gain the most information about the injury. The effectiveness of evaluation decreases dramatically after muscle spasm and injury guarding set in.

THE HEALING PROCESS

Tissue repair comprises processes that replace dead or damaged cells with healthy ones. Repair usually begins soon after injury, after enough cellular debris has been removed. The smaller the hematoma is, the more quickly repair can begin and the less there is to repair. Some consider repair part of the inflammatory response (J24, J67); others consider these to be separate processes (G76, J44, J48). I will use the latter categorization here.

Types of Repair

There are two types of repair: (a) reconstitution with the same type of cells that were injured, and (b) replacement with simpler cells. Reconstitution occurs in those cells that normally have a high rate of turnover, such as skin and liver cells. Perfect reconstitution means that the damaged cells are replaced by cells of the identical type, with no evidence that the injury occurred. Imperfect reconstitution occurs when most of the damaged cells are replaced by identical cells but some are replaced with connective tissue and thus forms some scar tissue. Replacement with simpler cells results in the formation of scar tissue. This occurs in connective tissue, muscle, and the central nervous system and in any area where the damage is extensive enough to disrupt the basic cellular framework. Also known as repair by connective tissue, this process occurs in two ways. Primary union occurs in an area with a small incision, which fills and heals very rapidly. Secondary union occurs when there is a large gap or hole to be filled in. It is much slower and leaves a larger scar.

■ CLOSING THE WOUND GAP

Lacerations must be sutured or steri striped to close the wound gap. This allows for faster healing and leaves less of a scar. For best results, these procedures should be done within 6 hours of injury.

Phases of Repair

As with the inflammatory response, the phases of tissue repair occur in a general sequence but may be occurring at the same time in different parts of a damaged area. The four phases of repair are as follows (J16, J26, J27, J32):

Phases of Tissue Repair

1. Cellular phase
2. Vascular response
3. Collagenization
4. Contraction and restructuring

Cellular Phase

The cellular phase is an extension of the phagocytosis phase of inflammation. During this phase, macrophages scavenge the cellular debris, and the circulatory and lymphatic systems drain away the liquified cellular remains, which are mostly small particles of free protein. This is very important, since the more protein that remains, the bigger the scar will be.

■ EXERCISE AND LYMPHATIC DRAINAGE

The lymphatic system is passive, which means that the walls of its vessels do not contract and that there is no pressure to cause fluid to move through the vessels, in contrast to the way in which the heart provides pressure to the blood system. The lymphatic system depends on external force to promote fluid movement—force such as muscular contraction. As a muscle expands during contraction, it squeezes the lymphatic vessels and forces their contents upstream toward the junction with the blood system. Moderate activity during the cellular phase thus promotes lymphatic drainage and hastens healing.

Vascular Response

The vascular response is a transient phase during which many new capillaries are formed. These vessels deliver to the wound area the great amounts of oxygen and nutrients that will be needed for repair. A process known as *capillary budding* is the primary mechanism of the vascular phase (Figure 3.19a). Endothelial cells of existing blood vessels at the edge of the wound begin to divide by mitosis. The new cells crawl away from, but keep in contact with, the existing vessel (Figure 3.19b). New cells force themselves between existing cells, thus forcing the end cells to advance into the wound area (Figure 3.19c). Bud sprouts adjacent to each other migrate toward one another, meet and connect, and create a *capillary arch* (Figure 3.20). Blood then begins to flow through the arch, and new budding begins from the arch. Soon a network of these arches, or a *capillary arcade,* is formed (Figure 3.21), which eventually develops throughout the entire wound area. This provides the wound area with abundant circulation, which is necessary to support collagenization, the next phase. Eventually, after collagenization has taken place and the need for abundant circulation has passed, many of the new vessels atrophy. Others form into arterioles or venules or remain as capillaries.

Collagenization

Collagenization is the process of manufacturing and laying down collagen in the wound space, which results in a scar. (Collagen, a fibrous protein found in all types of connective tissue, is the principal solid substance of ligaments, tendons, and scar tissue.) First, fibroblasts migrate along strands of fibrin into the wound area, but never very far beyond the capillary arcade. They then begin to manufacture strands of collagen, which are extruded haphazardly into the wound space (Figure 3.22a). Four to 6 days after the injury, the degree of vascularization and rate of collagenization are maximal. Most collagen is laid down by 15 to 20 days after the injury (J23). The wound is not very strong yet, however. Strength comes only after the collagen is realigned parallel to the lines of force (Figure 3.22b), a process that sometimes takes up to a year.

Collagenization requires great amounts of oxygen. Oxygen is needed to provide energy (through aerobic metabolism) for the fibroblasts and also as a substrate for collagen. Healing wounds normally do not have all of the oxygen that they could use (J69; Figure 3.23); research has shown that the amount of collagen accumulated in a wound area and the tensile strength

Figure 3.19 New blood vessels formed as the endothelial cells at a budding site on an existing vessel divide mitotically. They slide past each other (a) into positions distal from their place of origin (b) and form a bud (c). The process continues and the bud becomes larger until it joins with another bud to form a loop or capillary arch. Courtesy of Upjohn Corporation (G77).

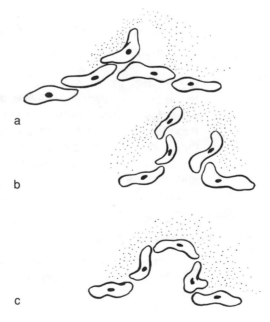

Figure 3.20 Capillary arches formed by numerous capillary buds along a vessel (a). Initially the buds grow randomly into the injured tissue (b), but eventually they move toward another bud, where they join to form a loop or arch (c). Once the loops form, blood begins flowing through them to supply fibroblasts and oxygen to rebuild the injured tissue.

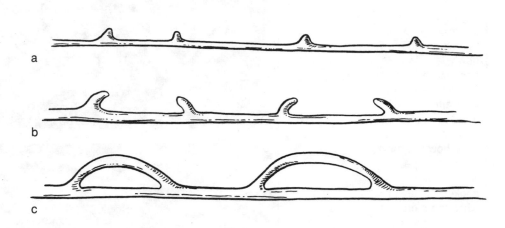

Figure 3.21 A capillary arcade develops as numerous capillary arches form from blood vessels on the periphery of the injured tissue. Most of these new vessels will collapse once the tissue is healed and the need for oxygen drastically decreases.

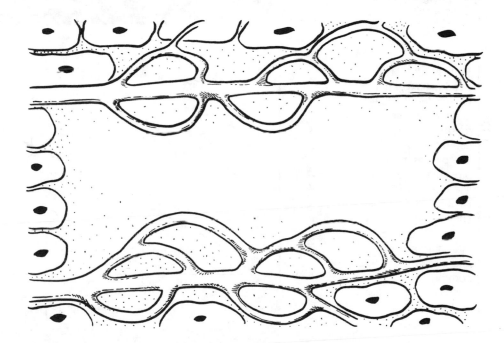

of skin wounds are linearly related to the amount of oxygen available to the wound. Niinikoski has shown that between 5 and 15 days following injury, the greater the percentage of oxygen in the air breathed by laboratory rats, the greater the tensile strength of their wounds (Figure 3.24).

Contraction and Restructuring

Contraction and restructuring are processes that cause the scar tissue to become smaller and more pale. A new scar will appear to be quite red (in lighter skinned people) and raised above the surrounding tissue. With time the appearance of the scar changes until it is pale and flat or sunken below the surrounding skin.

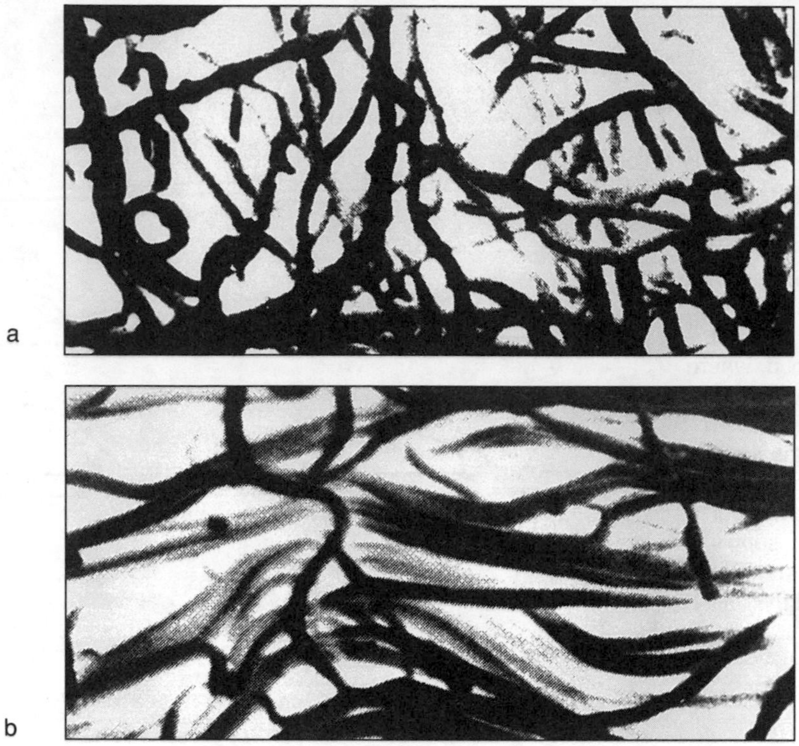

Figure 3.22 Electronmicrograph of human collagen (a) newly laid down in a haphazard fashion; (b) same site weeks later after the collagen has realigned in a parallel fashion. Note how the new collagen appears like a plate of cooked spaghetti, while the more mature collagen looks more like uncooked spaghetti right out of the box.
Photos courtesy of John Bergfeld, MD, Cleveland Clinic.

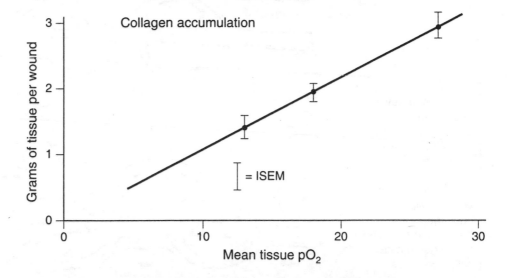

Figure 3.23 The need for oxygen in a healing wound is illustrated in this graph of collagen accumulation and tissue oxygen partial pressure. Note the linear relationship between collagen accumulation and pO_2 when pO_2 is less than normal, normal, and higher than normal.
Reprinted from Ehrlich (J83).

Because collagen is a relatively inactive tissue, it does not require much oxygen once it is laid down and therefore it does not need a great deal of circulation. Consequently, much of the capillary arcade collapses and is compressed by the surrounding collagen. This accounts for some of the contraction of the scar. Also, with less blood circulating through the wound, the scar appears paler.

Restructuring refers to the reorganization of collagen fibers from the haphazard fashion in which they were laid down to a parallel arrangement (J16). Although this process compacts the scar, the primary reason for rearranging the collagen fibers is to give the scar greater strength. Fibers running perpendicular to the lines of force (tissue stress) will not help keep the edges of the wound together. Only fibers parallel to the lines of force strengthen the injured tissue.

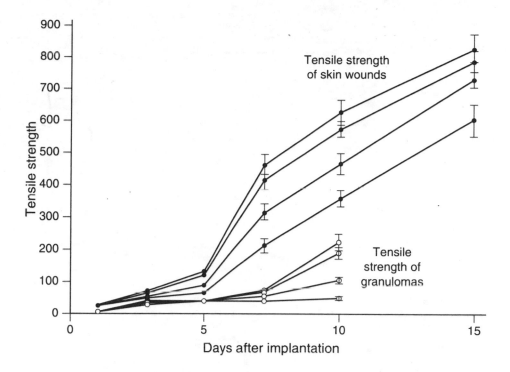

Figure 3.24 The effect of changing oxygen supply on wound healing. The more oxygen available, the stronger the wound becomes. Reprinted from Niinikoski (J57).

Restructuring of collagen occurs in response to force exerted on the scar. As the body part moves, the scar senses the direction of the movement and lines up the majority of the collagen fibers parallel to the lines of force (J23). Thus, active exercise is necessary to the final phase of wound healing, although activity that is too vigorous too early will tear an immature scar.

■ *EXERCISE IS ESSENTIAL DURING WOUND HEALING*

Exercise is essential during wound healing for two reasons. First, exercise stimulates the circulation and thus increases oxygen delivery to the healing tissue. Second, exercise stresses the tissue and thus guides the restructuring of collagen. Exercise must be controlled, however; overly vigorous exercise will disrupt the healing tissue. There is a fine line between the amount of exercise that optimizes tissue repair and that which tears down the repair.

SUMMARY

- Inflammation is the body's response to injury. Its purpose is to protect the body against invasion by foreign bodies and to prepare the injured tissue for repair.
- The repair process, also known as wound healing, follows the inflammatory response.
- Primary injury is tissue damage directly caused by trauma.
- Secondary injury is tissue damage that occurs in response to, and on the periphery of, the primary injury; it is caused by enzymatic and hypoxic changes in the tissue.
- Swelling is one of the signs of inflammation and should not be confused with the inflammatory process itself.
- Swelling is the result of both direct hemorrhaging (which results in turn from primary injury to blood vessels) and edema.

Sport Injury Rehabilitation

Rehabilitation is the process of restoring someone to a normal or optimal state of health. Since the optimum state of health for an athlete is a high level of conditioning, rehabilitation of an athletic injury is the process of returning the athlete to that high level of conditioning. But there is much more to rehabilitation than progressing through various phases of conditioning. For optimal results, rehabilitation must be planned and the plan executed systematically. Timing, goals, rate of progression, and criteria for progression are all important factors. There is also a significant psychological component to rehabilitation that you must understand and use.

In this chapter I look at the differences between rehabilitation and reconditioning and at some erroneous concepts of rehabilitation, present basic principles to guide rehabilitation, develop a rationale for a systematic approach to rehabilitation, list the 10 phases of rehabilitation, and discuss some psychological elements that can optimize rehabilitation.

REHABILITATION VS. RECONDITIONING

Injury rehabilitation is often called reconditioning because the athlete is being returned to his or her previously conditioned state. But the processes are different. The process of rehabilitation is based on principles of conditioning, but includes some very important modifications. For instance, an athlete who has torn a ligament cannot begin a reconditioning program until the ligament has healed, and so the processes involved in promoting healing must be considered as part of rehabilitation. Pain relief is also part of rehabilitation; since pain activates neural mechanisms within the body that inhibit strength, flexibility, power, and speed, pain must be dealt with before reconditioning can begin.

Another difference between rehabilitation and reconditioning is the rate of development of physical attributes during rehabilitation, which can be redeveloped much faster than they were developed originally (J37). Thus, it is possible to be much more aggressive during rehabilitation than during conditioning.

WHAT REHABILITATION IS NOT

The following are some erroneous concepts regarding sport injury rehabilitation.

Working With Weights

Some people talk of "rehab," "working with weights," and "strength training" as if all three were synonymous. The "rehab area" of many athletic training rooms and sports medicine clinics is the area that contains the weight equipment. This reflects an overly narrow concept of rehabilitation, however. Rehabilitation is not complete if the athlete only works with weights, no matter how intense this work may be.

Treat Then Rehabilitate

Another concept that is too narrow is the idea that an injured athlete is "treated" with various therapeutic modalities (whirlpools, ultrasound, etc.), and then "rehabilitated." Actually, rehabilitation is the entire process of returning an injured athlete to competition. It includes all activities which are designed to speed the healing process and to ensure that the athlete is in optimal health and conditioning before returning to competition.

Cookbook Approach

In the "cookbook" approach to rehabilitation, stages are established, each with a set length and specific exercises to be performed. For instance, Stage 2 might be defined as occurring from 2 weeks to 6 weeks following an injury and include isokinetic exercises, isotonic exercises, stair-climbing exercises, cycling, swimming, and light running. This approach does not take into account differences in the starting point (severity of injury) or the rate of progress of different athletes with the "same" injury. Rehabilitation of a certain type of injury can be different for athletes in different sports, because of the difference in demands placed on the injured body part during sport participation. A runner, for example, must spend more time developing muscular endurance than a golfer; a football player must develop more muscular speed than a distance runner.

The nature and severity of the injury affects the beginning point; the time of the season and the athlete's genetic makeup, general health, preinjury state of conditioning, psychological profile, and work ethic all affect the rate of progress through rehabilitation. Because every athlete and every injury are different, rehabilitation programs should be individualized. Optimal rehabilitation is not planned by the calendar or by specific exercises.

These erroneous concepts have developed because techniques tend to precede theory; that is, treatment or rehabilitation techniques are used and thought or known to be effective before it is known if or why they are effective. As a result, many professionals use an assortment of techniques that they have not brought together under an overall theoretical umbrella. This is changing, however. Athletic trainers (J36, J39) are beginning to look at the entire rehabilitation process and to take a systems approach to rehabilitation. I will discuss the principles of rehabilitation and then look at such an approach.

PRINCIPLES OF REHABILITATION

The following are 10 principles of rehabilitation. Each applies irrespective of the nature of the injury or the phase of rehabilitation.

Ten Principles of Rehabilitation

- The SAID Principle—Specific Adaptation to Imposed Demands
- Set Therapeutic Goals
- Continual Evaluation
- Functional Progression
- Pain Free
- Biofeedback

- Early Exercise
- Relatively Rapid Reconditioning Rate
- Immediate Initiation; Termination Only When Full Participation is Possible
- Athlete's Health Comes First

The SAID Principle

The SAID principle—(specific adaptation to imposed demands)—dominates rehabilitation. It means that the body responds to a given demand with a specific and predictable adaptation (J13). Stated another way, specific adaptation *requires* that *specific* demands be imposed. So, if you want to develop strength in a particular muscle group (the specific adaptation), you must require that particular muscle group to repeatedly contract against an overload (the imposed demand). Each physical attribute to be redeveloped (or developed, if the athlete was not properly conditioned before the injury) must be identified and specifically trained for. Complete or total rehabilitation can be achieved only if each aspect of conditioning is redeveloped through specific imposed demands.

Setting Therapeutic Goals

To take full advantage of the SAID principle, you must match the desired therapeutic goals with a specific therapeutic regimen that elicits the physiological and psychological responses required for achieving the goals. Plan your work, then work the plan.

Plan specific long-range, short-range, and daily goals (J18). Each long-range goal should encompass several short-range goals that progress to attaining it, and each short-range goal should have specific daily goals. Be flexible in adjusting goals or in adding additional ones as an athlete's needs change.

There are also psychological advantages of using goals liberally during rehabilitation (J18). These are discussed later in the chapter (J18).

Continual Evaluation

Proper application of the SAID principle requires both an accurate initial diagnosis of the nature and severity of the injury and continual—almost daily—reevaluation to determine the athlete's response to the therapeutic regimen and progress toward goals (Figure 4.1).

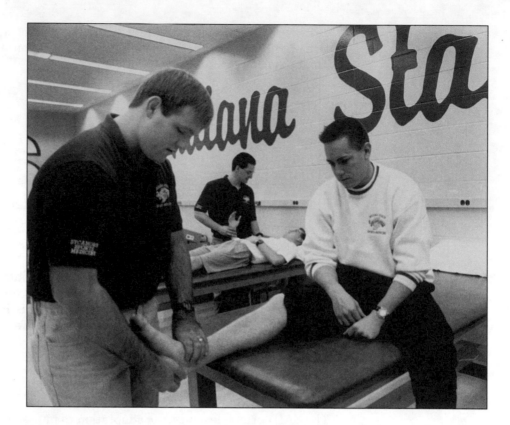

Figure 4.1 An accurate initial diagnosis and constant reevaluation are essential to good rehabilitation. Proper application of the SAID principle during rehabilitation requires matching rehabilitative procedures with the immediate need of the injured limb. The immediate need is calculated from specific information provided during evaluation and reevaluation.

Functional Progression

Progressive resistive exercise (PRE) was developed by Delorme (J17) as the key to strength development during rehabilitation. The concept of progression applies to all phases of rehabilitation. Athletes should progress from the easiest of activities to full sport participation. You usually progress from

- unloaded activities to
- loaded activities to
- overloaded activities

and from

- single-plane activities to
- multiple-plane activities.

Both of these progress from

- slow speed to
- normal speed to
- high speed

and with

- slow transition to
- normal transition to
- very quick transition.

Kegerreis (I26) referred to this concept with the phrases *progressive reorientation* and *functional progression*, which he defined "as an ordered sequence of activities enabling the acquisition or reacquisition of skills required for safe, effective performance of athletic endeavors." Each phase of the physical process is part of the larger picture of total rehabilitation and should proceed sequentially (J39).

The 10 phases of rehabilitation, described later in the chapter, are arranged so that athletes progress through a systematic program of physical reconditioning (J39). Although there will be some overlap, maximal development of any attribute usually requires prior development of the attributes that precede it.

Early Exercise

Exercise soon after injury is essential to rehabilitation (B36, H81, J41, J47). Not only does the proper use of early exercise speed healing, but lack of exercise during the early stages of rehabilitation may result in permanent disability (J18). A series of studies (J34-J35, J43) supports this theory. The researchers found that immediate mobilization following contusions to the legs of rats led to a more pronounced macrophage reaction (J43), quicker hematoma resolution (J35), increased vascular ingrowth (J34), quicker regeneration of muscle and scar tissue (J35), and increased tensile strength of the healed muscle (J33). Immobilization for as few as 2 or 5 days delayed contraction and maturation of the scar when measured 42 days later (J35). Others have shown that exercise during rehabilitation also results in stronger ligaments and tendons.

Caution must be observed, however. Exercise that is too vigorous can also result in permanent disability. The optimal conditions for healing apparently depend on a very fine balance between protection from stress and return toward normal function at the earliest possible time (Table 4.1; Figure 4.2) (J15). Sometimes pain is manifest long after the cause of the pain has been removed (E5, J15). In these cases interrupting the pain will allow full activity.

Rate of Reconditioning

Many physical attributes can be redeveloped much more quickly than the time it took to develop them originally (J35). Much performance loss attributable to injury is the result of pain-induced inhibition. Rehabilitation consists of systematically removing the inhibitions, rather than developing the attribute from the beginning.

Pain Free

All exercises should be pain free. Pain during an activity is an indication that the activity is too vigorous for the athlete and that he or she should back off. Residual pain (i.e., pain the next day) usually results from too vigorous activity the day before and indicates that you should have the athlete let up some. The concept of "no pain, no gain" has no place in rehabilitation. Use the athlete's pain reaction as an indication of being too aggressive (see Figure 4.2).

Biofeedback

Biofeedback can be very useful in rehabilitation, and you don't have to have fancy machinery to use it. Simply measure an athlete's performance in some meaningful way and then tell the athlete what his scores were. For instance, when you are trying to develop range of motion in a knee, tell the athlete to "move your leg so that your heel touches the wall and your toes touch my hand." Then count the repetitions, making sure the athlete knows that incomplete repetitions don't count. You can provide further biofeedback by timing the athlete's performance: "Let's see how long it takes you to perform 10 complete repetitions." Then share the time with the athlete. The second set of 10 will almost always be quicker than the first.

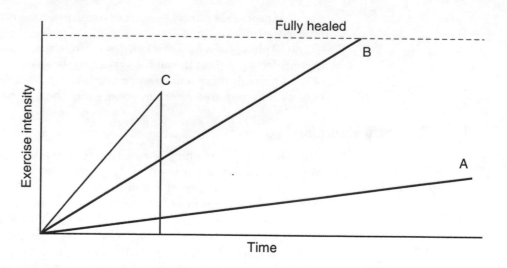

Figure 4.2 There is a fine balance between too little and too much exercise during rehabilitation. Too little exercise results in permanent disability (a), while too vigorous exercise will reinjure the healing tissues (b).

Time post injury	Walk naturally		Resumed work		Resumed sports	
	early	late	early	late	early	late
1 week	22	0	17	19	0	0
7 weeks	100	11	100	81	11	0
3 months	100	100	100	100	86	49
1 year	100	100	100	100	86	89

Table 4.1   Course of Function After Immobilizing (Late) and Early Mobilizing (Early) Treatment

Numbers are the percentages of patients of the group that could perform the activity at follow-up examinations. These data (from Konradsen et al. [J41]) illustrate the beneficial effects of early exercise.

Use your imagination to determine specific performance goals for every therapeutic exercise you have the athlete perform. Then measure the performance and report the results to the athlete.

When Does Rehabilitation Begin and End?

Rehabilitation should begin immediately after injury occurs and end only when the athlete can fully participate in his or her sport, with no limitations imposed by the injury. Obviously, the complexity of rehabilitation will depend on the magnitude and type of injury sustained, as well as on the requirements of the sport. A runner with a sprained finger usually will not have to worry about it as much as a quarterback would. But even for a quarterback, rehabilitation of a sprained finger would not be as complicated or take as long as rehabilitation of a sprained ankle. Whether the rehabilitation is simple or complex, though, it should follow the same general process, to ensure total and complete rehabilitation.

Make every effort to accomplish the rehabilitation process as quickly as possible, since there are many negative consequences of prolonged absence from participation. Inactivity can lead to atrophy of specific muscle groups, loss of overall conditioning, rusty skills, loss of one's sixth sense, and even emotional trauma. Athletes engage in sport to participate, not to sit on the sidelines. Often an injury is accompanied with feelings of frustration, discouragement, and self-doubt, which become greater the longer the athlete is out of commission.

Athlete's Health Comes First

The interests of the athlete must be the motivating factors for early rehabilitation. No matter how valuable an athlete is, the interests of neither the team nor the coach should take precedence over the health of the athlete. But athletes want to participate, not sit on the bench. As long as the athlete's health is the uppermost concern, rehabilitation should proceed as quickly as possible.

A SYSTEMS APPROACH TO TOTAL REHABILITATION: THE 10 PHASES

In a systems approach, you identify each phase of rehabilitation and establish criteria for developing each phase. In addition, you carefully analyze the limitations imposed upon the athlete by the injury. Based on the specific needs of the athlete, you determine which phase of rehabilitation to begin with and establish specific long- and short-range goals to guide the athlete in meeting the criteria for each phase. You then select specific techniques that will assist the athlete to progressively meet the established goals, as well as additional techniques and activities that enable the athlete to meet successive criteria and thereby progress through the remaining phases of rehabilitation.

There are 10 phases, or elements, of rehabilitation discussed in detail in the following sections. As noted previously, these are arranged so that athletes progress through a systematic conditioning program. Although some overlap is permitted, maximal development of an element usually occurs only if the elements that precede it have been developed.

Ten Phases of Rehabilitation

1. Structural integrity
2. Pain-free joints and muscles
3. Joint flexibility
4. Muscular strength
5. Muscular endurance
6. Muscular speed
7. Muscular power (strength and speed)
8. Integrated and coordinated movement (skill patterns)
9. Agility (speed and skill)
10. Cardiovascular endurance

Structural Integrity

Structural integrity means that the athlete's anatomical structures (joints, ligaments, muscles, etc.) are intact. Any disrupted structure must be repaired. Surgery and immobilization are usually required to repair a totally disrupted musculoskeletal structure. Immobilization and rest are used to protect less severely injured structures while the healing process takes place.

Immobilization can cause problems, however (J23, J54). It often increases neural inhibition and results in decreased neuromuscular function. Judicious use of exercise and thermotherapy increase circulation and metabolism, thus speeding the healing process.

Pain-Free Joints and Muscles

Immobilization, therapeutic modalities, cryotherapy, and exercise are all used to diminish pain. Graded exercise, especially important during this phase, helps overcome neural inhibition and gradually readjusts the body part to full pain-free activity (E82).

Pain must be monitored throughout the rehabilitation process. Pain during an activity indicates that the activity is too strenuous or complex and that the athlete should drop back to a lower level of activity. Residual pain, or pain the next day, indicates that the previous day's activity was too strenuous, so the current day's activity must be adjusted accordingly. Activities that result in pain during rehabilitation will hinder the rehabilitation process by inducing neural inhibition (B43).

Sometimes pain is the problem rather than a symptom of the problem. It sometimes happens that pain remains even after the cause of the pain has been removed or the injury has healed (E5, E77, J15). In this case, once you remove the pain, the athlete can resume full activity.

Joint Flexibility

Decreased joint flexibility results from either (a) muscle spasm, pain, or neural inhibition secondary to acute injury or (b) connective tissue adhesions and contractures secondary to surgery or immobilization. Therapeutic exercise is essential in improving flexibility, but can be facilitated by applying hot and cold packs. Cold packs are generally more effective with muscular conditions, while hot packs are preferred when connective tissue is involved (J66).

During periods of immobilization, limited motion helps maintain joint flexibility. After the immobilization period ends, static stretching and such proprioceptive neuromuscular facilitation (PNF) techniques as hold-relax (a static stretch interspersed with an isometric contraction of the involved muscle) and contract-relax (a static stretch interspersed with an isometric contraction of the antagonistic muscle) (J40) are effective (J36). In addition, exercises such as flexion and extension to the limits of the range of motion and riding a stationary bicycle (J11) are excellent ways to restore flexibility. For acute muscle spasm, the cryostretch technique (B22), which combines cold applications with hold-relax stretching, is very effective, as is electrical muscle stimulation if applied so as to cause successive maximal tetanic contractions. Providing resistance to the muscle contraction allows for an increased intensity of current flow and thereby a greater muscle contraction.

Muscular Strength

The athlete must perform some progressive resistive exercises on a regular basis using the involved musculature if an increase in strength is desired (Figure 4.3). Programs based on the daily adjustable progressive resistive exercise (DAPRE) technique are becoming increasingly popular (Tables 4.2 and 4.3). The DAPRE technique takes advantage of the fact that strength can be redeveloped much more quickly than it was developed initially. The key to the technique is that patients perform maximal repetitions during their third and fourth sets, with the number of repetitions performed used as a basis for adjusting the resistance for the fourth set and next day, respectively. In any event, the program is more important than the equipment used (no matter what manufacturers may claim).

Each side of the body should be worked independently. This prevents the injured limb from depending on the noninjured one, and establishes a functional strength-development goal for the injured side. Once strength in the injured side is 90% to 95% of the strength in the noninjured side, the

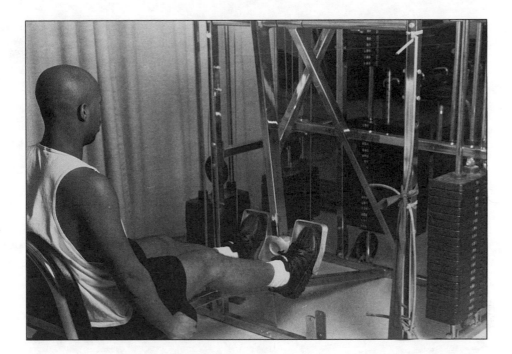

Figure 4.3 Aggressive isotonic strength training is an important component of most rehabilitation programs.

Table 4.2 The DAPRE Technique for Isotonic Strength Development		
Set	Portion of working weight used	Number of repetitions
1	1/2	10
2	3/4	6
3	Full	Maximum*
4	Adjusted	Maximum**

*The number of repetitions performed during the third set is used to determine the adjusted working weight for the fourth set, according to the guidelines in Table 4.3. **The number of repetitions performed during the fourth set is used to determine the adjusted working weight for the next day, according to the guidelines in Table 4.3.
Reprinted from Knight (J37).

strength development program is changed to one of strength maintenance and the rehabilitation emphasis moves to the development of muscular endurance. Strength can usually be maintained with one or two workouts per week at near maximal resistance.

Muscular Endurance

Some athletic trainers advocate using a stationary bicycle (Figure 4.4) for the muscular endurance phase (E59). Although this can be effective, running (or an equivalent upper body exercise for upper extremity injuries) is more specific to most sports and is therefore preferred. The athlete should jog 400 meters the first day and increase this distance by 400 meters each day or

Table 4.3 General Guidelines for Adjustment of Working Weight During the DAPRE Technique

Number of repetitions performed during set	Adjustment to working weight for:	
	Fourth set*	Next day**
0–2	Decrease 5–10 lb and perform the set over	
3–4	Decrease 0–5 lb	Keep the same
5–7	Keep the same	Increase 5–10 lb
8–12	Increase 5–10 lb	Increase 5–15 lb
13 to . . .	Increase 10–15 lb	Increase 10–20 lb

*The number of repetitions performed during the third set is used to determine the adjusted working weight for the fourth set according to the guidelines in Table 4.2. **The number of repetitions performed during the fourth set is used to determine the adjusted working weight for the next day according to the guidelines in Table 4.2.
Reprinted from Knight (J37).

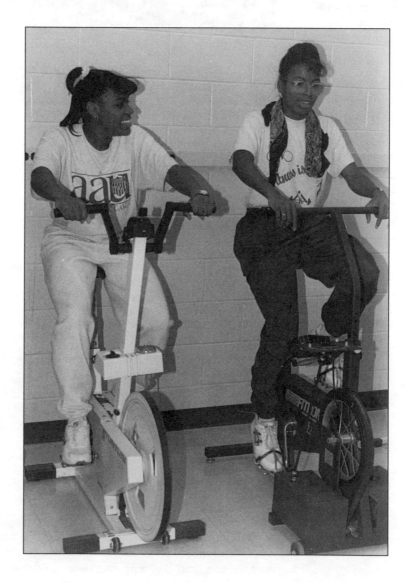

Figure 4.4 A stationary bike can be used to redevelop muscular endurance, but running or another type of repetitive exercise is equally effective if performed long enough.

two as tolerance increases. If there is any soreness from the previous day's activity, the distance should be decreased for a few days. After the athlete can run a mile, he or she should begin the next phase, but distance running should continue and progress to a level commensurate with the requirements of the athlete's sport. I do not advocate weightlifting for developing endurance. More than 100 to 200 repetitions would be necessary for developing significant levels of endurance, and this would be too time consuming.

Muscular Speed

Muscular speed can be developed by participation in team drills at half speed, then three-fourths speed, and finally at full speed, with emphasis given to explosive-type activities (Figure 4.5). Work on Cybex/Orthotron equipment also does a good job of developing muscular speed, but is not necessary if the athlete develops near maximal strength and then progresses through team drills at increasing speed.

Muscular Power

Power is a measure of the rate of doing work—a combination of strength and speed of movement. Muscular power can be developed with an isokinetic device or with high-speed resistive work.

Skill Patterns

Integrated and coordinated movement can be developed only by practicing sport-specific skill patterns (H82, J52, J65). This phase is developed along with muscular speed by using increasingly complex team drills (Figure 4.6). Observe athletes closely to ensure that they are performing the activities correctly. It is often necessary to isolate a specific part of the skill pattern and work on it independently. This involves returning to the joint flexibility

Figure 4.5
Develop muscular speed by performing explosive-type sport-specific skills as quickly as possible. Coaches usually design team drills to emphasize these skills.

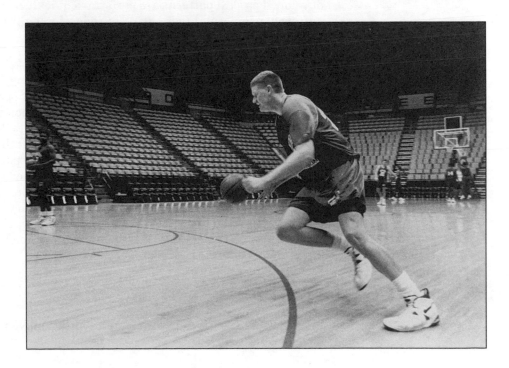

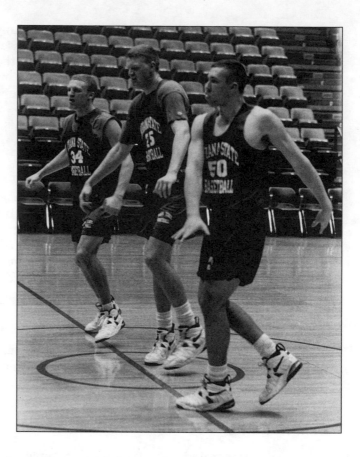

Figure 4.6 Proprioception and integrated skill patterns are developed as the athlete performs team drills of increasing complexity. The basketball players here are performing a carioca drill.

phase and progressing through strength, endurance, and speed development with the specific muscles involved in this part of the skill.

Agility

Agility is a combination of speed of movement and coordination. Agility is developed as skill patterns are performed quickly and speedily. As with skill patterns, use normal team drills to redevelop agility.

Cardiovascular Endurance

As muscular endurance develops beyond beginning levels, the activity will also develop cardiovascular endurance. Other sport-specific conditioning drills should also be instituted, gradually at first, and then increasing in difficulty.

Also, if it appears that it will take more than 2 to 3 weeks to complete the total rehabilitation program, you should try to limit the loss of cardiovascular endurance. How you do this depends on the body part injured. If the injury does not hinder the athlete's ability to perform normal conditioning activities, continue with normal activities. For example, a football or basketball player with an arm injury can still run. If the injury is such that it prevents normal activities, use a substitute. For example, a football player with a thigh injury can swim, run in a swimming pool in chest-high water, or ride a stationary bike (I31).

WHAT MODALITY IS USED WHEN?

If you use a systems approach in rehabilitation, you must have some basis for choosing which therapeutic modality to use during various phases of rehabilitation. As mentioned earlier, the proper therapeutic modality must be matched with the therapeutic goal. Obviously, a whirlpool treatment is not the best choice for improving cardiovascular endurance. In Table 4.4 various therapeutic modalities are rated according to their efficacy in promoting each of the 10 phases of rehabilitation. The most commonly used modalities are given one of three ratings for each of the phases of rehabilitation that they have some effect on:

| 1 | The modality has a direct effect and is a good choice during this phase of rehabilitation.

| 2 | The modality can be effective if used in a specific way. For instance, isotonic resistive exercises can be effective in developing muscular endurance if used with many repetitions. Using the equipment to perform 10 to 15 repetitions, however, will not develop significant muscular endurance.

| 3 | The modality is somewhat effective but is not the best choice to use for developing this phase. There are better modalities for developing this phase of rehabilitation.

THE PSYCHOLOGY OF REHABILITATION

Rehabilitation is usually discussed in terms of its physiological aspects; however, the psychological side cannot be ignored (I53). In fact, it has been said that rehabilitation is 75% psychological and 25% physiological. This is an exaggeration, but it emphasizes the psychological needs of rehabilitation. Some athletes seem to give up after an injury and must be constantly prodded to fulfill their rehabilitation objectives. The coach or athletic trainer must constantly check on them to make sure that they follow through with what they are supposed to be doing. Other athletes are overly aggressive and have to be held back to prevent overwork and possible reinjury. This athlete takes as much time and effort as the one who gives up does.

Another aspect to the psychology of rehabilitation is just beginning to emerge. There is a direct connection between a person's mind and his or her physiological processes (E71). The way people think is manifested in the way their bodies perform. There apparently *is* "power in positive thinking." Make every effort during rehabilitation to ensure that athletes don't give up on themselves or their ability to recover from the injury and perform once again. This can be done by pointing out even the smallest degree of progress.

SUMMARY

- Rehabilitation is the process of restoring an injured athlete to his or her preinjury state of conditioning, which involves progressive redevelopment of the physiological and psychological elements of total conditioning:

  1. Structural integrity
  2. Pain-free joints and muscles
  3. Joint flexibility
  4. Muscular strength
  5. Muscular endurance
  6. Muscular speed
  7. Muscular power (strength and speed)

Table 4.4 Efficacy of Therapeutic Modalities in Rehabilitation of Sports Injuries

Modality	Rehabilitation objective							
	Intact joints/muscles	Pain-free joints/muscles	Flexibility	Muscular strength	Muscular endurance	Speed of movement	Coordination/ sport skills	Cardio-vascular endurance
Cold packs		1*	2					
Ice massage		1	2					
Whirlpool (cold)		1	2					
Whirlpool (hot)	1	3	2					
Hot packs	1	3	2					
Paraffin baths	1	3	2					
Contrast baths	1	3	2					
Infrared	1	3	2					
Ultrasound	1	3	3					
Diathermy	1	3						
Low voltage muscle stimulation	?	1	2/3	2/3				
High voltage muscle stimulation	2	1						
Tens								
Exercise								
Passive		2	1					
Assistive		2	3	?				
Active								
Range of motion	2	2	3					
Jogging (or EUBA)†		2		3	1	1		1
Sprinting (or EUBA)		2		3	2	1		1
Agility drills		2		3	2	1	1	2
Team drills		2		3	2	2	1	2
Practice		2		3	2	2	1	2
Resistive								
Manual				2				
Isotometric				2				
Isotonic								
Free weights				1	2	2	3	3
Universal				1	2	2		3
Nautilus			2	1	2	2		3
Isokinetic				1	2	1		3

*1 = Direct effect—good choice; 2 = Effective under certain conditions; 3 = Somewhat effective—not the best choice; †EUBA = Equivalent upper body activity.

8. Skill patterns (integrated and coordinated movement)
9. Agility (speed and skill)
10. Cardiovascular endurance

- Rehabilitation cannot be separated from treatment. The rehabilitative process begins immediately after the injury and ends only when the athlete is fully participating in his or her sport.
- Understanding the healing process helps understand the need for early controlled exercise.
- Rehabilitation should be individualized for specific athletes and injuries and should be goal-directed. Numerous long-range, short-range, and daily goals help keep the athlete progressing properly through the physical elements of rehabilitation and provide psychological aid as well.
- The SAID principle is the dominant principle of rehabilitation. It establishes the needs for therapeutic goals, for evaluation prior to and throughout the process, and for functional progression.
- Specific performance feedback helps the athlete progress faster.
- The rehabilitation process should be aggressive, progressive, and pain-free.

5

Temperature Changes Resulting From Cold Applications

The primary physiological response of tissue to cold applications is a decrease in the temperature of the tissue to which they are applied. All other physiological changes occur in response to the temperature decrease. Surface temperature decreases more rapidly and to a greater degree than deeper tissues (Figure 5.1). Rewarming following application is slower than cooling during

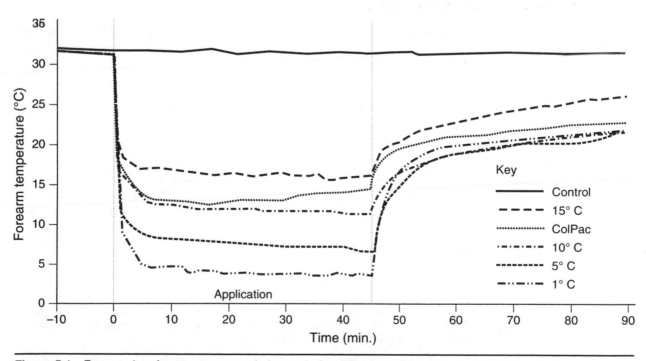

Figure 5.1 Forearm interface temperature during and after (45 min each) cold pack application and immersion in water of various temperatures. Data from Knight (C43).

application and usually takes more than 2 hours following a 30-minute ice-pack application.

All cold applications are not the same. The rate and magnitude of the temperature decrease and the subsequent rewarming following application vary greatly due to the cold modality used (e.g., ice pack, cold pack, ice massage, immersion in ice water), the tissue you are trying to cool, the environment, and the length of application. Also, since the device used to measure temperature changes affects what we think the temperature is, we cannot interpret temperature changes without an understanding of temperature measuring devices.

HEAT AND HOW IT IS MEASURED

Thermal energy is the result of random motion of the particles that make up all substances (C59). As the motion of the particles changes, the thermal energy of the substance changes proportionately. Changes in thermal energy occur at the same time as changes in other properties of the substance, including its

- electrical resistance, its
- volume and
- pressure (if it is a confined gas),
- any thermoelectromotive force (electrical current) going through the substance, and
- the radiation from its surface.

Each of these properties has been used as the basis for measuring the amount of thermal heat in a substance.

Heat, Cold, and Temperature

Heat is the quantity of thermal energy transferred between two substances or systems that are in thermal contact and are of differing temperatures (C59, C60). Heat is commonly measured in joules or calories. Unlike heat, cold is not a quantifiable physical entity. *Cold* is an arbitrary term that refers to the opposite, or lack, of heat (C59). For instance, if the temperature goes down to 60 °F in July we call it cold; yet when it gets up to 40 °F in February we call it warm (E18).

Temperature is the degree of "hotness" of a substance as measured on some definite scale (J73). It describes whether the substance will transfer thermal energy to another substance (thermal energy will not transfer unless there is a difference in temperature between the two substances and will always transfer when there is a difference in temperature between them).

Temperature Scales

Several scales have been devised to report temperature. The most common scale in use in the United States is the Fahrenheit (F) scale, on which the freezing point of water is 32 °F and the boiling point of water 212 °F. Most of the rest of the world, as well as the U.S. scientific community, uses the Celsius (C) scale, on which the freezing and boiling points of water are 0 °C and 100 °C, respectively. The following formulas give the relationship between the two scales:

$$°F = 9/5(°C) + 32 °F$$
$$°C = 5/9(°F - 32 °F)$$

Temperature Measuring Devices

Temperature is usually measured with thermometers, thermistors, thermocouples, or thermography (Figure 5.2).

Thermometers

Bulb thermometers filled with either alcohol or mercury are the oldest temperature-measuring devices and are based on volume changes (C15). A thermometer has a glass bulb attached to a long, thin glass tube. The bulb and tube are filled with alcohol or mercury. The fluid expands as it warms and contracts as it cools, causing the fluid to move up and down in the tube. The calibration marks on the glass tube allow you to read the temperature of the substance in contact with the thermometer bulb.

Thermistors

A thermistor is a temperature-sensitive resistor, generally composed of semiconductor materials. As the temperature of the thermistor changes, so does its electrical resistance. The temperature can be computed from the change in the resistance.

Thermocouples

A thermocouple consists of two dissimilar metals joined together at one end to form a junction (J59). For instance, J-type thermocouples are made of iron and constantan. Heat at the junction produces a small thermoelectric voltage between the two metals. As the temperature goes up or down from a calibration point, the voltage changes.

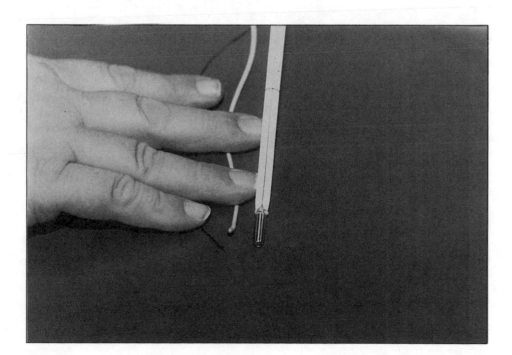

Figure 5.2 Three types of temperature measuring devices: thermocouple (left), thermister (center), and thermometer (right).

The electronic device to which thermistors and thermocouples are attached by wires is called a telethermometer. Simple telethermometers, such as those commonly used in hospitals to measure patient temperatures, are battery powered and thus portable. Older telethermometers had a dial with a needle from which to read the temperature; most newer models provide a digital readout. Devices commonly used for research are attached to a computer and provide various types of readouts depending on the software and desires of the operators.

Thermography

A substance emits infrared radiation at a rate proportional to its surface temperature (C31, J19). Thermography measures this infrared radiation and converts the measurement either to a color (a qualitative display) or to the corresponding temperature (a quantitative display).

Accuracy of Temperature Measurements

The accuracy of a measured temperature depends on the inherent accuracy of the device and how it is used. The precision and calibration of the device and how accurately the technician reads its output are the two most important factors. A digital readout telethermometer is easier to read than the stem of a bulb thermometer, and thus is usually more accurate. Different models of each of the four types of devices are manufactured with differing precision. Usually the less expensive models are also less precise.

To understand how precision affects a measurement, consider a device that has an accuracy of ±5%. A readout of 40 °C means that the temperature could be anywhere between 38° and 42 °C, a range of 4°.

But the most precise instrument is only as good as its calibration. A measuring device is calibrated by using it to measure a range of temperatures with a known standard. If it records a temperature different from that of the standard, the calibration is adjusted so that it reads the correct temperature.

Interface Temperature

When measuring an internal temperature, the substance surrounds the thermometer or temperature probe, so only the temperature of that substance is measured. When measuring surface temperature, however, only part of the probe is in contact with the surface. The rest of the probe is in contact with the surface's immediate environment (e.g., the air or water), which is usually at a temperature different from that of the surface you are measuring (Figure 5.3). Since the probe is influenced by both the surface and the environment, its temperature is somewhere between the temperatures of the surface and the environment and is called an interface temperature. The temperature of the environment around the body part is usually lower than that of the body part itself, so the recorded surface temperature is lower than the actual surface temperature. How much lower is unknown. Present work in our laboratory with infrared thermography should help to better understand this problem.

Lewis (C51) attempted to overcome this source of measurement error by applying plaster of Paris over the exposed portion of the thermocouple. This

Figure 5.3 . Thermocouple applied to the ankle with a small strip of tape. Note that the tape does not cover the tip of the thermocouple; therefore the thermocouple is influenced by both the skin temperature and whatever is placed over it (the atmosphere, in this case) so it measures an interface temperature. If a cold pack were placed over this ankle, the interface would be the skin and the cold pack.

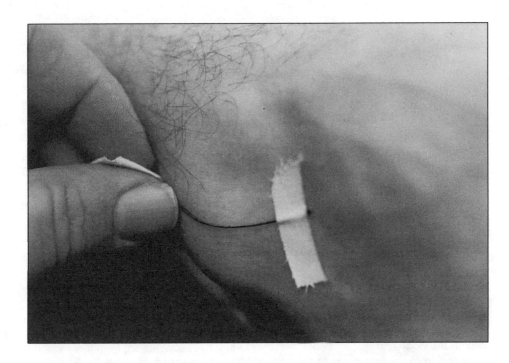

did not eliminate the error; it just changed it, since the plaster, now the immediate environment, had a temperature different from that of the body part.

The rapid changes in surface temperature upon cold application and immediately after removing the cold modality are exaggerated because of the change in the interface. When a body part is immersed in a water bath, for instance, the environmental temperature changes from that of the room to that of the water bath (sometimes a change of more than 20 °C). For example, if the surface temperature of an arm is 33 °C and is being measured in an atmosphere of 25 °C, the interface temperature would be (33 °C + 25 °C)/2, or 29 °C. (In this example, we divide by two because we assume the interface is equally between the surface and the bath.) If the arm were then placed in 1 °C water and measured before any heat exchanged the interface temperature would be (33 °C + 1 °C)/2, or 17 °C, an apparent decrease of 12 °C. I use the term *apparent* because the arm temperature didn't change at all; the environmental temperature changed, causing the measuring device to change.

Admittedly, this is an overly simplistic example. It doesn't include the effects of thermal gradients on interface temperatures. Keep this in mind as you read the following discussions of these temperature changes.

Thermal Gradients

A thermal gradient is a progressive change in temperature between two bodies of differing temperatures. Heat is exchanged between molecules. For instance, when a cold pack is placed on the arm, the molecules of the arm's surface conduct heat into the adjacent molecules of the cold pack (Figure 5.4). The second layer of molecules of the arm would now be warmer than the first, so they would conduct heat to the first. At the same time, the first layer of cold-pack molecules would conduct heat to the second. Now the temperature of the two bodies is no longer unequal (one gained heat; the other gave it up). So the first layer of the body again gives up heat to the

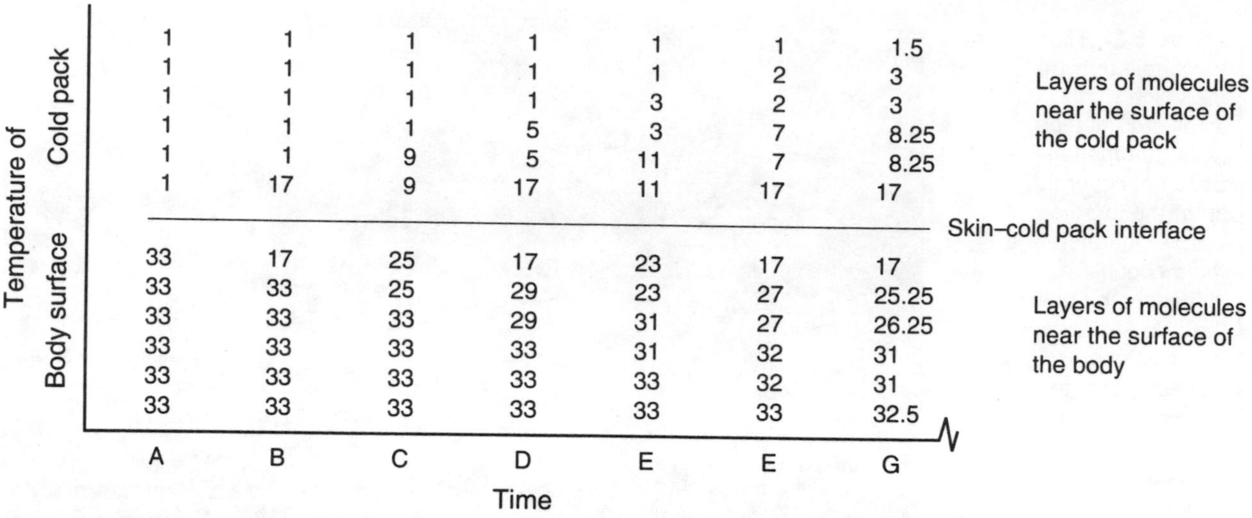

	A	B	C	D	E	E	G	
Cold pack	1	1	1	1	1	1	1.5	Layers of molecules near the surface of the cold pack
	1	1	1	1	1	2	3	
	1	1	1	1	3	2	3	
	1	1	1	5	3	7	8.25	
	1	1	9	5	11	7	8.25	
	1	17	9	17	11	17	17	
								Skin–cold pack interface
Body surface	33	17	25	17	23	17	17	Layers of molecules near the surface of the body
	33	33	25	29	23	27	25.25	
	33	33	33	29	31	27	26.25	
	33	33	33	33	31	32	31	
	33	33	33	33	33	32	31	
	33	33	33	33	33	33	32.5	

Temperature of — Time

Figure 5.4   Model of the development of thermal gradients in an ice pack and the body surface to which the ice pack is applied. At time A, a cold pack at 1 °C is applied to an extremity which is 33 °C. Because of the heat differential, heat is conducted from the body surface to the cold pack, resulting in the superficial molecules coming to temperature equilibrium (time B). The temperature differential between the surface and second layer of molecules in both the body and the cold pack result in further heat conduction; from the second to the superficial layer of the body and from the superficial to the second layer of the cold pack (time C). As the process continues, a temperature (or thermal) gradient is developed in both the cold pack and the body.

first layer of the cold pack. In time, the temperature of the layers of molecules in the cold pack will progressively increase from the cold pack's core temperature to a temperature near the surface of the body part. In the body part the temperature will progressively decrease from core to surface. In chapter 2, this concept is used as one of the explanations for the hunting response. This also is important when applying a cold pack (chapter 16).

■ *REMOVING THERMAL GRADIENTS*

Thermal gradients in air and water can be removed by circulating the air or stirring the water. A cold pack should be jiggled every 5 minutes or so to break up the thermal gradient in the melted water, thus making the modality interface colder.

The interface temperature between the body part and its environment is not midway between the "core" temperature of the two. Although each has a thermal gradient, the slope of the two gradients differs. Dissimilar rates of heat conduction within the two result in different thermal gradients.

HEAT CONDUCTION

During cooling, heat is transferred from the body tissues to the cold modality through a process known as *conduction*. Conduction is the exchange of heat between two substances that are in contact with each other; the heat always moves from the body of higher energy to the body of lower energy (C59, J30, J68). This causes the warmer body to cool and the cooler body to warm until they reach a common equilibrium (J68). The rate of conduction, and therefore the rate of temperature decrease of the tissue, depends on the interaction of many factors:

- *The temperature difference between the body and the cold modality* (A12, C5, D84). Heat from 34 °C tissue will conduct more quickly into a 10 °C cold pack than it will into a 25 °C cold pack.
- *Regeneration of body heat and modality cooling* (C5). As the tissue gives up heat to the modality, some lost tissue heat is replaced by circulating blood and conduction from surrounding tissues. Simultaneously, the heat given up to the cold modality either is held by the modality, whose temperature therefore rises, or is removed from the modality (e.g., as with a cryomatic unit), so that the lower temperature is maintained.
- *The heat storage capacity of the cold modality*. Different modalities can accept different amounts of heat before they begin warming. Consequently, a modality that can accept greater amounts of heat maintains a greater temperature differential between the modality and the tissue. (See "Heat Capacity," the following section.)
- *The size of the cold modality*. If two cold packs are identical except for their size, the larger one will have a greater heat storage capacity.
- *The area of the body in contact with the cold modality*. The body will suffer a greater heat loss if the entire body part is immersed in water than if a cold pack is applied to one side of the body part. This is why immersing the forearm in 10 °C water will cool it to the same degree as a –10 °C ColPac (see Figure 5.1). Also, if other things are equal, a large cold pack will cool a body part more than a smaller one because it covers a larger area of the body.
- *The duration of application* (C5). The longer the application of the cold modality, the more time there is for energy to be exchanged, so more heat will be removed from the body.
- *Individual variability*. People react differently to cold applications (C9).

HEAT CAPACITY

The amount of heat that equal sizes and shapes of various modalities can accept depends on their sizes, specific heats, and their latent heats of fusion. *Specific heat* is the amount of heat energy required to raise 1 kilogram of a substance 1 °C. Thus, the greater a substance's specific heat, the more heat energy it can withdraw (assuming that the substances being compared have equal masses). Water has a very large specific heat, greater than most substances, and so it is excellent for cold packs.

The *latent heat of fusion* is the amount of heat energy needed to convert a substance from a solid state to a liquid state without changing its temperature. It takes a tremendous amount of heat energy to change ice at 0 °C to water at 0 °C. This is one of the advantages of crushed-ice packs over cold-gel packs for cooling the body. (Cold-gel packs don't freeze solid because they are water mixed with a substance such as gelatin to give them body and an antifreeze to keep them from freezing solid.)

The following example illustrates the difference in heat energy extracted from the body by these two modalities.

HEAT ENERGY EXTRACTED FROM BODY BY COLD-GEL PACK AND CRUSHED-ICE PACK

Assumptions:

Both packs are 1 kilogram in mass and are applied to the same surface until they withdraw enough heat to warm to 5 °C (41 °F). The crushed ice came from a free standing ice machine that stored it at –1 °C (30 °F). The gel pack was stored in a freezer unit at –17 °C (–1 °F). Thus, we will be showing that (solid) ice at only –1 °C extracts four times as much heat as much colder liquid gel. (Note: kg = kilogram; J = joule.)

Cold-gel pack.

Requires a single step, to heat water from –17 °C to 5 °C, i.e., 22 °C.

$$\text{Heat required} = \text{mass} \times \text{specific heat} \times \text{temperature change}$$
$$= 1 \text{ kg} \times 4{,}186 \text{ J} \cdot \text{kg}^{-1} \cdot {}^\circ\text{C}^{-1} \times 22 \text{ }^\circ\text{C}$$
$$= 92{,}092 \text{ J}$$

Crushed-ice pack.

Requires three steps:

1. Heat ice from –1 °C to 0 °C, i.e., 1 °C

$$\text{Heat required} = 1 \text{ kg} \times 2{,}090 \text{ J} \cdot \text{kg}^{-1} \cdot {}^\circ\text{C}^{-1} \times 1 \text{ }^\circ\text{C}$$
$$= 2{,}090 \text{ J}$$

2. Change ice to water at 0 °C (heat of fusion)

$$\text{Heat required} = \text{mass} \times \text{latent heat of fusion}$$
$$= 1 \text{ kg} \times 333{,}000 \text{ J/kg}$$
$$= 333{,}000 \text{ J}$$

3. Heat water from 0 °C to 5 °C, i.e., 5 °C

$$\text{Heat required} = 1 \text{ kg} \times 4{,}186 \text{ J} \cdot \text{kg}^{-1} \cdot {}^\circ\text{C}^{-1} \times 5 \text{ }^\circ\text{C}$$
$$= 20{,}930 \text{ J}$$
$$20{,}090 \text{ J} + 333{,}000 \text{ J} + 20{,}930 \text{ J} = 356{,}022 \text{ J}$$

■ *USE CRUSHED-ICE PACKS INSTEAD OF COLD-GEL PACKS*

Crushed-ice packs are safer and longer lasting and cool the body more than cold-gel packs. As the example just showed, because of the tremendous amount of heat required to change ice to water at 0 °C, a crushed-ice pack can cool the body more than a cold-gel pack, even if the ice pack "wastes" some of its capacity by thawing partially during practice. Also, a cold-gel pack must be cooled much lower than 0 °C to have enough capacity to cool 1/4 as effectively as a crushed-ice pack, and thus it may cause frostbite during the first few minutes of application if applied directly to the skin.

SURFACE TEMPERATURE

Cold applications cause an immediate and rapid decline in the temperature of the surface to which the cold is applied (Figure 5.5). The rate of cooling

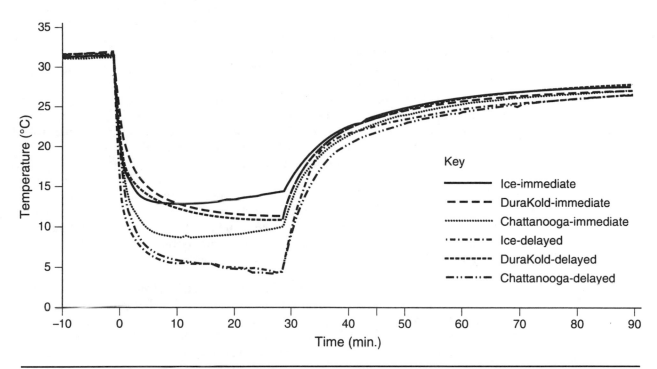

Figure 5.5 The effect of the heat of fusion can be seen in this comparison of cold packs. The crushed-ice and Dura*Kold packs cool the skin more than the Chattanooga frozen gel pack. The effect is even greater when application is delayed for 20 minutes after the packs are removed from their cooling devices. Data from Knight et al. (C46).

steadily slows until the surface temperature eventually plateaus a few degrees above the temperature of the modality (see Figure 5.1) (C42, C44, C45, C59, D83, D84, E13, E107, H48, H56, H74). Following application the temperature increases sharply, like the initial decrease but of lesser magnitude, and then begins a very gradual and prolonged return toward the preapplication temperature.

Much of the initial temperature change at the beginning of application and following application is due to the change in environment (see "Interface Temperature" earlier in this chapter).

The type of cold modality affects the magnitude of the difference between the modality temperature and the plateaued tissue temperature (C7), and whether or not the tissue temperature begins to rise before the modality is removed. For instance, compare the temperature curves for the ColPac (a cold-gel pack) to the 1 °C and 10 °C water baths in Figure 5.1. Although the arm treated with the ColPac was initially colder than when immersed in the 1 °C water bath, the ColPac does not have as great of a heat capacity and therefore cannot cool the forearm as much as the 1 °C water bath. In fact, it appears much like the 10 °C water bath during the first 15 or so minutes of application. After 15 minutes, the temperature of the arm treated with ColPacs began to increase, whereas the temperature of the arm in the 10 °C water bath continued to decrease slightly. After 15 minutes the ColPac had warmed to the point where it was extracting less heat from the arm than the circulation restored to the arm, and so the arm began to warm.

Commercial cold packs that freeze solid (such as Dura*Kold) are safer and generally perform better than frozen gel packs (Figure 5.5). The former cool the body more and can be out of the freezer unit (such as on the sidelines) without losing their effectiveness.

Another exception to the plateauing of temperature may be in the finger, where the "hunting response" is thought to occur. The "hunting response" may be a measurement artifact, however, and not a physiological response to cold-water immersion (see chapter 9).

The amount of cooling, but not the rate of cooling, is affected by previous activity (C59, H40). In research studies, stationary bike riding at a moderate intensity (enough to increase heart rate to 60% to 80% of the heart rate range) (J19) increased ankle (C59, H40) and thigh (C59) surface temperature almost 2 °C before, during, and following ice pack application.

The degree of cooling during a second application depends on the length of the first application, the time between applications (C59, H56), and the activity of the patient between the two applications (C59). Our studies of application (crushed ice bag and elastic wrap) versus rewarming (elastic wrap only) ratios (in minutes) of 20:60, 20:90, 30:60, 30:90, and 40:60 to the ankle (C59, H56) and thigh (C59) with and without 20 minutes of mild activity (crutch walking and showering) indicate the following:

- Mild activity causes a more rapid rewarming. Therefore, reapplication of cold packs should be sooner if the athlete is active between applications.
- Protocols with cooling-rewarming ratios of 1:2 (i.e., 30:60) and greater result in lower temperatures at the beginning and end of the second application–rewarming cycle. (A cycle consists of the beginning of one application to the beginning of the next application, so it includes both application and rewarming.) If additional reapplications have an additional cooling effect, tissue damage may result. Additional research is needed.

■ *ICE APPLICATION FOR IMMEDIATE CARE OF INJURIES*

Protocols for immediate care should include rewarming times at least twice as long as cooling times. Rewarming ratios less than this may result in excessive cooling during the third or fourth application-rewarming cycle.

Owing to the extent of rewarming during and following showering, changing clothes, and returning home, immediate-care protocols should call for ice packs to be applied before and immediately following these activities.

A compression wrap over an ice pack causes a greater decrease in both surface and deep temperatures during application than an ice pack alone, as well as less of an increase in temperatures following removal of the ice pack (Figure 5.6). This decreased temperature may result from decreased blood flow due to the compression (J75).

DEEP-TISSUE TEMPERATURE

The response of deep tissue to surface cooling depends on the depth and type of the tissue (C34, C66, C72). The reaction of subcutaneous tissues (those just below the skin) is the same as that of the skin itself, except decreased in magnitude (C36, D1, D33, D38): Temperature initially decreases sharply, then more gradually, then plateaus (Figure 5.7). Like skin temperature, subcutaneous temperature immediately begins to increase following the application.

Deeper tissue temperatures, on the other hand, do not begin decreasing until minutes after the cold application (C8, C9, C13, C72, D103) and then

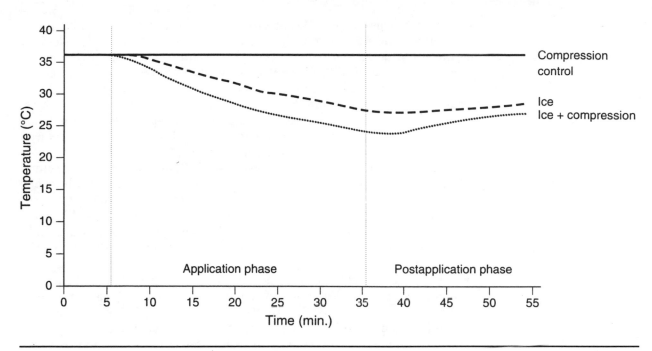

Figure 5.6 Compression wraps insulate the skin against the atmosphere, so cold packs cool more and the tissue rewarms less quickly following cold pack application.
Reprinted from Merrick et al. (C57).

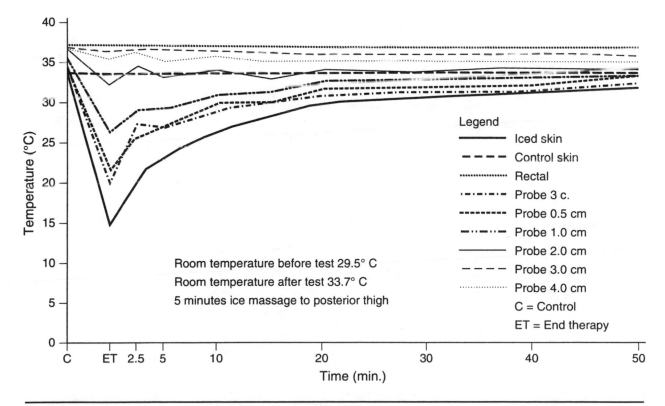

Figure 5.7 Effect of 5 minutes of ice massage to the human posterior thigh on various surface and internal temperatures.
Reprinted from Waylonis (C72).

decrease much more gradually and to a lesser magnitude than the subcutaneous temperature does (Figure 5.8) (C8, C72, C75, D84). Both the delayed response and decreased magnitude of temperature changes in the deeper tissue are the result of the time it takes for heat to be conducted between various layers of molecules in the tissue. Following cold application, deep-tissue temperature continues to decrease (C8, C9, C13, D84, I61). The duration of the decrease depends on the depth of the tissue (C72). In one study (C72), following 5 minutes of ice massage to the calf, temperatures decreased for an additional 2.5 minutes at a depth of 1 centimeter, 10 minutes at 2 centimeters, 30 minutes at 3 centimeters, and 50 minutes at 4 centimeters.

The magnitude of the temperature change in deep tissues (at all levels) is dependent upon the magnitude of cold application—the amount of heat removed from the body. This relationship can be seen in the data of Waylonis (C72), who investigated the effects of 5 and 10 minutes of ice massage. Skin temperature was basically the same following the two procedures, but the temperature at 4 centimeters decreased more than twice as much following the 10-minute ice massage. This difference in deep-tissue temperature reflects a greater conduction due to the longer application of ice. (This point must be borne in mind when interpreting a study [C53] that concluded there was no additional significant decrease in intramuscular [2.0 cm] temperatures with ice massage for longer then 5 minutes. The conclusion was based on temperature changes during application; Waylonis based his conclusion on changes following application.)

Tissue surrounding the area of cold application also decreases in temperature, although not to the extent of those tissues directly cooled. Heat is conducted from adjacent tissues into the cooled tissue. The degree of temperature decrease in peripheral tissues is directly related to the distance from the area of cold application (C9).

Thus, it appears that as cold is applied superficially to a specific tissue, heat is conducted from both deep and peripheral surface tissues in an effort to replace the heat lost to the modality. This establishes a thermal gradient. Heat conduction continues following removal of the modality. Heat from both the atmosphere and the deeper, warmer tissues is conducted to the coldest area, the surface that was in direct contact with the modality. This results in a rapid increase in skin temperature and a continued but lesser decrease in deep-tissue temperatures.

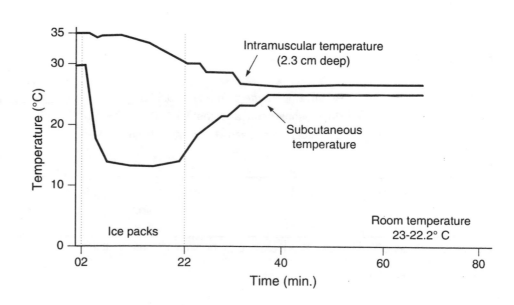

Figure 5.8 Intramuscular (gastrocnemius) and subcutaneous temperatures during and after a 20-min ice pack application. Note that intramuscular temperature declined much more slowly than subcutaneous temperature, and continued to decrease after the ice pack was removed. Reprinted from Hartviksen (F12).

Adipose tissue (fat) insulates deeper tissues and thus diminishes the effect of cooling on them. Changes in deep-tissue temperature correlate with the amount of adipose tissue over the biceps brachii muscle (C53) and the thigh (A25) when cold is applied to the skin over these muscles and to the percent of fat of the entire body when application and measurement involve the lower leg (C37). Changes in rectal temperature during whole body immersion are related to percent of subcutaneous fat (C39).

INTRAARTICULAR TEMPERATURE

Studies in humans (C13, C32, C35, C58), dogs (C11, C19, C70, G28), cats (C24), and steers (C40) indicate that intraarticular (within joints) temperatures behave much like other tissues in that the temperature seems to be a function of the magnitude of heat lost. Studies report the following observations:

- Cold-water immersion results in a greater temperature decrease than application of crushed-ice packs; the temperature decrease with ethyl chloride spray is even less (C11).
- Intraarticular temperatures decrease more than adjacent muscle (C13, C70).
- As with other deep tissues, the minimum temperature is reached after the ice pack is removed (C11, C40, C54).
- The longer the application, the greater the decrease in temperature (C11).
- Rewarming following cold applications is delayed for hours (C40, C58). A frozen gel pack (–23 °C) applied over a thin towel to the knees of 10 young healthy bulls for 30 minutes resulted in a decrease of 6.6°±1.0 °C in intraarticular knee temperature that lasted for 215 minutes (C40). A 30-minute crushed-ice pack application to 42 human knees resulted in a decrease of 9.4°±0.7 °C in intraarticular knee temperature that was still depressed 4.4 °C 150 minutes after the application (C54).

The only conflicting study (C35) reported that intraarticular temperature in humans increased with the application of cold packs even as surface temperature decreased.

One study (C19) reported that blood flow to the knee joint of dogs decreased substantially during a 10-minute application of crushed ice.

REWARMING FOLLOWING COLD APPLICATIONS

Following cold applications, the cooled body part rewarms due to heat conduction from the atmosphere, surrounding tissue, deep tissue, and circulating blood. *Rewarming* has been evaluated in two ways: return to the temperature of the body part prior to cold application, and return to contralateral–body part temperature (e.g., the temperature of the unaffected right ankle when the left ankle is undergoing cold treatment). There are problems with both definitions. In some long-term (> 2-hour) studies, the body part did not return to preapplication temperature, even in control conditions that employed no cold application at all (C43, C44, C74). This discrepancy is presumably due to the interaction of two factors: extended inactivity of the body part and exposure of the body part to an unnatural environment. The best example of exposure to an unnatural environment comes from research involving the ankles of subjects who normally wear socks and shoes (C44, C45). The ankle adapts to the environment of the sock, which is warmer than normal room temperature. Therefore, when a sock is removed and the ankle exposed to "normal room temperature," it is actually being exposed to a temperature colder than normal for the ankle. This phenomenon is shown in Figure 5.9, in which the temperature of the control (contralateral or opposite) ankle is 3° to 4 °C lower than the control arm.

Extended inactivity of a body part results in decreased metabolism and decreased heat production in the body part; such inactivity may therefore result in a gradual decrease in temperature (see control condition in Figure 5.1 and contralateral limbs of Figure 5.9) (C20).

Because of these problems, we have chosen to use the contralateral limb temperature as a control and to evaluate rewarming in relation to the contralateral limb (C42-45). This choice is not above criticism, however. For example, measuring rewarming in comparison with the contralateral temperature would not be valid if application of cold to the experimental limb caused temperature changes in the contralateral limb. Although I do not believe that such a change occurs, other researchers do (C37, C74). If indeed there is a systemic effect, much past rewarming research would be suspect and will have to be reevaluated.

How long does rewarming of the tissue take? Rewarming is probably related only to the interaction of two factors: the amount of heat removed from the body (which in turn depends on the magnitude and duration of cold exposure) and the amount of heat available to rewarm the area. There are some subtleties involved in the amount of heat available to rewarm the area. For instance, the fingers rewarm much more quickly than the ankle,

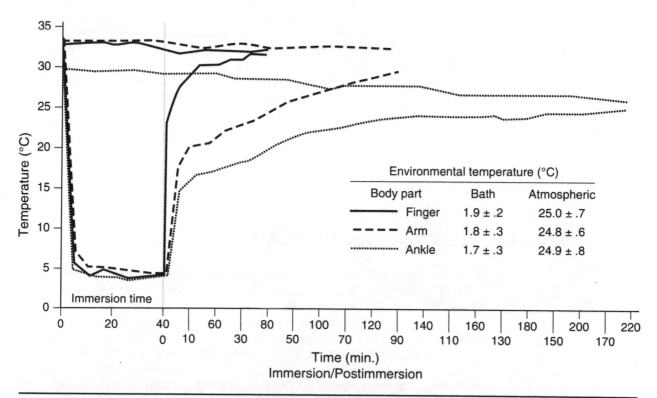

Figure 5.9 Experimental and contralateral (control) finger, forearm, and ankle temperatures during and after 40 min of immersion in 2 °C water. Note: misinformation from a pilot study resulted in a decision to measure forearm rewarming for only 90 min.

Reprinted from Knight and Elam (C45).

forearm (see Figure 5.9) (C42, C45), and knee joint (C40, C58). This is presumably due to the increased circulation in the fingers and therefore the increased amount of heat brought to the area.

In two studies (C42, C45), finger temperature returned to preimmersion levels within 15 minutes in 13 of 15 subjects. However, in the forearm (C45), ankle (C42, C45), and sheep thigh (C71) rewarming took more than 2 hours. In a later study, an average of 175 minutes were required for the ankle and forearm to rewarm to within 0.5 °C of the temperature of their contralateral counterparts following 30 minutes of immersion in 1 °C water (C44). Similarly, following immersion of the calf in 12.5° to 15 °C water for 30 minutes, skin temperature was 3.6 °C less than the preimmersion temperature after 180 minutes of rewarming and still about 2 °C less after 6 to 7 hours of rewarming (D84). Rewarming is also delayed following applications of other types of cold modalities, including ice massage (E13), ethyl chloride (C13), and crushed-ice, Blue Ice, and Chattanooga packs (C60).

Activity during rewarming increases the rate of rewarming (C59). Even mild activity like walking on crutches and standing in a shower for 20 minutes significantly increases the rewarming rate. The tendency for deep-tissue rewarming, however, is not as straightforward as that for surface temperature rewarming. Some authors (D84, F12) have reported an intramuscular temperature after extended "rewarming" lower than the temperature immediately after application (see Figures 5.8 and 10.15). Others (C37) have reported an increase of deep-tissue temperature following cooling, while one researcher (C67) reported both increased and decreased temperatures, depending on the depth of measurement and the length of application. In general, the longer the cold is applied, and the deeper the tissue, the slower the rewarming. Measurements of tissue at 2 centimeters and less demonstrated a gradual increase following 10 minutes of ice massage, while temperatures at 3 and 4 centimeters continued to decrease for 50 minutes (Figure 5.7) (C67).

Delayed rewarming following cooling may be due to the diminished blood flow that accompanies tissue cooling (A24).

Rewarming times following a second application of an ice pack are generally the same as following the first application as long as the application times and the activity level during both rewarming times are the same and as long as the ratio of application time to interval between applications is greater than 1:2 (C59, H56). In two studies involving two cycles of 30- or 40-minute applications to the ankle and thigh and 60 minutes of rewarming, the second rewarming was less than the first (C59, H56). (Rewarming following a third ice pack application or the second application of other cold modalities has not been investigated.)

CONTROVERSY OVER CONTRALATERAL LIMB TEMPERATURES

Cold applications cause temperature changes only in the tissue to which they are applied. Reports (C37, C74, E60) that cold applications cause a decrease in temperature to the contralateral limb, owing to an alleged internal physiological adjustment were based on an incomplete interpretation of the facts.

The first to challenge the idea of a contralateral effect was DonTigney (C20), who felt that the decrease in the contralateral limb temperature measured by Johnson et al. (C37) was due to the 5 hours of inactivity of the seminude subjects during the testing protocol. Two studies (C44, C45) from our laboratory have shown decreases in the surface temperature of the contralateral ankle but not in the contralateral forearm or in the contralateral finger during 4- to 5-hour testing protocols involving 30 and 40 minutes of immersion of ipsilateral limbs in 1 °C water. In addition, Coppen et al. (D16) reported no change in contralateral forearm temperatures after the ipsilateral forearm and hand were immersed for 30 minutes in 10 °C water. We concluded that since the ankle is normally covered and therefore in an environment warmer than laboratory ambient temperature, exposure resulted in a progressive cooling with time. The steeper decrease reported by Johnson et al. (C37) was probably due to the cold radiating from the large stainless steel tank into which the experimental leg was immersed. Their protocol required the contralateral limb to be fairly close to the tank.

Wolf (C74) measured the extensor digitorum muscle of the arm, so the explanations just noted will not account for his results. But the contralateral limb temperatures decreased during control as well as during experimental procedures during his experiments. The difference between the experimental and control contralateral temperatures reveals no effect of the experimental procedures on the contralateral limb.

Bing et al. (C9) reported no change in the temperature of the contralateral biceps brachii muscle or the brachioradialis muscle of the same arm due to ice application to the biceps brachii muscle. The temperature effects of cold applications are only local.

ADAPTATION TO A COLD ENVIRONMENT

Lewis (C51) observed that decreased environmental temperature caused a decrease in the surface temperature of the extremities. Others (C10, C17, C55, C64, C65) have confirmed this effect of environmental temperature on surface temperatures of the finger, cheek, ears, calf, thigh, and forearm.

The body adapts to chronic exposure to a cold environment, such as working out of doors in a cold environment for an extended period (E36, E59, E60, E63). For instance, the average indoor finger temperature of groups of soldiers changed from 31.7 °C to 29.3 °C following 2 weeks of drills in the Arctic (E63). The application also applies to cooling during immersion. Their average finger temperature during immersion for 30 minutes in 0.1 °C water decreased about the same amount (2.3 °C); it was 9.7 °C prior to and 7.4 °C following the drill period.

LeBlanc et al. (E59, E60) have demonstrated adaptation in a number of physiological responses resulting from chronic exposure to cold. Such adaptation is characterized by a decline in the specific responses and reactions normally experienced by acute exposure to cold. Following adaptation, acute exposure to cold resulted in decreased caloric cost of activity, decreased psychological disturbance of shivering, an increased ability to sleep, decreased sympathetic response to the cold presser test (less increase in blood pressure and heart rate when the hand is immersed in cold water), and a reduced decrease in skin temperature.

SUMMARY

- Cold packs that freeze solid have a greater cooling capacity than gel packs because of the heat of fusion.

- It takes 80 times as much heat to transform ice into liquid without a change in temperature as to raise the same amount of water 1 °C; 160 times as much heat than to raise ice 1 °C.
- Cold applications result in a marked and immediate decrease in surface temperature and a slower decrease in deeper tissue temperature.
- Rewarming is much slower than cooling, usually requiring 10 to 20 minutes for fingers to return to the temperature of their contralateral counterparts, and hours for ankle and forearm temperatures to return.
- The temperature effects of cold are apparently confined to local responses, due to conduction of heat from the body to the cold modality during cooling and to cooled tissue from the atmosphere and warmer tissue during rewarming.

6

Metabolism and Inflammation

One of the most important effects of cold application is decreased metabolism, or a decreased need for oxygen. Application of this principle has allowed great advances in organ transplantation: A longer time between harvesting the organ from the donor and insertion into the recipient is possible when the organ is cooled, and cooling the organ and recipient allows for a longer surgical procedure.

Decreased metabolism is the primary benefit of cold application during immediate care of acute trauma. But because of decreased metabolism, cold application during rehabilitation must be combined with other therapy. To understand these effects we must understand more about the metabolic effects of cold applications. The purpose of this chapter is to present the pathophysiology of metabolism during cold application.

DECREASED METABOLISM AT LOWER TEMPERATURES

"In most instances in which hypothermia is used, the primary aim is to reduce the body's metabolic activity so that an organ which has been severely injured, or is receiving an insufficient amount of blood, will have a better chance of survival. This is true because when the body temperature is kept at a subnormal level organs require less blood" (G64; see also G10). "[Hypothermia] is used clinically to protect tissues and organs from ischemia during a decrease or interruption of the circulation" (G69). Delorme (G25) explained how controlled cooling of tissues can lower the respiratory activity of cells without depressing the function of essential tissues below a level compatible with life. He stated that "cooling brings a higher organism to the level of the more resistant lower organism, and in so doing, enables it to withstand otherwise lethal ischemia." Although laboratory research has demonstrated conclusively that hypothermia decreases metabolism, specific mechanisms by which it occurs and clinical application of this information are still being debated.

Hypothermia reduces cellular energy needs (C62, G10, G29, G45, G63), thereby reducing the tissue requirements for oxygen. The deeper the cooling of an organism, the more profound is the depression of metabolism (G21, G36, G43, G59, G69, G72). This relationship is shown in Figure 6.1 (G10; original data from G21) for whole-body oxygen consumption in dogs at various temperatures. Does skeletal muscle react similarly? Apparently so. Oxygen consumption in perfused rat hind-limb muscle at 15°C was one third the value at 35°C (C62). And oxygen consumption in 21 human forearms immersed in water baths of 45°, 32°, and 17°C decreased an average of 2.5 times per 10°C decrease in temperature (G63).

Michenfelder and Theye (G59) reported that glucose consumption paralleled oxygen consumption in the canine brain. Rao et al. (G73) found significantly higher levels of ATP, creatine phosphate, and glycogen in canine hearts maintained at 5°C during 1 hour of no blood flow than in hearts maintained at normal temperature. This difference indicates less of a breakdown of the high-energy phosphate bonds, apparently because of less demand for energy by the cooled tissues. The effects of hypothermia on carbohydrate metabolism, proteins, fats, water balance, potassium, sodium, chloride, calcium, and magnesium have also been reviewed (G10).

Anoxic (no oxygen) hearts protected with local hypothermia have less histological disturbance, higher levels of ATP and AMP, and better myocardial contractility than anoxic hearts maintained for a similar time by other types of ventricular protection (G23, G74). Nonperfused canine hearts maintained at 37°C for 1 hour used 4 times as much glycogen, produced 3 times as much lactic acid, and had an ATP level one-half that of hearts maintained at 17°C (G37). Profound local hypothermia also fared better than other methods in protecting left ventricular function (as measured by length-tension, force-velocity, and diastolic pressure–volume relationships) during occlusion of the ascending aorta (G32).

There is less muscle (G44, G78, G94) and testicular (G48) damage during ischemia with cooling than during ischemia at normal temperatures. Mechanistic studies indicate that metabolic deterioration (G80), cellular acidosis (G68), and the normal increase in serium albumin that occurs following tourniquet use (G44) are all moderated with hypothermia. Also, less oxygen is necessary to store mitochondria at lower temps (C62, G83).

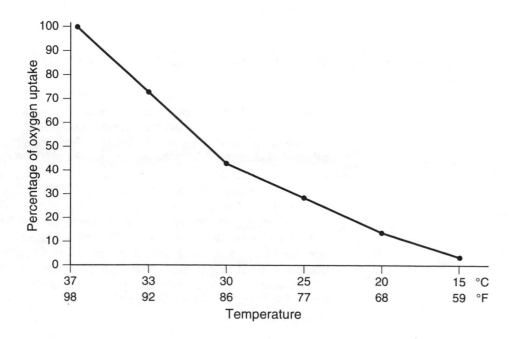

Figure 6.1 Oxygen consumption values during progressive hypothermia induced by extracorporeal cooling (dog). Reprinted from Blair (G10).

CRYOTHERAPY IN CARDIAC SURGERY AND TRANSPLANT SURGERY

Dramatic advances were made in cardiac and transplant surgery in the 1950s as a result of clinically induced hypothermia (G27, G56, G81, G90). Surgeons discovered that during arterial bypass surgery they were able to occlude circulation for a longer period of time if they lowered the body temperature (G27, G81). Initially, temperature was lowered to 26° to 30° C; however, Swan and Patton (G89) suggested in 1961 that more profound cooling would permit circulation to be safely arrested for longer periods of time. This has indeed been true (G38, G53, G56). Later studies (G62) demonstrated longer survival following cardiac surgery with deep local hypothermia and total occlusion than following cardiac surgery with either moderate systemic hypothermia and total perfusion, or with normothermic perfusion.

For temperatures between 15° and 37° C, Angell et al. (G6) demonstrated a linear relationship between the logarithm of the temperature and the length of time the heart could survive anoxia. At 37°C, hearts remained viable following anoxia for up to 35 minutes; at 15°C, they survived anoxia for 230 minutes. Similar results have been demonstrated in the brain (G39), liver (G52), lung, kidney, and pancreatic islets (see G69 for references). And kidneys can now be stored successfully for up to 5 days (G85).

Hypothermia is a vital part of preserving organs that are awaiting transplantation (G7, G84). When metabolism is reduced by hypothermia, the rate of perfusion of physiological fluids can be reduced to between one fifth and one third of that required when the organ is at normal temperatures. Preservation of the unperfused dog liver for 3 hours at 18°C to 20°C resulted in disturbance of the integrity of cell membranes and carbohydrate metabolism became dysfunctional (G52). When the liver was preserved at 4°C to 6°C metabolism was preserved.

In addition to decreasing metabolism, hypothermia may also enhance the solubility of oxygen, thus increasing the amount of oxygen in physical solution (G2). This would add to the protective effect during circulatory arrest.

STUDIES OF INDUCED INJURIES

A number of scientists have attributed to decreased metabolism the decreased morbidity in experimental animals treated with cold following crush wounds, lethal burns, and spinal cord trauma.

Crush Wounds

Blalock (G11) experimentally traumatized 50 dogs using blows with a blunt instrument to induce lethal soft tissue injury in the hind leg. Half the dogs were then treated with heat and half with cold. The dogs treated with cold lived about twice as long as the heat-treated dogs (11.4 vs. 5.8 hours). Cold applied during 5-hour traumatization of animals in a mechanical press exerted a definite protective influence (G30). However, if applied after the 5-hour trauma, no benefit was gained, possibly because anoxia had already exerted its deleterious effects.

Burns

One study on mortality following extensive burning (G65) used rats immersed in 83°C water for 30 seconds. When the burns covered approximately one fifth of the surface area of the body, all control rats died after 30 days. In contrast, all rats that were immersed in 25°C water for 30 to 45 minutes following the scald lived. Others (G14, G35, G49, G54, G57, G70, G93) have obtained similarly impressive results in reducing mortality from burns by treatment with cold-water-induced hypothermia. In another study, 20°C water was more effective than either 40° or 30°C water in reversing mortality in rats that had 40% of their body surface burned (G51). But there is evidence that cooling below 10°C causes damage to tissue (G33). Subsequent research (G26) indicated that the beneficial effects of cold were negated if the application of cold to an injury was delayed by even 2 minutes, a finding with significant practical implications. Overall research on burns shows that immediate treatment of burn injuries with hypothermia causes a reduction in pain, edema, local fluid loss, tissue injury, and fall in blood volume during the first 48 hours following the injury and a decrease in pyrexia and peptic ulceration during the later postinjury period (G12, G13).

Cooling decreases the magnitude of the injury—that is decreases the amount of necrotic tissue (G15, G33, G71, G92, H7, H8). The effect of cold applications is apparently to decrease the nonthermal cell death that results from local ischemia and occurs long after the initial injury (G79, G92). This concept is consistent with the thesis presented later in this chapter that the major effect of cold during immediate-care procedures is to decrease and retard secondary hypoxic injury.

Spinal Cord Injuries

Albin and associates (G4, G5) were able to reverse paralysis resulting from experimental spinal cord injuries in dogs treated with 5°C saline for 2.5 hours and in monkeys treated with 10°C saline for 3 or 6 hours. Animals that were treated recovered fully, while those untreated remained paralyzed. The protective effect of hypothermia seemed to be partially the result of marked reduction in metabolic activity in the cooled tissue. Early treatment is essential (G40, G41). Hypothermia must be applied soon after the injury to be effective (G40, G41, G60). Hypothermia applied to dog kidneys after one hour of ischemia exaggerated the deleterious effects of the ischemia rather than reversing its effects (G60). Neurons in the brain suffer irreversible damage after 3 to 5 minutes of ischemia (G39), while 1 to 2 hours of ischemia is required to reduce irreversible damage to liver cells (G76). Jennings and associates (G46, G47) report irreversible injury occurs in the myocardium within 20 to 60 minutes of total ischemia. Vogt & Farber (G91) reported no renal cell death as a result of 20 minutes of total ischemia, but widespread death after 30 minutes.

At least 10 studies have demonstrated the effectiveness of cooling the traumatized segments of spinal cords in cats, dogs, and monkeys (see G16 for references). Humans with spinal cord injuries also have benefitted from local hypothermia treatments. Bricolo et al. (G16) reviewed 30 cases from the literature and presented the results of 11 of their own patients. Six of their patients achieved at least partial recovery, even though cooling did not begin until at least 7 hours following injury. The researchers began using hypothermia after a review of the literature indicated that (a) the complete destruction of the spinal cord, which is responsible for irreversible paraplegia or quadriplegia, often does not occur at the moment of impact, but is related to a self-destructive process in the cord that may be evolutionary in character and (b) neurological degeneration is hypoxic in nature, secondary to profound vascular alterations (G16, G66).

CRYOTHERAPY AND INFLAMMATION

The effects of cold on traumatically induced inflammation have apparently not been investigated. Research involving cold and the inflammatory response has concentrated on either healing of surgically induced wounds or inflammation induced by injection of various substances. These studies indicate that cold acts in different situations to delay, stimulate, or retard the inflammatory response (A3, G82). Much more work is needed in this area, especially to determine the effect of cold on various phases of traumatically induced inflammation.

Brooks and Duncan (G18) administered three sets of wounds to the backs of rabbits. Each set of wounds contained a subcutaneous injection of oil of turpentine and next to it a subcutaneous injection of a culture of *staphylococcus aureus*. One set of wounds was treated with nothing, one with 40°C hot packs, and one with 10°C cold packs. After 34 hours the inflammatory response was greatest in the wounds treated with 40°C and almost nonexistent in those treated with 10°C. Twenty-four hours after the treatments were discontinued, the wounds that had been treated with cold appeared much as the untreated wounds had appeared 24 hours after the initial injury. Thus, it appears that cold did not alter the inflammatory response but only delayed it (G87, G88). Abakumova (G1) also reported the inflammatory response delayed by hypothermia. In studies of lip mucosa wound healing in rats, both the leukocytic and macrophagic phases occurred much later in hypothermic rats than in those exposed to normal conditions.

Schmidt et al. (G82) concluded that cold applications can significantly inhibit some types of inflammation, while stimulating other types. Cold stimulates cellular prostaglandin–mediated inflammations. Formol induced inflammation (an acute necrotizing inflammation thought to act similarly to traumatically induced inflammation) was significantly inhibited by cold applications. These anti-inflammatory effects occurred only after prolonged application, however. Short application, such as with ice massage, did not effectively suppress it. The researchers felt that their data confirmed clinical experience that acute exudative inflammations (those involving blood or serum) react well to cold.

The effects of histamine on the vascular membrane is lessened by cooling (G15, G75). The normal increase in fluid filtration caused by histamine was largely prevented by cooling the perfusate (the fluid containing the histamine) and immediately reversible by rewarming the perfusate.

Harris and McCroskery (G42) applied synovial collagenase, an enzyme that is produced in joints by rheumatoid synovium and that destroys articular cartilage collagen, to synovial cartilage at temperatures of 30°, 33°, and 36°C. At lower temperatures the collagen fibril degradation was greatly decreased (Figure 6.2). Does cold exert a similar effect on other degradative enzymes (i.e., lysosomal enzymes) involved in the inflammatory process? If so, this would be beneficial in decreasing secondary enzymatic injury and in chronic inflammatory states, but detrimental to macrophage phagocytosis hematoma resolution. I could find no evidence to indicate that such an effect does or does not occur, however, except for a marginally related study by Dorwart et al. (G28).

Dorwart et al. (G28) injected monosodium urate crystals into the knee joints of dogs to induce inflammation and immediately applied ice or heat packs to one joint for 4 hours (the opposite joint served as a control). Synovial fluid was then aspirated and studied. Synovial fluid leukocytes exposed to cold performed less phagocytosis and less inflammation than controls. This may have been due to increased viscosity of the synovial fluid, which may have impeded the movement of leukocytes toward the crystals.

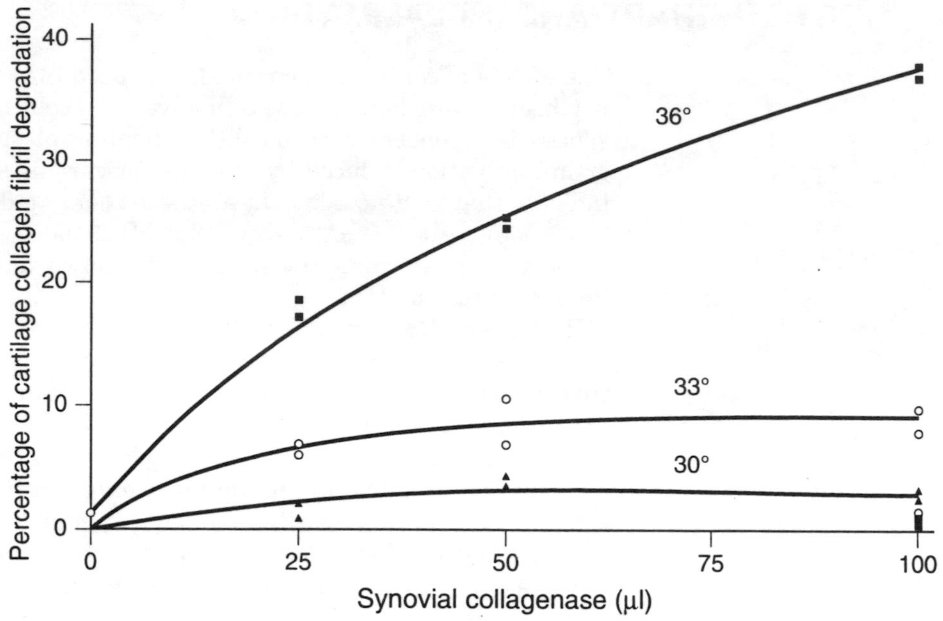

Figure 6.2   Degradation of human articular cartilage collagen fibrils by functionally purified rheumatoid synovial collagenase at different temperatures as a function of time. Reprinted from New England Journal of Medicine 290:1-6, 1974 (G42).

EFFECTS OF COLD ON WOUND HEALING

Hypothermia depresses wound healing (G1, G52, G55), but can be helpful in the healing of some infectious wounds (G8, G9). Apparently, depressed healing is the result of decreased metabolism and circulation. Abakumova (G1) reported a sharp reduction in endogenous respiration of the regenerating lip mucosa of rats under hypothermia. The decreased oxidative metabolism lead to depressed carbohydrate and protein metabolism.

Lungren et al. (G55) reported that the tensile strength of healing incisions on rabbits' backs was decreased by lowering their environmental temperature from 20° to 12°C for 5 days. This decrease was eliminated, however, when the skin was denervated prior to inflicting the wounds. The authors concluded that vasoconstriction in the skin was the principal factor responsible for impairment of healing during hypothermia.

The two studies just mentioned involved extended periods of hypothermia and so are not directly related to the extended use of short-term applications of cold. The effect of 20- to 40-minute cold applications during wound healing is unknown. It is the opinion of many who advocate the use of cryotherapy during rehabilitation, however, that exercise must accompany the cold applications (B14, B18, C46, E101, H36). This view is based on clinical observation that the earlier exercise is initiated, the faster rehabilitation will be. The detrimental effects of cold are overshadowed by the overwhelming benefits of exercise.

Bingham (G8) felt that cold packs were an effective adjunct to rest, immobilization, and antibiotic therapy in treating three types of infection: acute osteomyelitis, wound infections, and joint infections. Ice packs were applied over a moist towel almost continuously until 1 or 2 days after the patient's temperature returned to normal. The ice packs were removed for 1 hour to allow observation of the limb circulation and to examine the inflammation. Patients treated with ice packs were more comfortable, recovered more quickly, and experienced fewer complications. Bingham (G9) felt that cold therapy inhibited the rate of growth and reproduction of bacteria, made the bacteria more susceptible to attack by the body's immune system and antibiotics, and reduced the output of bacterial toxins and metabolic substances such as penicillinase (which destroys the activity of penicillin). He also felt that the decreased metabolism in the tissue resulted in less tissue death and autolysis and that the decreased pain reduced sympathetic vasospasm and thus improved deep circulation.

SUMMARY

- Local hypothermia decreases tissue metabolism and thereby allows the tissue to survive long periods (up to 5 days) of hypoxia. Great strides in transplant and open heart surgery have been made because of cooling tissues during surgery.
- Prolonging tissue survival during periods of oxygen deficit is the basis of using cold applications following soft tissue injury.
- Local hypothermia decreases, increases, or delays inflammation induced by various injected substances.
- The effects of histamine and synovial collagenase are decreased by cold, while the effects of antibiotics are enhanced.
- Uncomplicated wound healing is also decreased by local hypothermia.
- Much more research needs to be done to elucidate the effects of cold on the inflammatory response induced by acute trauma.

7

Rest, Ice, Compression, Elevation, and Stabilization for the Immediate Care of Acute Traumatic Injuries

Ice, compression, elevation (ICE; also known as RICE, ICES, RICES, and RICSE*) is the universally accepted procedure for immediate care of acute sport injuries, at least among sport medicine clinicians in North America (Figure 7.1) (B3, B44, G50, H9, H31, H59, I32). Unfortunately, some other medical and allied medical personnel (such as those in hospitals) continue to use older methods that are not as effective. Moreover, the technique is not well-established in other parts of the world, particularly where crushed ice is not as readily available as it is in North America.

When used properly, RICES reduces the total amount of damaged tissue, swelling, muscle spasm, and pain, thus reducing disability time and allowing for quicker healing of the injury. Whereas there seems to be no doubt about using RICES, there is confusion about the pathophysiological response to, and specific protocols for, using these modalities.

---

*Variations on this acronym exist, depending on the steps included or the sequence used by the researcher or clinician. We will use RICES throughout this book.

85

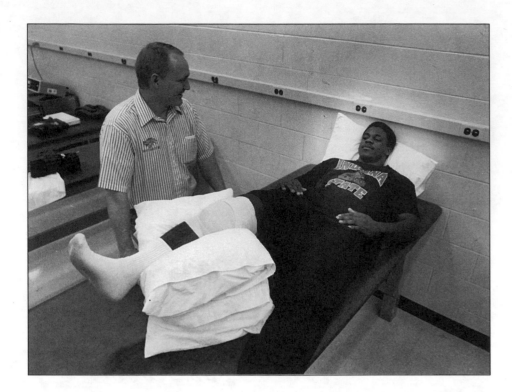

Figure 7.1 Application of ice, compression, and elevation to the knee. Note how the pillows support the entire lower leg; such support contributes to muscular relaxation and results in less pain.

The aims of this chapter are to explore the various controversies concerning RICES, why cold applications are necessary in treating acute injuries, and how cold applications help decrease swelling and pain; to develop a theoretical basis for RICES; and to review available research concerning application procedures. Based on the information in this chapter, specific application techniques are presented in chapter 16.

CLINICAL STUDIES

It is the impression of most sports medicine clinicians that RICES used immediately following an injury (within the first 10-60 minutes after it occurs) will control swelling and other negative sequelae of acute musculoskeletal injuries. Not all agree with this opinion, however. Matsen et al. (H47) claimed that an extensive review of the literature revealed no scientific support for the practice. In addition, they concluded from a study on experimentally injured rabbits that cold and compression increased rather than decreased swelling. Two clinical studies since then, however, support the use of cryotherapy in the immediate care of acute musculoskeletal injuries.

Basur et al. (H5) treated 30 patients in each of two groups. One group was treated with cryotherapy for 48 hours followed by crepe bandaging. The therapy consisted of applying a cryogel cold pack every 4 hours. The second group was treated with crepe bandaging only. After 2 days, recovery was complete in 42% of the cryotherapy-treated group but in only 29% of the control group. After 7 days, recovery was complete in 84% and 60% of the respective groups. It is important to note that the patient population was from a hospital, so patients probably did not receive treatment within the 1st hour after the injury, the time during which cold applications are most effective. If this had been done, the results may have been more impressive in favor of cryotherapy. The same can be said about the report of Sloan et al. (B41), who treated 143 patients in a hospital emergency room within 24 hours of injury. They concluded that a single 30-minute application of a cryopac (which is not as cold as ice) has little clinical significance. Agreed; but repeated applications, begun much earlier, are effective.

Hocutt et al. (H26) compiled data on 18 patients with second-degree ankle sprains and 19 patients with "second-degree-plus" ankle sprains. (They categorized patients who could stand but not walk without pain as having a second-degree sprain and those who were unable to bear weight without pain, but whose ligaments were intact, as "second-degree-plus.") They divided each group of patients into three treatment groups:

1. Early-cryotherapy patients were treated with cryotherapy (cold packs or ice water immersion) for 12 to 20 minutes one to three times per day and their ankles wrapped with an adhesive or an elastic bandage. Treatment was applied within the first 36 hours following injury.
2. Late-cryotherapy patients were treated with cryotherapy as in Group 1, but treatment did not begin until at least 36 hours following injury.
3. Early thermotherapy patients followed the same timetable as Group 1, except that they were treated with a heating pad or with soaks in a warm bath instead of with cryotherapy.

Patients using cryotherapy rehabilitated more quickly than those who used thermotherapy, and early cryotherapy was almost twice as effective as late cryotherapy (Table 7.1). These data must be interpreted with caution, however. The authors have been criticized because of a lack of random assignment of subjects to treatment groups, of objective evaluation criteria, and of long-term follow-up, but not for their conclusions (H19).

EFFECTS OF ICE DURING IMMEDIATE CARE

There are two major theories to explain how cold limits swelling following an

Table 7.1 Immediate Care/Rehabilitation of Ankle Sprains*

Treatment schedule	Age of patients (number)	Day on which patients were able to _____ without pain			
		Stand	Walk	Climb stairs	Run and jump
Moderate sprains					
Early** Cryotherapy	28.0 (10)	0	2.6	3.7	6.0
Delayed*** Cryotherapy	24.7 (4)	0	5.2	6.8	11.0
Early** Thermotherapy	24.0 (4)	0	7.8	9.0	14.8
Moderate plus sprains					
Early** Cryotherapy	25.3 (11)	2.7	4.2	5.7	13.2
Delayed*** Cryotherapy	25.2 (5)	6.2	12.0	13.6	30.4
Early** Thermotherapy	23.7 (3)	5.7	9.7	9.7	33.3

*Adapted from data of Hocutt JE, et al. (H26). **Treatment was applied within 36 hours postinjury. ***Treatment was not initiated until at least 36 hours postinjury.

acute injury: a circulatory theory and a metabolism theory. The circulatory theory, the older, traditional one, states that as cold applications lower tissue temperature, blood vessels are cooled and constrict, decreasing vessel permeability and therefore limiting hemorrhaging into the tissue. Less hemorrhaging means less swelling.

The strengths of the circulatory theory are that cold does cause vasoconstriction and decreased vascular permeability. Its weaknesses are that hemorrhaging does not occur as a result of increased vascular permeability and that hemorrhaging via torn vessels is usually stopped before cold packs are applied. It usually takes at least 5 minutes to evaluate an injured athlete, get him or her out of the playing area, and get an ice pack applied, and an additional 10 to 20 minutes to cool the deep tissues enough to cause vasoconstriction. But the clotting mechanism generally seals torn vessels within 5 minutes (H28, H44)—usually before the injury is even evaluated. Thus, the beneficial effects of ice on swelling cannot be attributed to decreased circulation.

According to the metabolism theory, cold applications have little effect on hemorrhaging; rather, they limit the amount of secondary hypoxic injury and edema (G50). Without cold, cells within the injured tissue that escaped ultrastructural damage from the trauma, and many cells on the periphery of the primary injury undergo metabolic changes that lead to secondary hypoxic injury because of inadequate oxygen. Cold applications, however, decrease the metabolic needs of these cells, so that they require less oxygen; they are put into a state of "temporary hibernation." These cells are therefore more resistant to the period of hypoxia brought on by the compromised circulation. The result is less secondary hypoxic injury (Figure 7.2).

Ice application has no effect on primary traumatic injury. Nothing can be done about such injury once it has occurred. Early applications of ice or cold packs decrease the amount of secondary hypoxic injury, although they do

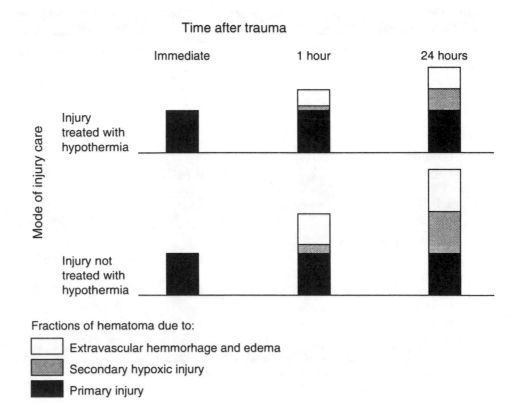

Figure 7.2 Development of the three major fractions of a hematoma following an acute musculoskeletal injury. In contrast to the lower model, which represents normothermic treatment, the upper model illustrates that the early use of local hypothermia acts to decrease secondary hypoxic injury and edema, but not primary injury. Reprinted from Knight (G50).

Time after trauma

Immediate   1 hour   24 hours

Mode of injury care

Injury treated with hypothermia

Injury not treated with hypothermia

Fractions of hematoma due to:

☐ Extravascular hemmorhage and edema

▨ Secondary hypoxic injury

■ Primary injury

not totally eliminate it. With less secondary hypoxic injury, the total amount of damaged tissue is less, and therefore there is less edema (as explained in the next section).

Thus, although cold decreases circulation, it has little to do with controlling swelling. It is by decreasing secondary hypoxic injury and thus limiting edema formation that cold controls swelling (A18, A29, A41, A44, H34).

■ *APPLY COLD PACKS QUICKLY AFTER INJURY*

Cold packs should be applied as quickly as possible following the injury. Blood flow is compromised by primary injury, so the events that lead to secondary hypoxic injury begin immediately after the injury. The more quickly you counteract these events by decreasing metabolism, the less secondary injury will develop. Haste decreases waste in this situation.

Heat applications during this period have just the opposite effect. Heat causes an increase in metabolism and therefore increases the oxygen consumption of the tissue. This causes greater secondary hypoxic injury, which leads to greater edema.

The major benefit of ice applications during immediate care results from decreased metabolism. Decreased circulation probably has no beneficial effect during immediate care.

EFFECTS OF ICE ON SWELLING

Swelling occurs from two sources: direct hemorrhaging into traumatized tissues and edema formation (H67). Ice, compression, and elevation, if used properly, are all effective in reducing edema but probably have little effect on hemorrhaging.

How Could Cold Decrease Hemorrhaging?

Cells stick together

Cold applications induce vascular spasm and increase adhesiveness in endothelial cells (those that line blood and lymphatic vessels) (H64); compression decreases underlying blood flow (H27); and elevation reduces blood pressure (H23). These measures would decrease hemorrhaging, except they rarely are taken soon enough to do so. Under normal conditions, clotting occurs within 5 minutes of the injury (H28, H44). With most sport injuries (i.e., sprains, strains, and contusions) the initial concern is to determine the extent of the injury; clotting will have already stopped the associated hemorrhaging.

How Does Cold Decrease Edema?

The majority of swelling occurs due to edema rather than hemorrhaging, and edema can be controlled with cold applications. Cold application cannot decrease tissue oncotic pressure, but it can limit the amount of the increase of such pressure following injury by limiting the amount of tissue debris (Table 7.2). This is done in two ways: by decreasing metabolism and by lowering permeability. Decreased metabolism results in decreased secondary hypoxic injury and so less tissue debris. With less tissue debris, there is less free protein and therefore a lower tissue oncotic pressure.

Capillary filtration pressure component	Average normal pressure (mmHg)	Change in pressure due to			
		Injury	**Ice**	**+ Compression**	**+ Elevation**
Capillary hydrostatic	+23	~	~	~	↓
Tissue oncotic (osmotic)	+10	↑ ↑ ↑ ↑	less ↑	~	~
Tissue hydrostatic	−1 to 4	↑	~	~	~
Capillary oncotic	−25	~	~	~	~
External	−0	~	~	↑ (—)	~
Net (overall)*	−4 to 7	↑ ↑ ↑ ↑ ↑	↑ ↑ ↑	↑ ↑	↑

Table 7.2 Effect of Changes in Capillary Filtration Pressure Components on Edema Formation Following Acute Injury

*If sum is +, fluid moves into tissue; if −, out of tissue.

Increased permeability of the blood vessel wall is a necessary part of the normal inflammatory reaction. Chemical mediators (e.g., histamine, serotonin, and the kinins) that initiate and control the inflammatory response are released from dead or dying cells (G53, G61, H78). One of the actions of these mediators is to cause blood vessel endothelial cells to separate, creating gaps in the vessel wall. This allows leukocytes to pass through the vessel wall and into the tissue spaces. It also allows great amounts of protein-rich fluid to escape, which contributes to increased tissue oncotic pressure. Rippe and Grega (G75) demonstrated that cooling (to 10°-15 °C) largely prevented the marked increases in fluid filtration and the capillary filtration coefficient induced by histamine at normal temperature. They theorized that this was due to decreased development of venular gaps, which lessened protein and fluid losses from the vascular system.

So ice applications, when used immediately after the injury, limit not only the extent of the injury but also the amount of edema that develops as a consequence of the injury. But once secondary hypoxic injury has occurred, ice applications will have no effect on edema or swelling. Ice must be applied within minutes after the injury for maximal results.

Preventing or Controlling Swelling vs. Reducing or Removing Swelling

There is a difference between preventing swelling from occurring and removing swelling once it has occurred. Although both are accomplished by controlling excess tissue oncotic pressure, the effects of ice on these two processes are dramatically different. Misunderstanding this distinction has led many clinicians to use cold applications to "treat" or remove swelling, a technique that is both ineffective and delays proper therapy. Cold prevents swelling but doesn't decrease it once it has occurred (A29).

Ice is effective in partially preventing swelling by limiting secondary hypoxic injury, the increase of free protein in the tissue, and tissue oncotic pressure, as discussed in the previous section. Decreasing the injury-elevated tissue oncotic pressure involves removing the excess free protein from the tissue, an active process that requires intermittent physical pressure. External force from massage, from compression or edema boots such as the Jobst pump, or from the "muscle pump" of active exercise physically forces the excess free protein into and along the lymphatic system (see Figure 3.18, page 34). Neither heat nor cold applications by themselves affect removal of excess free protein, and therefore have no effect on removing swelling. They can be helpful, however, in facilitating one of the other modalities. For instance, with cryokinetics, ice applications decrease pain so that active exercise can begin sooner and be more vigorous.

Some advocate combining high volt pulsed electrical stimulation with ice immersion for initial care of sports injuries (B25, B46). Among patients with ankle sprains, however, pain, edema, and range of motion were no different than control patients who used traditional ice, compression, and elevation (B28).

This differentiation is especially important when interpreting research involving the effects of cryotherapy on swelling (B34). For instance, Prentice and associates (B38, G24, H60) conducted three studies of edema control following first- and second-degree ankle sprains. Their subjects had been injured 24 or more hours prior to experimental intervention, so they were studying swelling removal, not limiting swelling with immediate applications.

EFFECTS OF COMPRESSION ON SWELLING

Compression (external pressure) acts to increase pressure outside of the vasculature (see Table 7.2). Since external pressure is on the right side of the capillary filtration pressure formula (see chapter 3, pp. 33-34), compression helps control edema formation and reduce the swelling by promoting reabsorption of this fluid. External pressure is most beneficial once edema begins occurring and is effective as long as edema is present.

External pressure has no effect on normal fluid exchange between capillaries and tissue. An analogy using a balloon illustrates this. When a balloon is filled with water, it expands. If the end of the balloon is not held tightly, the elasticity in the balloon will force the water out. If, however, the balloon is first filled with rocks, the water will occupy spaces between the rocks. As long as just enough water is added to fill the spaces between the rocks, it will not be forced from the balloon—the rocks overcome the balloon's elasticity. Squeezing the balloon (or putting an elastic bandage around it) will similarly have no effect on the water. As more water is added, however, and the balloon swells beyond the rocks, pressure is exerted on the water by the elasticity of the balloon. An elastic bandage around this swollen balloon would increase the external force, forcing the water from the balloon. Also, if the elastic bandage were placed around the balloon before the additional water was added, it would be much harder (i.e., take more force) to add the additional water. The same is true with the human body. An elastic bandage around a normal ankle will have no effect on fluid exchange, but it would tend to retard or cause reabsorption of swelling.

Wilkerson (H79) believed compression must be focused rather than generalized. He reasoned that general compression allows excess edema to accumulate in the area of the anterior talofibular ligament. Subsequent healing then leads to increased synovial thickening and fibrotic scar tissue in the lateral gutter (J25). Pressure measured with a 1-inch diameter, .15-inch thick manometer air cell over the anterior talofibular ligament was no different with or without focused compression (i.e., a felt horseshoe under an elastic wrap) (J20). Further research with smaller pressure sensors is needed to definitively answer this question.

Since it has not been determined exactly how long after injury edema begins developing, it is recommended that compression be applied within minutes and remain for a minimum of 24 hours.

EFFECTS OF ELEVATION ON SWELLING

Elevation lowers capillary hydrostatic pressure and therefore decreases the major factor (in a noninjured state) in forcing fluid out of the capillary.

Hydrostatic pressure results from the weight of water (J29). In a swimming pool, lake, or ocean, the deeper one dives, the greater the hydrostatic pressure becomes, as there is more water above pushing down. The same is true in the body with the fluid portion of blood. Capillary hydrostatic pressure is greater when a body part is in a dependent position than when it is elevated because there is more water weight above it (H23, H37). Elevation, then, retards swelling during immediate-care procedures by lowering capillary hydrostatic pressure (see Table 7.2), which decreases capillary filtration pressure. Although elevation also lowers tissue hydrostatic pressure, the normal value of this pressure is so much less than capillary hydrostatic pressure that the effect of capillary hydrostatic pressure to decrease edema predominates.

REST

Rest, when used in sports injury management, means decreased activity, not inactivity. Some clinicians use the term *relative rest* (H18). There is a thin line between aggravating the injury because of too much activity and complications due to too little activity. Too much activity may stress the injured tissue and result in further stretching or tearing (B5). Reduced activity is necessary to protect the injury from being aggravated and to allow healing to take place (B5).

Another problem with activity following an injury is pain—not the discomfort itself, but the changes in the body due to the pain. The body responds to pain by shutting things down. It attempts to protect itself by eliminating any activity that causes pain—by inhibiting normal musculoskeletal functions, such as strength and range of motion, that is, most activity. Often these neural inhibitions continue long after the injury itself has healed (J15) and thereby prevent the athlete from engaging in sport activities. By resting immediately following an injury (i.e., keeping activity below the level at which it causes pain), the complications of neural inhibitions are avoided.

The primary rationale for using crutches following a lower extremity injury is to remove pain. Limping results from pain. Even though patients may think that they can "hobble along," to do so invokes pain and thus neuromuscular inhibitions, which is bad. Patients should always use crutches until they can walk with a normal gait. (Patients on crutches should use the three-point, or walking, gait and should seldom use the swing gait, in which all weight is removed from the injured limb. As the injury heals, the crutches support less and less weight.)

■ **AVOID PAIN LIKE THE PLAGUE**

Two rules of thumb for rehabilitation are "If it hurts, don't do it" and "Work up to the level of pain, but don't go beyond it." The concept of "No pain, no gain" is all right during conditioning exercises but totally wrong during rehabilitation. Pain causes neural inhibitions that prolong rehabilitation. It's not a question of how tough an athlete is, but how smart he or she is. Athletes must work around their pain, not fight their way through it.

Too little activity can be as detrimental as too much activity. Complications due to insufficient activity include delayed healing, development of adhesions, muscular atrophy, loss of conditioning, "rusty" skills, and loss of confidence (H34). The loss of skills is also probably due to neural inhibition.

Keep an injured athlete as active as possible without causing further problems. Usually this means exercising noninvolved body parts to the maximum extent possible and exercising the involved body part to a level just under that which causes pain.

STABILIZATION

Do not confuse stabilization with compression or rest; its purpose is quite different. Although stabilization may provide compression and may force the injured body part to rest these benefits are secondary. The purpose of stabilization is to provide enough support to the injured limb that the surrounding muscles can relax.

Muscle guarding, in which the muscles surrounding an injury contract or spasm in an attempt to splint the injured area and protect it from further injury, is an unwanted response to injury. Muscle guarding causes pain, which causes more muscle spasm, which causes more pain, and so on. Thus a pain-spasm-pain cycle is perpetuated. Early stabilization allows the muscles to relax and thus decreases the pain-spasm-cycle. There are numerous braces and splints that can be used for stabilization (see Figure 7.3).

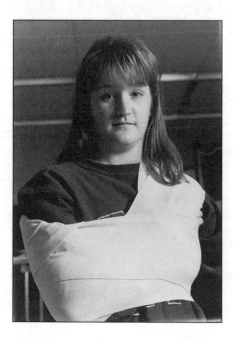 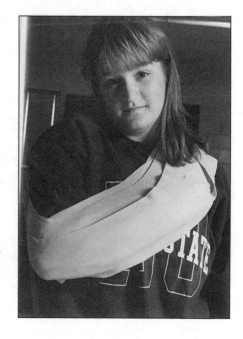

Figure 7.3 Stabilization with a sling and swath allow the muscles of the shoulder to relax (left). Contrast with a nonstabilized condition, where the muscles must stabilize the shoulder following injury (right).

WHAT TYPES OF INJURIES ARE TREATED WITH RICES?

All acute musculoskeletal injuries should be treated with RICES. Whenever there is tissue damage, there is the potential of secondary hypoxic injury. Failure to treat with RICES results in greater soft tissue damage and thus delays final resolution of the injury.

Among clinicians outside of sports medicine, it is common to treat sprains, strains, and contusions with RICES; care of fractures, abrasions, and dislocations usually does not include ice and compression (H22, J56). One popular first-aid text advocates ice, compression, and elevation for sprains and dislocations, but only ice packs for strains (H22). There is no logic to these recommendations. RICES should be used for immediate care of all acute musculoskeletal injuries.

ICE APPLICATION PROTOCOLS

Various protocols have been suggested for applying cold during immediate care of injuries. Mlynarczyk (H48) reviewed the recommended length, frequency of application, and duration of therapy of over 30 published protocols and found only two instances in which two recommendations were the same. I hope the following sections resolve some of the confusion.

Apply Ice Directly to the Skin

Apply crushed-ice packs directly to the skin (A19, H9, H47, H66). Some clinicians have claimed that this will cause frostbite and so advocate applying oil to the skin (A11) or putting a towel or elastic wrap between the skin and the cold pack (A46, B8, B47, H14, H25, H69, I7). But a towel or wrap between the skin and cold pack insulates the skin against the full effects of the cold, thereby decreasing the effectiveness of the cold application. Therefore, other clinicians have suggested using wet (B8, H12, H14, H34, H45) or frozen (H75) elastic wraps between the skin and cold pack, thinking this method allows the cold to penetrate while still protecting the skin against frostbite. Although wet or frozen wraps are better than dry ones, they too insulate the skin against the cold (Figure 7.4) (C7, C50, H73).

Urban and I (H73) studied the insulating effects of wet, frozen, and dry elastic wraps on an ice pack applied to the lateral ankle (Figure 7.4). After 5 minutes of application the surface temperature of the ankle had decreased from 32 °C to 13.9 °C when the ice was applied directly to the skin, to 18.1 °C when applied over a wet wrap, to 15.5 °C when applied over a frozen wrap, and to only 26.7 °C when applied over a dry wrap. After 30 minutes of application, the skin temperatures were 3.2 °C for no wrap, 8.9 °C for the wet wrap, 10.8 °C for the frozen wrap, and 19.5 °C for the dry wrap (all temperature figures are average temperatures). As the numbers indicate, frozen wraps are no more effective than wet wraps, and, while both wet and frozen wraps are more effective than dry wraps, neither are as effective as ice applied directly to the skin. Any type of material between the ice pack and the skin will insulate the skin against the full effects of the ice pack.

What about the frostbite problem? Mirkin (H47) supported his practice of applying ice packs directly on the skin reasoning that living tissue will not freeze until its temperature drops below 25 °F (–3.9 °C). Since the

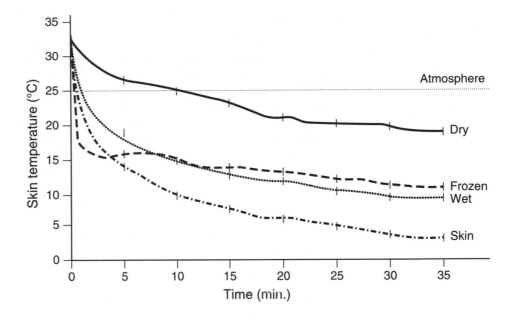

Figure 7.4 Mean skin temperature recorded each minute during application of crushed ice packs to the lateral ankle. The four conditions represent application of the ice pack directly to the skin or over dry, wet, or frozen elastic wraps (H73).

temperature of an ice pack is 32 °F (0 °C), it is incapable of causing frostbite. Although Mirkin probably is 2° to 3 °C low concerning the freezing temperature of skin (see chapter 14), he is correct in stating that ice packs can be applied safely to the skin as long as they are not left on longer than 30 to 60 minutes. Long-term application can lead to tissue damage (see chapter 14).

The same cannot be said about frozen-gel packs. The temperature of a gel pack can be many degrees below freezing, depending on the temperature of the freezer unit in which it is cooled. Do not apply a frozen-gel pack directly to the skin (H71).

I could find no reference to any occurrence of frostbite as a result of a short-term (30-minute) ice application. Also, in 25 years of clinical experience I have not observed frostbite after applying ice packs directly to the skin of athletes for up to 45 minutes at a time.

Some are opposed to applying the cold pack directly to the skin because they fear that applying the elastic wrap over the cold pack will result in less compression than if the wrap was applied directly to the skin. Such is not the case, however. Pressure under a sealed ice pack and a 6-foot long, 6-inch wide elastic wrap applied over the thigh and ankle of human volunteers is the same whether the wrap was applied over or under the ice pack (H74). Apparently, by tying a knot in the ice pack, the volume remains constant and the pressure of the wrap is transmitted through the pack to the skin underneath.

■ *DON'T USE A TOWEL UNDER YOUR CRUSHED-ICE PACK*

Apply crushed-ice packs directly to the skin. A towel or elastic wrap between the ice pack and the body insulates against the full effects of the cold and makes the treatment less effective. This will not cause frostbite if used for less than 30 to 60 minutes. *Do not place frozen-gel packs directly on the skin, however.* Their temperature may be many degrees below zero, and they could cause frostbite.

Length of Application

The question of how long cold packs should be applied involves not just the initial application, but the repeated applications and time between the applications as well. Suggested durations for applying cold packs have varied from 6 minutes to continuously for 24 to 48 hours. Proulx (I51) reported on a patient who applied ice packs continuously for 72 hours and caused frostbite. Most clinicians, however, use intermittent applications for various reasons.

Some use intermittent application because they believe cold-induced vasodilation (CIVD) increases blood flow to the area if they apply cold for longer than 10 to 12 minutes (A46, B3, B8, B18, B31). Chu and Lutt (C16) felt that initial cold applications should last at least 20 minutes so that the body part could pass through a 3- to 5-minute period of vasodilation and be in a second period of vasoconstriction. Others fear frostbite (A46, H25, I51) or nerve palsy (I10) if they apply cold too long. Boland (H9) felt that the application of ice packs for longer than 30 minutes was too painful and should not be done.

Most advocate intermittent application because continuous application is unnecessary—the beneficial effects of cold applications (depressed tissue temperature) remain after the cold packs are removed (chapter 5); thus, tissue metabolism remains depressed (chapter 8).

There is no direct research on the effects of length of application on the amount of tissue damage or on subsequent resolution of the injury. We must look to expert opinion and research on peripheral issues, primarily tissue temperature changes during various protocols.

After reviewing the literature, McMaster (A31) claimed that cold should be applied for at least 20 minutes and preferably for 30 minutes. Applications of less time than this would not effectively lower the temperature of deeper tissues and therefore would not have a beneficial effect at the site of injury. The same logic was used by Laing et al. (B24), who felt that a 20-minute application was adequate but that a 10-minute one was not.

Studies from our laboratory shed some light on this topic. Mlynarczyk (H48) studied the cooling and rewarming characteristics of the ankle for 3 hours following ice pack applications for 10, 20, 30, 45, and 60 minutes. During the initial 2 hours of rewarming, the ankle was significantly warmer following the 10- and 20-minute applications than following the three longer application times. Rewarming following the 45-minute application was not significantly different than following either the 30- or the 60-minute conditions. These data indicate that, as far as rewarming of the ankle is concerned, an ice pack must be applied for at least 30 minutes, but that longer applications provide no additional benefit.

The activity level of the patient determines how quickly subsequent applications should be administered. Generally, following the first application athletes will shower and go home. Cold packs should be reapplied immediately (C59). If the athlete is inactive, however, applications of more than 30 minutes every 2 hours will cause a progressive decrease in the temperature of the ankle (H56).

The area of the body also affects the length of application. Thick muscular tissues, such as in the thigh, require longer to cool than bony areas, such as in the ankle (C59, H74).

The ankle and forearm temperatures remain depressed for hours after application, while the finger rewarms within minutes (see Figures 5.5 and 5.9). The thigh cools more slowly and rewarms faster than the ankle and forearm (C59, H74). Preliminary results from current research indicate that the knee reacts like the ankle and forearm.

■ *LENGTH OF APPLICATION*

Ice packs should be applied intermittently. Continuous application is both unnecessary and potentially dangerous. You could cause frostbite with continuous application; besides, the majority of the body's parts rewarm quite slowly following ice pack application. So you can keep the body part cool by applying an ice pack for 30 minutes (40 minutes for a large muscle mass like the thigh) every 2 hours (every hour if the patient is active between applications; such as showering or walking on crutches).

Duration of Therapy

Duration, as used here, refers to the length of time that intermittent 30-minute applications of cold packs should be continued. I could find no data to indicate an optimal duration. Most clinicians (see H48 for references) recommend applications for 12 to 72 hours, or until the tendency for swelling has passed. A guideline, part of the answer, lies in the severity of the injury. You can terminate immediate-care procedures earlier when treating a mild injury than when treating a severe injury. Also, you can switch from immediate-care to rehabilitation procedures earlier when using a cryotherapeutic technique for rehabilitation than when using a thermotherapeutic technique. But a definitive answer to the question of the optimal duration of cold applications during immediate care awaits further research.

■ *TYPES OF COLD PACKS*

Recommendations on the types of cold packs to use depends on convenience and budgetary factors. Crushed-ice packs and frozen-gel packs responded similarly in studies involving 30-minute applications to human subjects. Crushed-ice packs are cheaper but somewhat more messy. Also, in a situation in which a great number of athletes may have to be treated within a few hours, the frozen-gel packs will not have enough time to rechill.

Chemical ice packs have no place in athletics. They neither get the body cold enough nor last long enough to be used in place of crushed ice. There also is a danger of chemical burns when using these—if the contents of a chemical pack leak onto the skin, serious damage may result.

■ *RECOMMENDED PROTOCOL FOR APPLYING AN ICE PACK*

Make an ice pack by placing slightly more than 1 kilogram (2-1/2 pounds) of crushed or cubed ice in a plastic bag. Suck out as much air as possible from the bag and tie the end in a knot. Place the ice pack directly on the injured part and secure it with a 15-centimeter (6-inch) elastic wrap. Elevate the injured part 15 to 25 centimeters (6-10 inches) above the level of the heart. After 30 to 45 minutes, remove the ice pack, replace the elastic wrap, and continue elevation. Reapply the ice pack in the same manner and for the same duration every 1 to 2 hours until the athlete goes to bed. The elastic wrap should be worn throughout the night.

SUMMARY

- Rest, ice, compression, elevation, and stabilization (RICES) are each important in controlling swelling following an acute musculoskeletal injury.
- RICES procedures do not exert their beneficial effects through altered circulation as clinicians have believed in the past.
- Ice limits the increase in tissue oncotic pressure because lowered metabolism decreases secondary hypoxic injury, thus limiting the amount of tissue debris; compression increases external pressure; and elevation decreases capillary hydrostatic pressure. Each of these factors decreases the transvascular pressure, thus limiting edema formation.
- Immediate care of acute sports injuries includes RICES.
- Apply ice packs intermittently (30-45 minutes every 1-2 hours) directly to the skin for the first 12 to 24 hours following injury.
- Compression and elevation should be applied continuously during this period, except when changing the ice pack.
- Compression is achieved with an elastic wrap applied over the ice pack or directly to the body part when the ice pack is not in place.
- Stabilize the injury with a brace or splint and rest the body part.

8

Orthopedic Surgery and Cryotherapy

The postsurgical application of cold packs is well established but its use has been questioned. For many years the theory was that cold decreases swelling and pain. Questions arose when research using long-term applications with animals and on humans following dental surgery revealed little or no decrease in swelling. Recent research has focused on pain relief, drug consumption, hospital stay, and return to activity. These parameters all are positively influenced by cryotherapy and they indicate a definite place for cryotherapy following orthopedic surgery.

The use of cryotherapy before and during orthopedic surgery has been proposed, but is still being investigated. The proposal is based on the benefits of cryotherapy during thoracic and abdominal surgery—namely, a decrease in metabolism and thus a reduction in tissue death resulting from secondary hypoxic injury. In this chapter, I review these effects and recommend that cryotherapy be used before and during orthopedic surgery.

POSTSURGICAL CRYOTHERAPY

Cold compresses were a recognized adjunct to surgery as early as 1881 (A11) to decrease pain. A 1945 study (H61) reported that cold application (ice caps) following orthopedic surgery and manipulation cases was associated with fewer postsurgical complications (Table 8.1). Among 345 patients treated with ice caps over their casts or dressings for 48 hours, fewer casts were split; patients' temperature, pulse, and respiration were lower; leukocyte counts were closer to normal; narcotic consumption was lower; and there were fewer postoperative complications of other kinds in the 72 hour period following surgery than in the over 450 patients not treated with cryotherapy.

Drug use was lower among patients treated immediately following surgery with ice caps over inguinal hernia and appendectomy incisions (H68). Unsolicited remarks from floor nurses indicated the cold-treated patients experienced less pain and ambulated more easily than control patients who had experienced the same surgery.

99

Table 8.1   Effects of Ice Caps Used Following Orthopaedic Manipulation and/or Surgery

	Ice used for 48 hours post operatively	Ice not used post operatively
Total cases	345	479
Number casted	207	312
Casts split	5.3%	42.3%
Elevated white cell count		
1st day P.O.	12.4%	33.4%
2nd day P.O.	3.2%	12.3%
3rd day P.O.	1.4%	5.6%
Temperature higher than 38.3°C (101°F)	11.3%	23.2%
Pulse rate over 115/min	11.3%	25.1%
Respiratory rate over 20/min	2.6%	14.6%
Use of narcotics (avg. dosage/case)		
Codeine	1.4 mgm	4.2 mgm
Morphine	1.9 mgm	.4 mgm
Complications	5.5%	12.5%

*Data taken from Schaubel (H61).

Bingham (G8) applied ice compresses postoperatively in chronic osteomyelitis patients. All patients treated with ice healed without recurrence, which was not so in those who were not treated with ice, and the need for postoperative draining was lower. Bingham also reported that the need for surgery was decreased among patients with acute hematogenous osteomyelitis who were treated with cold compresses. The length of hospitalization was less than half that of a similar group of patients treated identically except for cold applications.

Numerous clinical research projects on cryotherapy have been reported. These are summarized here for type of surgery, type of cryotherapy, and results:

TYPE OF SURGERY OR PATIENT

- Outpatient arthroscopy (E20, H6)
- Retinacular release (H6)
- Anterior cruciate ligament reconstruction (H10)
- Total knee arthroplasty (H24, H38, H50, H52)
- Podiatric surgery (H62)

TYPE OF CRYOTHERAPY

- Outpatient treatment for 3 hours (E20, H6)
- Dura*Kold (E20, H10)
- Icy/Hot or similar machine (H6, H10, H50, II52)
- Cryo Cuff (E20, H38, H62)

RESULTS

- 30% to 50% less blood loss (H38, H50)
- Less swelling (H24)
- Less medication (H10, H38)

- Less pain (H26, H38, H62)
- Patients more compliant with therapy (H10)
- Subjective evaluation by nurses indicated preference for cryotherapy (E20, H10)
- No difference in hospital stay (H10)
- More active (E20, H10, H38)

One group of surgeons reported no difference in swelling, pain, or medication use (H50). They used a cryotherapy machine with no compression. In contrast, those who did use compression with cold reported positive results (E20, H38, H62).

Another group reported cryotherapy was beneficial in decreasing swelling in total knee arthroplasty patients, but they did not use the cold until 14 days following the procedure, and then only as an adjunct to rehabilitation (H24). Cryotherapy's effects were probably secondary to less pain and more activity. As with initial care of sprains and strains, the sooner cryotherapy is used following the trauma the better it prevents swelling. After a few hours have passed, cryotherapy is effective only as an adjunct to other therapy (the most effective being active exercise).

Postpartum Cryotherapy

Cold applications are more effective than thermotherapy for treating postpartum pain and return to normal activities (B17, E66, H15, H57). Cold was significantly more effective among 40 postpartum patients who compared heat and cold sitz baths for relief of episiotomy pain (although 119 patients refused to participate in the study, 58 saying that they would not sit in a cold sitz bath, no matter how severe their pain became [H57]). Droegemueller (H15) also advocated cold (rather than hot) sitz baths for relief of postpartum perineal pain, as well, his patients experiencing less pain and swelling and having a quicker return to normal activities with cold sitz baths, as opposed to hot baths.

Cold packs can be used rather than cold sitz baths. My wife has given birth to eight children. After birth of the first five she used the standard protocol of hot sitz baths and heat lamps; after the last three she applied crushed-ice packs to the perineum. The difference in recovery was so dramatic (25% to 35% quicker) that she now recommends the technique to every pregnant woman of her acquaintance.

Temperature Changes Under Surgical Dressings

Omer and Brobeck (H53) measured forearm temperatures under plaster casts and under bulk compression dressings. Their cold packs consisted of frozen rubber water bottles changed every 4 hours. Temperature was measured every hour for 24 hours. Average temperature due to cold pack application dropped a few degrees, but these differences were not significant. Although patients consistently felt more comfortable when treated postsurgically with ice packs, the authors considered this response to be subjective. However, this conclusion seems unwarranted in light of the data of others (C46, H61) and our own clinical experience dealing with acute sport injuries. It is possible that the bandages were so thick that they almost totally insulated the area against the cold; that the ice packs were changed too infrequently; or that the temperature measurements were taken so infrequently that the major decreases in skin temperature were missed.

Research from our laboratory indicates that cold packs are capable of lowering temperatures under surgical dressings consisting of two layers of gauze pads, two thicknesses of 1/8-inch surgical dressing, and an elastic wrap (C46, E20). Knee surface temperatures decreased during Dura*Kold pack application to normal volunteers (Figure 8.1) and athroscopy patients (E20). And cold-gel packs applied over short arm casts (plaster and fiberglass; .85 = .9 cm thick) decreased skin temperatures over the wrist joint (H33).

Does Cryotherapy Decrease Postsurgical Swelling?

Finding little quantitative documentation in the literature for the use of cold application to minimize posttraumatic swelling Matsen et al. (H47) studied the effects of cold application on rabbits in which they produced a standardized midshaft femoral fracture. Limbs cooled to 5°, 8°, 10°, and 15°C all showed an increase in swelling that began to be apparent at 6 hours following the 24-hour cooling period and was maximal at 24 hours after this treatment. Limbs cooled to 20° to 25° C showed no difference from control (controls were fractured contralateral limbs treated with water at 32°C). Dissection following the procedure revealed the swelling to be in the subcutaneous tissue. The authors hypothesized that in limbs cooled to 15°C or colder, vessels in the subcutaneous tissue were damaged by cold-induced ischemia and that perfusion of these vessels following cooling produced local exudation.

Matsen et al. concluded that their results do not prove that ice applications have no place in orthopedics, but rather challenge those who use ice to objectively demonstrate its effectiveness. Perhaps that challenge should be modified—the challenge should be to objectively determine the proper protocol for the use of ice postsurgically. The protocols studied by Matsen et al.

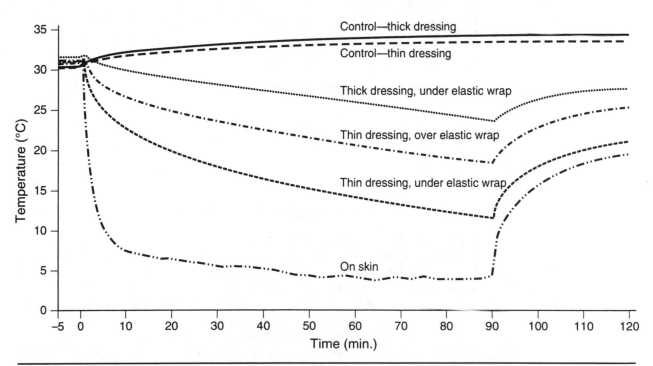

Figure 8.1 The thicker the surgical dressing between a cold pack and the skin, the less effective the cold pack is in decreasing temperature. These data are knee surface temperatures in normal subjects under thick (2 ABD pads + a 6" × 6 yd elastic bandage) and thin (2 4 × 4 gauze pads + 6" × 6 yd elastic bandage) surgical dressings. Two thin dressings conditions were investigated: one with the ice pack over the gauze pads but under the elastic bandage, the other with the ice pack over both the gauze pads and the elastic bandage. Data from Knight (C46).

were not judicious therapeutic protocols (H46). The application times were much too long, and some of the temperatures to which they cooled the limbs were much lower than would occur clinically during extended continuous application.

Improper technique also could have accounted for Rembe's (H58) failure to demonstrate a statistically significant decrease in swelling during postsurgical cryotherapy in the rheumatoid hand. Patients received only two 4-minute treatments (immersion in 10°C water) beginning 48 hours following surgery. Treatments must begin earlier (within 30 minutes following surgery), last longer (30 to 60 minutes), and be more numerous (every 2 hours for the first 24 or more hours following surgery).

Jedzinsky et al. (H29) reported that cold applied immediately following injury exerted an unfavorable effect on the development of traumatic edema. Again, one must question their application protocol. Rat paws were mechanically traumatized (crushed) and then placed between two rubber tubes filled with cold water (11.5°-12.5°C) at a pressure of 7.5 or 10 cm of water for 2 to 10 hours. There were no significant differences from cold during cold application, but in most cases there was an increase in edema following the application. Both the length of application and the lack of compression present a basis for questioning the authors' conclusions.

Farry et al. (H16) countered the conclusions of Matsen et al. (H41) by demonstrating that ice applications result in subcutaneous tissue swelling even in the absence of injury. They applied crushed-ice packs to both injured and uninjured pig forelegs for 20 minutes, removed the packs for 1 hour, and then reapplied the ice packs for an additional 20-minute period. After 48 hours, the legs were examined for swelling and biopsies taken for blind evaluation of the inflammatory reaction by a pathologist. They found, like Matsen et al., that injured limbs treated with ice were more swollen than those not treated with ice.

These results, however, were tempered by three additional findings:

- Noninjured limbs treated with ice swelled. In fact, the difference between iced and noniced noninjured limbs was greater than the difference between ice and noniced injured limbs.
- In 9 of 10 injured limbs treated with ice, the inflammatory reaction was reduced, as was microscopic evidence of edema in the injured ligaments.
- The swelling occurred in the soft tissue overlying the injured ligament, rather than in the ligament itself.

The authors concluded that ice application was beneficial, even though it would cause some unwanted swelling. They felt that the associated swelling could be minimized if the injured area was treated with compression and elevation after ice was removed. More recent research indicates that compression during cryotherapy is important (H79-H81).

Not If, But How?

Postsurgical cryotherapy is underutilized (E66, H43). Perhaps this is because crushed-ice packs are messy and labor-intensive for nurses (H52), because they were evaluated following inadequate application (e.g., through a bulky dressing only many hours following surgery), or because the early research questioned its use. But there are too many positive reports of its use to discount the value; many are presented earlier in the chapter. The question concerning postsurgical cryotherapy should be "How is it most effective?" not "Is it effective?"

Peterson (personal communication) is emphatic about the use of ice post-surgically because the use of pain medication was greatly reduced and his patients became active much sooner.

PRESURGICAL CRYOTHERAPY

Local hypothermia has been used presurgically to produce surgical anesthesia prior to amputation of gangrenous limbs (H1, H13, H65), to reduce postoperative morbidity, mortality, and length of hospital stay (G17); to lower an elevated bodily temperature caused by some neurological diseases (H65); for tissue preservation during abdominal and thoracic surgery (see chapter 13); and to suspend the spread of infection and absorption of toxins in gangrenous patients when an inevitable amputation had to be delayed for some reason (H20).

Allen and associates (H1, H13) used ice as an anesthetic in poor-risk patients requiring amputation. Limbs were either immersed in ice water (preferred) or packed in crushed ice for 1 to 5 hours (depending on the thickness of the tissue) prior to surgery. Not only did this method allow surgery with no other anesthesia, but it provided a number of other benefits:

- The surgical shock response was eliminated.
- Most patients were able to return directly to the ward and eat a full meal following surgery.
- Postsurgical morphine was unnecessary.
- The tendency toward thrombosis, infection, and tissue infection was suppressed.
- General strength was preserved.

Muscle injury during tourniquet ischemia is decreased in limbs cooled prior to tourniquet application (H55, H84). Levels of serum myoglobin, a protein released by damaged muscle cells, were decreased in patients whose arms were immersed in ice water for 20 minutes prior to hand and wrist surgery.

Although I could find nothing in the sports medicine literature about the use of cryotherapy prior to orthopedic surgery, the Sports Medicine Clinic of Seattle, Washington (personal communication), has used a Cryomatic unit in what they termed a "fact-finding experiment." The unit was applied for one hour presurgically, as well as immediately postsurgically. The clinicians were encouraged by this protocol because their patients had much less pain and seemed to recover faster. Drug use was reduced to aspirin only. Additional clinical research is in progress.

There is a strong theoretical argument for presurgical cryotherapy. Since organ viability is preserved during surgically induced hypoxia (see chapter 16), it is reasonable to assume that musculature and connective tissue viability would also be preserved during surgery. Precooling of these tissues would decrease the amount of secondary hypoxic injury during and after orthopedic surgery. Decreased secondary hypoxic injury would mean less total injury (see chapter 7). This result, combined with decreased pain, would allow ambulation sooner than usual. The negative sequelae to immobilization would therefore be decreased. Much more research needs to be conducted in this area. Precooling may be of even more benefit than postsurgical cooling.

CRYOANALGESIA

Cryoanalgesia—cold pain relief—involves a cryosurgical probe whose tip is cooled to –60°C by circulating nitrous oxide gas (E7, E62, E64). The probe is applied to nerves for 1 minute, causing them to freeze. The nerve is allowed to thaw out and is then refrozen by applying the probe for another minute. Among 64 patients with pain from assorted pathology, cryoanalgesia produced pain relief for a median of 11 days (range = 0-224 days) (E64). A comparison between two matched groups of 29 postthoracotomy patients, one of which was treated with cryoanalgesia, revealed less of a demand for postoperative analgesic medication among the cryoanalgesic group (E31).

SUMMARY

- Local hypothermia has been used before and after orthopedic surgery to decrease pain, decrease secondary hypoxic injury, and control edema. Its use for controlling edema postsurgically has been challenged, but the experimental data supporting those challenges have used protocols that are suspect.
- Clinical research indicates that cryotherapy following an orthopedic procedure leads to use of less pain medication and quicker ambulation.
- Investigation of various protocols of postsurgical application is needed to determine the most effective use of cryotherapy following surgery.
- Compression must be combined with cryotherapy. Although we can't explain all the *why*'s, clinical and experimental evidence is mounting that cryotherapy is much more effective when combined with compression.
- There is a strong theoretical basis for presurgical local hypothermia. Its use could decrease cellular necrosis, tourniquet ischemic injury, postsurgical pain, and narcotic use. Ambulation would be possible sooner, which would decrease the negative sequelae to immobilization.

Circulatory Effects of Therapeutic Cold Applications

There is much confusion about the circulatory response to cold application during both immediate care and rehabilitation. Many believe that the major benefit of cold during immediate-care procedures is that it decreases circulation at the site of the injury and thereby limits hemorrhaging and swelling. Cold does cause vasoconstriction, but, as noted in chapter 8, cold is usually not applied until after the damaged vasculature clots. Furthermore, the changes in circulation during immediate-care procedures probably have little effect on resolution of the injury.

The confusion about rehabilitation concerns cold-induced vasodilation (CIVD). There is a common belief that therapeutic cold applications cause an *increase* in blood flow that is greater in magnitude and longer lasting than that brought about by hot packs (A47, C16, C22, C67). However, the professional literature does not support this contention. There are numerous opinions as to what CIVD is, and when and how it occurs, but no direct statement as to its magnitude. On the other hand, there is ample evidence that therapeutic cold applications cause vasoconstriction and *decreased* blood flow.

So what does it matter? People still use cold, isn't that all that counts? No! Many athletes are treated improperly during both the periods of immediate care and rehabilitation, because of their athletic trainer's, therapist's, or physician's beliefs about CIVD. For example, during immediate care, many therapists apply ice, compression, and elevation only for 20 minutes because they fear that CIVD will occur after that, thus increasing blood flow and hemorrhaging. For most injuries, however, 20 minutes of cooling isn't enough to lower metabolism sufficiently to decrease secondary hypoxic injury (see chapters 6 and 7), so many athletes receive less-than-optimal care.

But the negative implications of the CIVD concept have been worse with regard to rehabilitation. People are treated with cold immersion and sent on their way with an explanation that this has stimulated a great increase in blood flow. In reality, it has decreased blood flow, so the athlete gets nothing more than a placebo effect from the treatment.

Contrast bath therapy, a popular technique for treating ankle and other sprains, is based on a flawed theory involving circulatory changes. The theory involves alternately immersing the injury in hot and cold water baths. The theory is that during the procedure the tissue will alternately vasodilate and vasoconstrict and that this action will flush injury debris from the tissue and deliver increased amounts of nutrients to rebuild the tissue. The theory is flawed, however, as will be discussed later in this chapter.

In this chapter I will also discuss the definition of CIVD, review the reasons for and against it, and explain why the concept as applied to sport injury management has been helpful, even though it is wrong.

WHAT IS COLD-INDUCED VASODILATION?

The term *cold-induced vasodilation (CIVD)* means blood vessel dilation as a result of cold application. The phrase was coined by Lewis (C51) in 1930 as an explanation for two phenomena that he observed while measuring finger temperatures during and after immersing a hand in cold water: a "hunting response" during immersion and an "aftereffect" following it. Lewis observed that immediately after immersing a finger in ice water there was a sharp decrease in its temperature (Figure 9.1). After 8 to 16 minutes in the water, the temperature increased a few degrees. This was followed by a nonrhythmical decreasing-increasing pattern of 2°C to 6°C per oscillation, which Lewis called the hunting reaction. In another experiment, Lewis attributed these oscillations in temperature to CIVD. Subsequently, writers have assumed that the hunting reaction was a circulatory phenomenon (A47, C6). Lewis also observed that upon removing the cooled finger from the

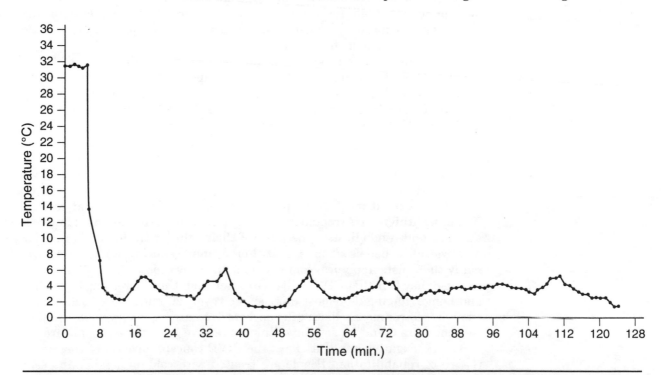

Figure 9.1   Finger temperature during immersion in crushed ice. Oscillations in temperature during application were termed the "hunting reaction."
Reprinted from Lewis (C52).

water, its temperature rose abruptly many degrees above that of the control finger (Figure 9.2). This aftereffect of cooling, he wrote, "is clearly a vasodilation." Clinicians mistakenly inferred from this that CIVD causes or is a net increase in blood flow similar to the increase in blood flow caused by heat applications (B4, B21, B35, C6, C16, C22, H35). But Lewis's (C51) own data do not support this conclusion, a point that will be discussed later.

By the mid 1970s the idea that CIVD was either an increase in blood flow during (Figure 9.3) or following (Figure 9.4) cold applications was firmly established among sports medicine clinicians. But these later definitions are filled with contradiction and were based on incorrectly interpreted research, probably because they provided a ready theoretical explanation for some rather new and dramatic therapeutic techniques (cryokinetics, cryostretch, etc.).

I don't argue that CIVD occurs, only that its effects have no bearing on cryotherapy during sport injury management—neither during immediate care nor rehabilitation. First, since CIVD occurs after 20 to 40 minutes of cold application, it probably does not occur during most sport injury cryotherapy; but its effects are negligible if it does. Second, cryotherapy is beneficial during immediate care because it decreases metabolism and during rehabilitation because it decreases pain. Circulatory effects are inconsequential.

What is Dilation?

Dilation is an expansion of an organ, orifice, or vessel. It is relative and depends on your perspective. For instance, a vessel with a diameter of 5 (arbitrary units) that decreased to 3 has constricted (Figure 9.5). An increase to 8 would be dilation. On the other hand, if you began at 5, constricted to 1, and then increased to 3, would the last phase be dilation or a partial reversal of the initial constriction? Either would be correct.

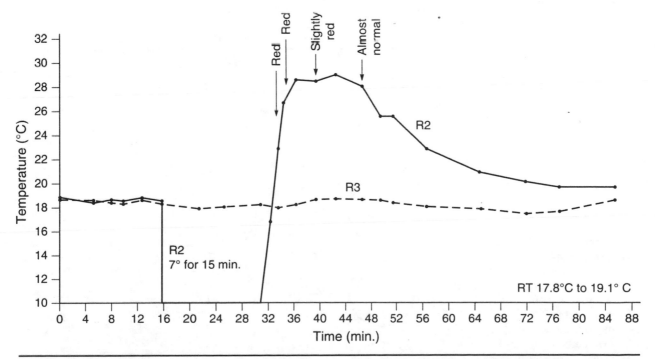

Figure 9.2 Finger temperature following 15 minutes of immersion in 7 °C water, showing an aftereffect which was thought to be due to cold-induced vasodilation. Note, however, the artificially low temperature (approximately 19 °C) of the control finger (R3).
Reprinted from Lewis (C52).

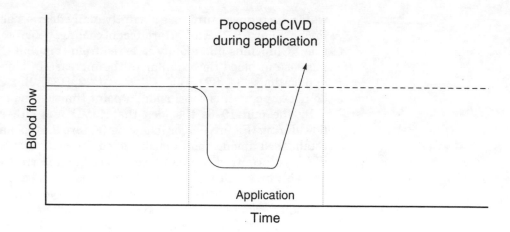

Figure 9.3 Cold-induced vasodilation during cold application. This proposed phenomenon does not occur during therapeutic applications of cold.

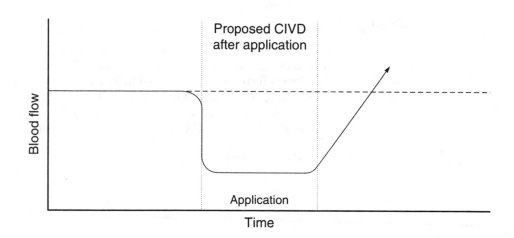

Figure 9.4 Cold-induced vasodilation following cold application. This proposed phenomenon does not occur as a result of therapeutic applications of cold.

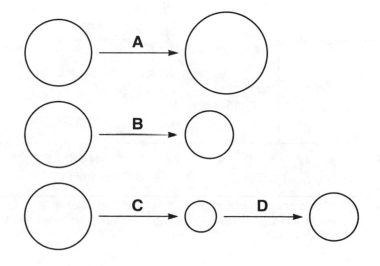

Figure 9.5 Dilation and constriction are processes, not end results. For instance, if a vessel changed diameter from a to b, it would be dilation; but if it changed from c to b, it would be constriction.

What Is CIVD?

CIVD, cold-induced vasodilation, means blood vessel dilation (opening) as a result of cold application. Many incorrectly believe the term means either an increase in blood flow during (Figure 9.3) or following (Figure 9.4) cold applications; an increase they think is greater than resting or heat-induced blood flow. But dilation (whether cold-induced or not) is a process—not a result. Consider, for instance, a blood vessel that first constricted (decreased) to 20% of its usual size and then dilated (increased) to 25% of its usual size. Even though the vessel dilated, blood flow through it would only be 25% of its regular amount. So just because a vessel dilated does not mean that it is carrying more blood than it usually would.

COLD DILEMMA

The initial vascular response to cold is vasoconstriction and decreased blood flow (C3, C5, C12, C21, C25, C30, C43, C46, D1; see also Figures 9.11 and 9.13, pages 118, 119). The response is gradual, resembling deep tissue temperature changes rather than the steep, immediate plunge of surface temperatures.

Do cold applications result in both increased and decreased blood flow? The literature leads us to believe so—specifically, to believe that if cold is applied to the musculoskeletal system immediately after an acute injury it controls swelling by decreasing circulation, but if applied during rehabilitation of the injury (24 to 48 hours following an injury) it promotes healing by increasing circulation. It seems absurd that cold would decrease circulation one day and then increase it the next just because the reason for applying it has changed. Yet this is what the clinical literature seems to be saying (A35, A47, B8, B11, B21, F5).

Many clinicians have attempted to resolve this dilemma by explaining that cold causes an initial vasoconstriction and then later vasodilation (A46, A47, B3, B21, C16, F5). They advocate applying cold for various time periods, depending on the intended result (C16). For instance, during immediate-care procedures, when the intent is to control swelling, they recommend removing the cold packs before the vasodilation occurs. During rehabilitation they recommend applying cold long enough to achieve the increased circulation through reflex vasodilation. There are, however, various opinions on when during the application vasodilation occurs, ranging from 1 to 30 minutes (A47, B3, B18, C6, C16). Others report that vasodilation occurs after the cold is removed (C22, C51). This contradiction would present a problem during immediate-care procedures. If there is increased blood flow following removal of the cold pack, the benefits of the decreased flow during application would be canceled. There clearly is a great deal of confusion.

HOW CIVD CAME TO MEAN INCREASED BLOOD FLOW

The idea that CIVD resulted in a net increase in blood flow during sport injury rehabilitation started as an attempt to explain the dramatic success of cryokinetics. (See chapter 2.) As the popularity of cryokinetics grew, ever more authors attributed its success to increased blood flow during CIVD, until in time CIVD meant increased blood flow induced by cold (B21, C1, C6, C16, C22). However, none of these authors presented original data to support this theory; rather, their writings were based on the research and opinions of others.

Evidence Cited in Favor of Increasing Blood Flow as a Result of CIVD During Sport Injury Care

- Lewis's aftereffect
- Lewis's hunting response
- Clarke, Hellon, and Lind's research
- Feeling of warmth during application of cold
- Redness of body parts during/following cold applications
- Quickness of injury resolution with cryokinetics

Lewis's Aftereffect Reexamined

Although Lewis coined the term *CIVD*, he did not claim that it resulted in blood flow greater than usual, nor can his data be used to infer such during therapeutic applications. First, Lewis was measuring temperature, not blood flow. The two are related, but not quantitatively; that is, a 30% increase in temperature does not mean blood flow increased 30% (A9, C23, C26, C30). Second, sports medicine authorities have tried to generalize Lewis's results beyond the bounds of his experiment. Lewis's results are accurate, but their application to sports medicine has been inaccurate. Only part of the heat in tissues is brought to the tissue by blood flow (C23). Heat is lost during cooling (and absorbed during heating) when the thermal capacity of the tissue changes due to average tissue temperature changes. Unless the tissue is maintained at a steady state temperature during measurements, heat changes due to changing heat capacity will overshadow the heat changes due to circulation. Since the physiological state is one of continual transition during most cold research, blood flow changes cannot be inferred from temperature changes.

Lewis reported a series of individual experiments in which data were neither combined nor statistically analyzed. A typical experiment involved one of the fingers, with adjacent fingers as controls. The fingers rested on a cork platform above a beaker of ice water while control readings were made. The experimental finger was then immersed into the beaker through a hole in the cork. Figure 9.2 presents the data from one such experiment, which involved immersing the right second finger in 7°C water for 15 minutes (room temperature was 19.2°C). Ten minutes after it was removed from the cold, the experimental finger was 10°C warmer than the control (R3) finger. It remained at this level for 10 minutes and then gradually returned toward control; however, it was still 2°C above control 1 hour after immersion.

Many have accepted these data as unquestionable support for the concept that CIVD results in increased blood flow. But take a closer look at Lewis's data. The control finger was maintained at 19°C (probably because the room temperature was quite cold), and the experimental finger rose to 29°C. Normal finger temperature is 30° to 34°C. So the experimental finger warmed toward normal but began cooling without ever reaching normal temperature.

Lewis recognized that the aftereffect occurred only when the fingers and room were at a "suitable" initial temperature (i.e., were much cooler than normal). He stated that reflex vasodilation requires, "without fail," a suitable initial temperature both of fingers and room, and that if the fingers were 32° to 34°C (which he considered very hot, but which is actually normal) at the start of the observation, they would not respond to the stimulus (i.e., not vasodilate). In other words, in a cold room the temperature of the fingers will be below normal. Therefore, after removing a finger from ice water, its temperature will increase many degrees above that of the control finger (which is below normal) as it approaches normal.

We (C42) replicated Lewis's study with room temperature at 25.1°C and initial finger temperature at 31.8°C (Figure 9.6). The finger was immersed for 40 minutes in 3.0°C water. The finger temperature rose to 31.6°C 10 minutes following immersion and to 33.7°C 20 minutes following immersion; it decreased to 32.4°C 15 minutes later. Similar results were obtained in a second replication of Lewis's study (Figure 5.9). We (C42) also observed that although the fingers returned to normal temperature quite rapidly, ankle temperature rose to only 19.2°C after being immersed in 3°C water for 40 minutes (Figure 9.6). Subsequent work confirmed the slower response in the ankle and the forearm (Figure 5.9) (C44, C45); both the ankle and forearm require more than 2-1/2 hours to return to within 1°C of the contralateral control limb (C44).

So Lewis's aftereffect, which he attributed to CIVD, cannot be used as evidence that blood flow increases following therapeutic cold applications during sport injury management. The aftereffect is a temperature effect—not blood flow, and it occurs only when the fingers have been cooled to approximately 21°C before the experiment, and the experiment takes place in a cold room (18°C–21°C).

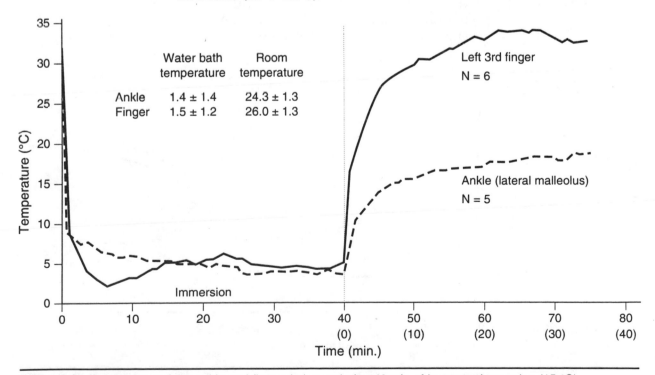

Figure 9.6 Temperature of the ankle and finger during and after 40 min of ice water immersion (15 °C). Reprinted from Knight et al. (C42).

Lewis's Hunting Response

The "hunting response" is a nonperiodic oscillation in temperature, first observed by Lewis (see Figure 9.1). It always followed a massive initial temperature decrease, and temperature usually changed only a few degrees. The hunting response is thought to occur from a cyclical opening and closing of arteriovenous anastomoses (A5, C6, E60, I35) as the activity of vasoconstrictor chemicals in the blood vessels changes (A9).

The hunting response has been accepted as a general phenomenon, but we (C42, C44, C45) have failed to demonstrate it in the ankle and forearm, although we demonstrated it in the fingers of the same subjects (C42, C45). Similarly, Petajan and Daube (D83) simultaneously measured a number of sites in the hand and arm and reported that the hunting response occurred on the surface of the finger but not on the surface of the thenar eminence, the volar forearm, or deep in the thenar muscle. The absence of the hunting response in deep tissue can be observed in the data of others (C8, C72) as well.

In any case, the hunting response may be no more than a measurement artifact caused by the development of a thermal gradient next to the body during immersion (E79, C42, C45). As the body gives up heat to the water, it warms the water next to the body. If the water is not vigorously stirred, a thin layer of water next to the body will eventually warm enough to affect the temperature probe. Since all surface temperature measurements are in actuality a measurement of an interface temperature between the skin and its immediate environment, changes in both the skin and water temperatures would be reflected in this measurement. Although he did not elaborate on the point, Lewis (C51) did state that the extent of the hunting reaction was greatest if the ice water remained unstirred.

To test this hypothesis, we measured the temperature at a number of sites on the foot and ankle during 20 minutes of ice-water immersion (Figure 9.7) (B39). The water was unstirred for 20 minutes, and temperature was measured regularly. We then stirred the water and again measured the temperature. At three sites (the big toe, Achilles' tendon, and base of fifth metatarsal) the average temperature at 20 minutes was 1.0°C warmer than

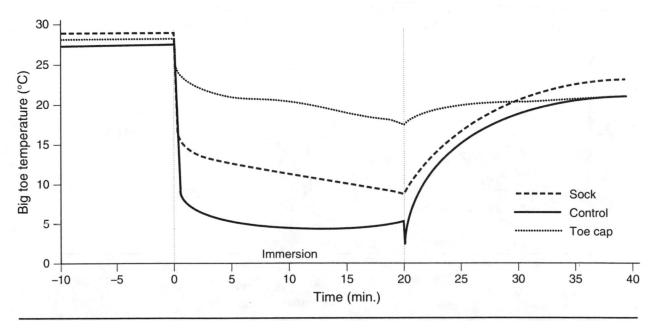

Figure 9.7   Effect of a toe cap on the temperature of the big toe during foot and ankle immersion in ice water. Reprinted from Nimchick and Knight (E79).

the minimum temperature during the 20-minute session. Stirring caused a drop of 2.1° ± 2.8°C. At two other sites (extensor hallicus longus tendon and over the anterior talofibular ligament) the minimum temperature was the same as the 20-minute temperature. The average temperature drop with stirring was 1.6° ± 2.0°C indicating that the increase in ankle temperature during the last 3 to 4 minutes of immersion was due to a blanket of warmer water around the ankle that the stirring removed. Thus, we concluded that much or all of the hunting reaction is a measurement artifact, not an actual increase in temperature in the cooled limb. And definitely the hunting response is not evidence of increased blood flow during cooling.

Taber et al. (C68) reported a fluctuation in blood flow during cold-gel pack application that reached a minimum at 13.5 minutes and then increased slightly (Figure 9.8). Interpreting this as a cold-induced hunting response would be erroneous, however, since a similar fluctuation occurred at the same time during unchilled (room temperature) gel-pack application.

Clarke et al. Revisited

Clarke et al. (C18) used strain gauge plethysmography to measure blood flow to the forearm of 4 subjects during 45 minutes of immersion in 1°, 6°, and 10°C water (Figure 9.9). In Figure 9.10 the data from the 4 subjects have been averaged. (This should be viewed as a rough approximation, since the data points were interpolated from Figure 9.9 rather than being derived from the original data.) At 10°C the changes in blood flow were variable, but in no case was there a marked increase or decrease from the preimmersion blood flow measured at room temperature. At 1°C and 6°C there was a gradual increase in blood flow throughout the 45-minute period, the increase being greater at 1°C. These data remained unchallenged for 20 years, but research in the early 1980s cast doubt on them (C43, C46).

A study from our laboratory (C46) was the first to challenge the validity of using the data of Clarke et al. to explain the success of cryokinetics for rehabilitating sport injuries. Large Hydrocollator ColPaCs, chilled to –7°C, were placed on either side of the ankle of 12 healthy subjects for 25 minutes. Blood flow was measured with strain gauge plethysmography 5 centimeters above the malleolus. [See Knight (C41) for a more complete discussion of

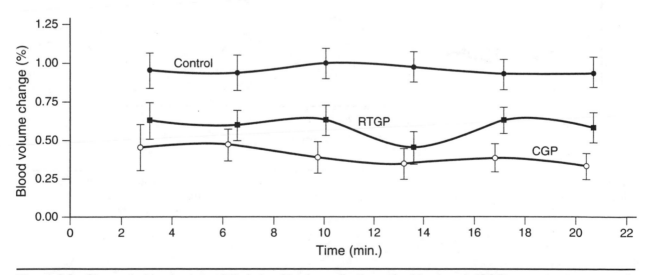

Figure 9.8 Change in blood volume (%) during 20-min applications of cold-gel pack (CGP), room temperature gel pack (RTGP), and control. There is no vasodilatation during these applications.
Reprinted from *Physical Therapy Journal* (C68) with the permission of the American Physical Therapy Association.

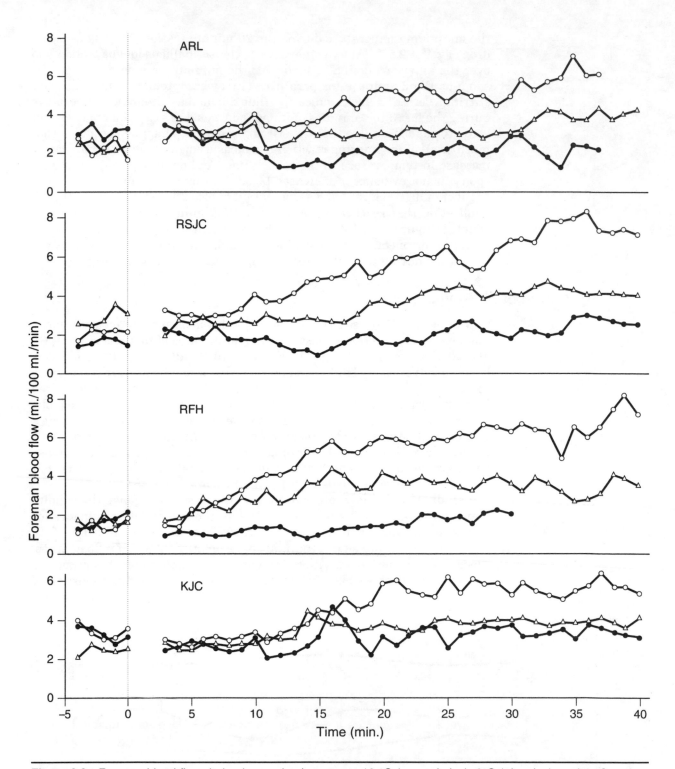

Figure 9.9   Forearm blood flow during immersion in water at 10 °C (open circles), 6°C (triangles), and 1 °C (closed circles). The initial measurements were in room air; immersion began at time 0.
Reprinted from Clarke et al. (C18).

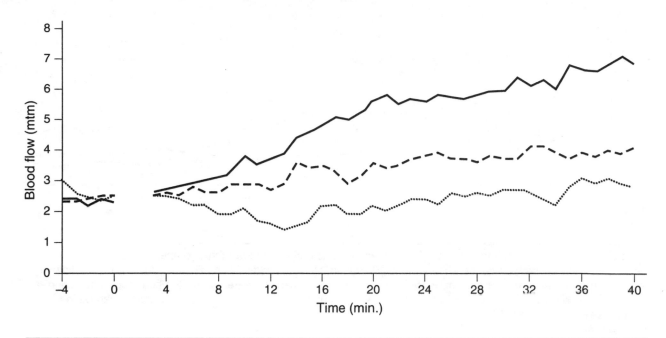

Figure 9.10   Alternative graph of the data in Figure 9.9. Individual data points were interpolated from the original graph, and the four subjects' data were averaged for each of the three conditions.

plethysmographic techniques.] Blood flow decreased progressively during the 25-minute ColPaC application and stayed at the depressed level for 20 minutes after the ColPaCs were removed, at which time blood flow measurements were discontinued (Figure 9.11).

Two improbable reasons for the difference between the two studies are that ankle blood flow responds differently to cold than forearm blood flow and that blood flow responses to cold immersion and cold-pack application are different. Although there may be differences in the magnitude of response, the general pattern of response appears to be the same, as reported in various studies (C43, C45, D1, J3).

Nine additional studies also contradict the results of Clarke et al. (C4, C33, C43, C56, C61, C68, C73, D1, J75). Abramson et al. (D1) measured forearm blood flow during immersion in 4°C water for 192 minutes (see Figure 9.12). Blood flow decreased to about 45% of control within the first 20 minutes, increased to about 75% of control, and then fluctuated between these levels for the duration of the measurement period. Average blood flow during the entire experiment appeared to be about 60% of control.

Minimal decreases in blood flow were reported by Schuster (C61) and by Baker and Bell (C4) but neither included a control group. Meeusen & De Meirleir (C56) reported a decrease in superficial blood flow during ice pack application which reversed during application and rose above control following application. Taber et al. (C68) reported that ankle blood flow was about 50% of control during 20 minutes of chilled-gel pack application using occlusion impedance plethysmography (see Figure 9.8). Arterial blood flow to the knee decreased 38% ± 5% and soft tissue blood flow decreased 29% ± 2% following a 20-minute application of a Dura*Kold ice pack to the knee (C33). Blood flow was measured in control and experimental knees of 21 subjects by technetium scintigraphy; a technique where a radioactive substance is injected into the bloodstream and the radioactivity of the target structures is monitored.

We (C43) also measured blood flow to the forearm during application of cold packs and immersion in 1°, 5°, 10°, and 15°C water baths for 45

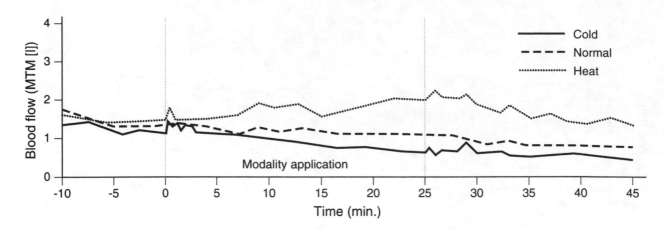

Figure 9.11 Blood flow in the ankle of 12 uninjured subjects during and after three temperature conditions (hot pack, cold pack, control). Note the absence of CIVD during and after cold-pack application. Average blood flow during 25-min application and for the entire 45-min period was significantly greater during the heat application condition than during either control or cold pack, and was significantly less during cold-pack application than during control (see also Figure 9.17).
Reprinted from Knight and Londeree (C47).

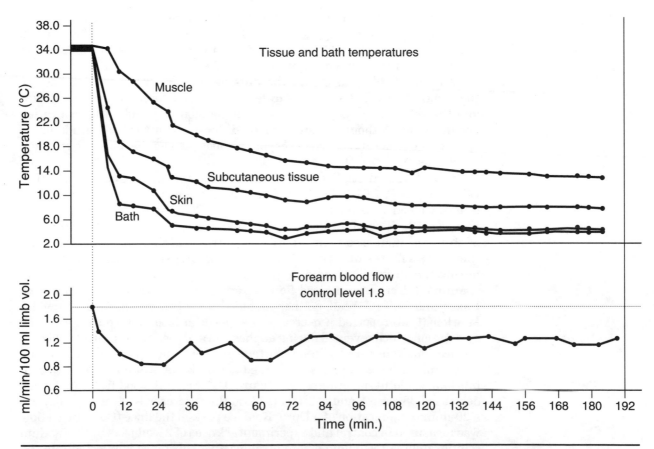

Figure 9.12 Forearm blood flow (lower graph) and temperature of muscle, subcutaneous tissue, skin, and bath during 192 min of forearm immersion in water bath (single "typical" subject).
Reprinted from Abramson et al. (D1).

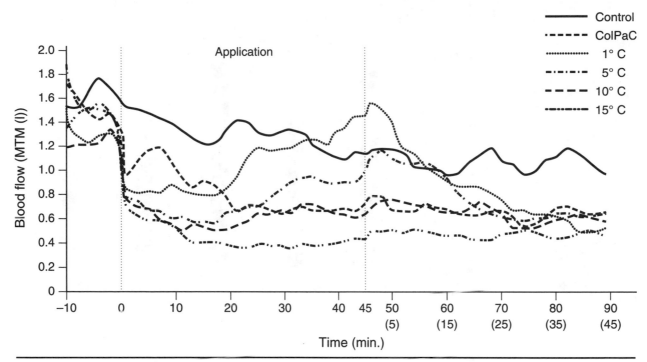

Figure 9.13 Instantaneous forearm blood flow during 45 min of application and for 45 min following application of Chattanooga cold packs and immersion in ice-water baths of 1 °C, 5 °C, 10 °C, and 15 °C. Vasoconstriction occurred during all conditions except control and reversed during the 1 °C and 5 °C conditions. The same data are averaged in Figure 9.14. Data from Knight et al. (C43).

minutes (Figures 9.13 and 9.14). Average blood flow was 69% of control during immersion in 1°C water, 45% during cold-pack application and immersion in 5° and 10°C water, and 25% during immersion in 15°C water. The pattern of blood flow in this study may give a clue to the data of Clarke et al.

During the 1°C condition, blood flow decreased during the first 20 minutes and then subsequently increased (see Figure 9.13). There was some increase in the 5°C condition also, but none in the 10°C condition. These data confirm the premise of Clarke et al. that blood flow is greater during immersion in very cold temperatures than during immersion in moderately cooled water. But our data contradicts the conclusion of Clarke et al. that blood flow at 1°C exceeds control conditions. In our study there was an initial vasoconstriction during all conditions. None of the subjects in the study of Clarke et al., however, exhibited initial vasoconstriction (see Figure 9.9). Under 1°C and 5°C conditions, the subjects' blood flow began immediately to increase. This is contrary to most other research (C3, C5, C21, C25, C30, D1). The initial response to cold is vasoconstriction. Another curiosity about their data is that blood flow during the first 2 minutes following immersion is not reported. Why?

Is it possible that Clarke et al. shifted their data upward (Figure 9.15)? When the strain gauge of a strain gauge plysthomograph is cooled the baseline of the plysthomograph shifts downward. This shift can be corrected by an electronic adjustment called "zeroing the bridge" prior to measuring blood flow (C41). For a time in the 1950s some thought the proper correction was to leave the baseline depressed and shift the resulting data upward. Whether or not Clarke et al. shifted their data is unknown. If they did, it would have been an honest mistake in keeping with scientific theory of the day, and their data would be in agreement with others. If they did not, we cannot

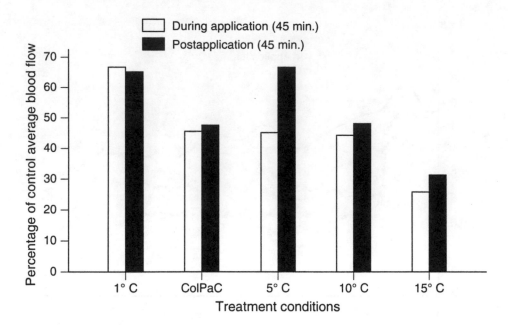

Figure 9.14 Data from Figure 9.13 expressed as average blood flow and percent of control. Even though vasoconstriction reversed during immersion in 1 °C water (see Figure 9.13), the average blood flow was still less than 70% of control. Note the inverse relationship between temperature and blood flow.

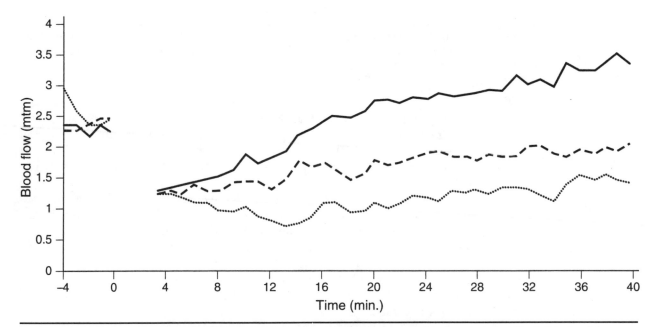

Figure 9.15 Data of Clarke et al. (Figure 9.10) as they may have appeared before being shifted, if indeed they were shifted to compensate for the effects of cold on the strain gauge. Note that the shape of the curves is similar to the shapes of curves of the same temperatures in Figure 9.13.

explain why their data are so different from others. In either case, the preponderance of the data indicate that blood flow during cold-water immersion (even in 1°C water) is less than control. Furthermore, it is inaccurate to conclude that cryokinetics is effective because it causes a greater average blood flow than heat packs do; it does not.

Feeling of Warmth

Early writers reported that during cold applications, most people experience four sensations: (a) pain; (b) warming or burning; (c) aching, tingling, or "pins and needles"; and (d) numbness (a relative skin anesthesia). The warming sensation was attributed to CIVD (B3, B10, C22) and thought to correspond to the hunting reaction. Other research supports the conclusion that the warming sensation is a psychological phenomenon (B11, E40, E49, E110). In an effort to determine if this is the case, we (C36) monitored surface and subcutaneous temperatures in the ankles of subjects during ice water immersion. Subjects were asked to indicate when they began feeling warm and when numbness began. There was no temperature increase at the time that warmth was perceived by the subjects (Figure 9.16). On the contrary, temperature decreased gradually during the warming sensation. We concluded that warming was a perceived sensation rather than a physiological sensation, perhaps due to the diminution of the pain sensation.

In a recent study (E91), blood flow to the arm was arrested with a sphygmomanometer cuff applied to the upper arm and inflated to 80 to 100 mm Hg. Cold was then applied to the thenar eminence. Most subjects reported cold and then hot or burning, and then pain. Associated data convinced the researchers that cold and pain are separate sensations that are transmitted to the brain on separate nervous pathways. Cold and pain coexist, but pain persists after the cold sensation is gone and changes so that it "becomes endowed with a burning quality."

In a pilot study we divided a group of high school students who had never been treated with cold into two groups and immersed their ankles in ice water for 20 minutes. We told one group that they would experience pain, warming, tingling, and numbness and that they should tell us when they experienced each. We did not tell the other group what to expect, just to write down whatever sensations they felt and the times they felt each. Most of the first group told us when warming occurred; few in the second group mentioned warming as a sensation. Warming has been absent from other studies in which subjects were asked to record their sensations but not told beforehand what to expect (E16, E39, E80). Evidently, if the brain is conditioned to expect a warming sensation, it thinks that the body part is warming when cold pain decreases; if it is not preconditioned, it calls this decreasing pain something else.

Redness of Body Parts

Some feel that the bright red color of the skin that occurs during cold applications is the result of increased blood flow caused by CIVD (C22). Two alternative explanations were given by Licht (A25):

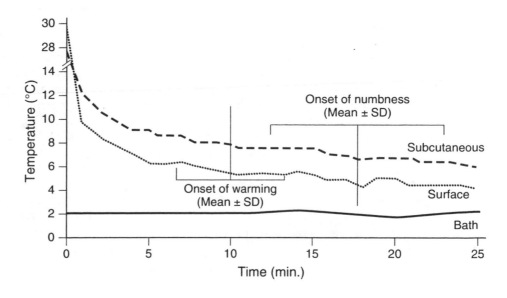

Figure 9.16 Correlation of minute-by-minute temperature changes with subjective reports of warming and numbness during ankle immersion in ice water. Unpublished data from Johannes and Knight (C36).

1. Cold application causes a greater decrease in venous return than in arterial inflow, resulting in arteriolar hyperemia in the skin
2. Because of decreased tissue metabolism during cold applications, oxygen exchange between the tissues and capillaries is decreased. This decreased exchange results in more highly oxygenated blood (which appears redder) in the skin's venous system (C28).

Research observations by Lewis and Love (I30) and Goldschmidt and Light (C27) confirm the second theory and led Lewis and Love to state that the tint of skin at low temperatures is largely independent of the rate of blood flow.

Increased Rate of Healing

Cryokinetics caused quite a stir because patients treated with cryokinetics returned to normal activity much sooner than they would have with traditional thermotherapy (B10, B16, B20). The basic assumption of thermotherapy is that heat applications cause an increase in blood flow, which in turn increases the delivery of materials to rebuild the tissue (A12, B9, H25). The apparent increase in healing rate due to cryokinetics tended to buttress the CIVD–increased blood flow theory. Since both heat applications and cryokinetics increased the healing rate, and heat applications did so by increasing blood flow, the assumption that cryokinetics increased blood flow seemed reasonable.

Actually, the success of cryokinetics is due to the combination of exercise and cold, not to cold alone. The only benefit of cold is that it diminishes pain so that exercise can begin sooner and be more vigorous than would be the case without cold analgesia. Cryokinetics treatment causes a greater increase in blood flow than heat treatment does (Figure 9.17), but this increase is due to the exercise, not the cold (C46).

Evidence Against the Concept that CIVD Results in Blood Flow Being Increased Beyond a Usual Amount

- Little of the research quoted in support of this theory has involved therapeutic applications of cold.
- Lewis's aftereffect
  - is a temperature response, not blood flow—temperature and blood flow are not directly related;
  - occurs in the hands, toes, and face—not in areas of the body that typically are the sites of sport injuries, such as the ankle, knee, and large muscles; and
  - occurs only under extreme circumstances when the fingers have been abnormally cooled, and then its magnitude is only up to usual finger temperature.
- Lewis's hunting response
  - may be mostly a measurement artifact, and

  - increases much less than, and follows, an initial decrease.
- Clarke, Hellon, and Lind's results are flawed because there is no initial vasoconstriction. And there is ample evidence that therapeutic applications of cold result in decreased blood flow; evidence from a variety of body parts and using a variety of measuring instruments.
- Feeling of warmth during application of cold is a psychological phenomenon.
- Redness of body parts during/following cold applications may be due to oxygen content of the cooled blood in the skin.
- Quickness of injury resolution with cryokinetics is the result of exercise. Cold only decreases residual pain so that exercise can begin more quickly and be more vigorous.

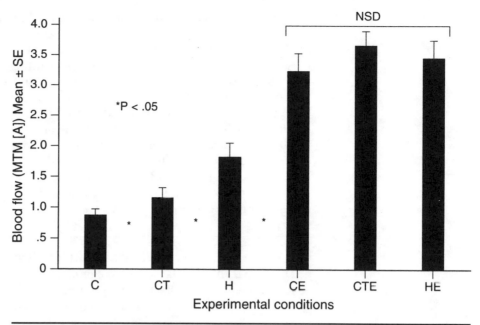

Figure 9.17 Comparison of the effects of heat, cold, intermittent exercise, and intermittent exercise combined with both heat and cold applications on blood flow. Blood flow represents average blood flow during a 45-min period that included application and postapplication of modalities. Heat and cold were applied for a total of 25 min; first 25 min of conditions C&H, and for the first 13 min and then for four periods of 3 min each interspersed with exercise in conditions CE and HE. Exercise consisted of five bouts of three min each (total of 15 min) interspersed with four periods (3 min each) of cold (CE), control (CTE), or heat (HE) applications. The differences between the three conditions and each of the nonexercise conditions were significant. All data from Knight and Londeree (C47).

CIVD: A RED HERRING

The vast body of literature on CIVD has overshadowed the importance of the exercise component of cryokinetics. Grant (B10) postulated that exercise was the key to the clinical success of cryokinetics, and many of the proponents of CIVD–increased blood flow theory write that exercise must follow cold applications (B3, B8, B21, B24, C1, C22). Values for exercise-induced blood flow found in the literature (C46, C50, J7, J10, J28, J31, J71, J72, J77) are much greater than any value found in the literature that resulted from heat applications (C2, C5, C46, J1, J2, J28, J62) or cold applications (A13, C18, C21, C23, C25, C26, C29, C30, C46, E1). Our data (C46) support the theory that the success of cryokinetics is due to exercise and that ice applications act only to allow relatively pain-free exercise in an injured joint or muscle (B10, B12, B24, B29, C2, C54).

Confusion in Clinical Practice

The CIVD–increased blood flow concept has caused confusion in clinical practice. Management of acute musculoskeletal injuries includes immediate-care procedures to limit the amount of swelling and hematoma and later rehabilitation procedures to accelerate the body's resolution of the hematoma and repair of the damaged tissue through delivery of essential nutrients. If cold somehow both increases and decreases blood flow, its effects would be counterproductive during one phase or the other. This seeming conflict has been rationalized in a number of ways by various clinicians. Some (B8, B18, C6) claim that vasoconstriction occurs for 10 to 20 minutes and is followed by vasodilation. Therefore, if the aim is immediate care, ice must be applied no longer than 10 to 20 minutes; if the aim is rehabilitation, it must be applied for at least 20 minutes to be beneficial (i.e., to increase blood flow). Other theorized time frames (with corresponding variations in immediate-care vs. rehabilitation protocols) add to the confusion: at one extreme, 5 to 7 minutes of vasodilation with ice application followed by vasoconstriction (C16); at the other, CIVD with 30 to 45 minutes of ice application (B21).

Searching for an answer to this confusion led me to the hypothesis that the benefits of cold application to acutely traumatized tissue are due to the metabolic effects of cold and are independent of circulation effects (G50). We (C47) further proposed that the beneficial effects of cold during rehabilitation are due to earlier active exercise, which is possible because cold decreases pain in the injured body part (A14).

What Should You Do?

Disregard the circulatory effects of cold and concentrate on either the metabolic or pain effects. When using cold for immediate care try to maximize the decrease in metabolism by applying the cold packs for 30 minutes (40 minutes for large fleshy areas such as the thigh). When treating the knee, elbow, or other area with superficial nerves, monitor motor function distal to the cold pack (i.e., in the hand and foot) for any evidence of palsy, and discontinue the cold pack if palsy occurs. To help reduce metabolism, reapply the cold pack following any activity, and at least every 2 hours during the first 16 to 24 hours after the injury. Wrapping the area with an elastic bandage between applications will also help reduce metabolism.

When using cold for rehabilitation, apply it only until the body part is numbed (or for 20 minutes maximum). The goal is to facilitate active exercise. Also, remember that new patients who have not yet adapted to the cold will experience extreme pain during the first cold application. Help them to cope by explaining that they will get used to the cold and by distracting them during the initial cold application.

BENEFITS OF THE CIVD–INCREASED BLOOD FLOW THEORY

Commenting on the gate control theory of pain, Nathan (J55) stated that ideas need to be fruitful, but don't necessarily have to be right. The same can be said about the theory that CIVD causes increased blood flow during therapeutic applications of cold. It is an idea that has proven to be false, but has been very fruitful. It has led to a greater understanding of the physiological basis of cold and rehabilitation and, therefore, has served us well. In one of the "classic" papers on cryokinetics, Moore et al. (B29) wrote that one of the purposes of their paper was "to stimulate competent researchers to pursue further study of the physiological mechanisms involved" with cryokinetics. Even though their paper has stimulated some work, much more needs to be done.

CONTRAST BATHS

A discussion of circulatory changes during rehabilitative cryotherapy is incomplete without mention of contrast baths, which involve alternating hot and cold immersions. The traditional theory for this therapy is that it reduces edema through a "pumping mechanism," that is, alternating vasoconstriction and vasodilation (B1, B37). If indeed the value of contrast baths is in providing a pumping action, cryokinetics would be a better treatment. Research has not yet been done to support this conclusion, but rather it is based on the following logic.

Numerous ratios (minutes of heat vs. minutes of cold)—4:1, 3:1, 3:2, 5:2, etc.—have been recommended for contrast baths (B37). There would be one "pump" per cycle and 8 to 15 cycles per hour. With cryokinetics, you get one pump with each muscle contraction: 30 to 40 "pumps" per minute. A typical cryokinetic session lasts approximately 1 hour and includes five 3-minute exercise bouts (see chapter 18). So an athlete would perform 450 to 600 pumps per hour of cryokinetics, considerably more than an hour of contrast baths.

In addition, edema reduction requires that free proteins be removed from the injury site, a process that occurs via the lymphatic, not the circulatory, system (see chapter 4). Because the lymphatic system is assisted by mechanical action and not by heat or cold, contrast baths would be of no value, whereas the muscle pump of cryokinetics would.

There is another possible application for contrast baths. The body often accommodates to sensory stimulation so that the effects of the stimulation are diminished. If during cryokinetics the body accommodates to the cold so that it no longer removes pain and allows exercise, a change in stimulation may be indicated. The same concept has been suggested for other situations, such as the use of ice for low back pain in place of transcutaneous electrical nerve stimulation (TENS) when the body has accommodated to the TENS (E7) and the use of TENS in place of cold if the body has accommodated to the cold (B32).

SUMMARY

Based on the current information available, I have concluded the following:

- Dilation is a process, not an end result.
- Vasodilation probably does occur during or following therapeutic applications of cold. If it does, it is only at the end of long-term applications, and its magnitude is minimal enough that average blood flow is still much less than no application at all.
- The benefits of therapeutic cold applications during both immediate care and rehabilitation are unrelated to the circulatory effects of cold.
- During rehabilitation procedures, the only purpose of cold applications is to facilitate exercise. This is done by decreasing pain and muscular spasm, thereby allowing exercise to begin earlier and progress at a faster rate.
- Exercise is the key to rehabilitation. Without properly executed therapeutic exercise, cold applications hinder rather than promote rehabilitation.
- The commonly accepted theory for contrast bath therapy is flawed for two reasons: (a) any vascular pumping resulting from contrast baths is hundreds of times less than that which occurs during cryokinetics, and (b) the need during rehabilitation is for lymphatic pumping, not vascular pumping. Cryokinetics also causes lymphatic pumping.

10

Neurological and Neuromuscular Effects of Cold Applications

Much of the therapeutic value of cryotherapy, as well as some of the problems, result from neurological changes during cold applications. Some nervous pathways are stimulated and others repressed as the nerve and surrounding tissue are cooled. In this chapter I review the effects of cold on various neurological tissues and systems. This information will then serve as the foundation for subsequent chapters on muscle spasm, pain, and problems and precautions.

EFFECTS OF COLD ON SENSORY NERVE FUNCTIONS

The effect of cold on sensory nerve fiber transmission depends on the function and purpose of the sensory fiber and also where the cooling takes place. Cooling a cold receptor increases the firing (or transmission) rate of the nerve fibers that carry impulses from the cold receptors to higher centers (primarily A-delta and C-fibers; see Table 10.1). Cooling the nerve fibers themselves causes a decrease in the rate of impulse transmission along the nerve fiber, regardless of the type or function of the fiber.

Cold Receptors

A cold receptor in a cat's nose is a dermal papilla containing a single small myelinated nerve fiber that branches into several unmyelinated terminals, which in turn penetrate the basal epidermal cells (D41). These cells are sensitive both to absolute temperature and to the temperature gradient, or rate of change of temperature (A6, D41, D104). Typically, the cells produce a transient burst of impulses with a frequency that is related to the rate of

Table 10.1   Classification, Diameter, Conduction Velocity, and Function of Afferent Nerve Fibers

Type	Group	Subgroup	Diameter (μ)	Conduction velocity (m/sec)	Presumed function
A	I	Ia	12–20	72–120	Signal muscle velocity and length change
A	I	Ib			Signal muscle shortening of rapid speed
A	II	Muscle	6–12	36–72	Signal muscle length changes
A	II	Skin			Convey information from touch receptors or pacinian corpuscles
A	III	Muscle	1–6	6–36	Convey information from pain-pressure receptors
Aδ	III	Skin			Convey information from pain, temperature, or touch receptors
C	IV	Muscle	1	0.5–2	Convey information from pain receptors
C	IV	Skin			Convey information from pain, temperature, or touch receptors

Reprinted from Mannheimer and Lampe (J48), using data from Willis and Grossman (J81).

fall of temperature, followed by a steady discharge of impulses whose frequency is related to the absolute temperature (D49). Experiments in rat skin (D49) and cat tongue (D106) have shown that cold receptors begin firing at about 36°C, rapidly increase to a maximum firing rate at temperatures between 25° and 28°C, and then decrease to minimal firing at 10° to 12°C (Figure 10.1). Human (D43) and rat (D44) C-fibers discharge maximally between 16° and 27°C when temperatures were held constant. The details of their functioning and their connections with the hypothalamus (the major cold-stimulation reflex center) have been reviewed by others (A42, D41, D42) and will not be further explained here.

The number of cold receptors varies throughout the body (A6). The face, fingers, and ears have the greatest number of cold sensory endings, while the feet and thighs have the least. Other fibers also respond to thermal stimulation, such as mechanoreceptors (pressure receptors) and polymodal nocioceptors (pain receptors that respond to many different modes of stimulation), and they influence the response to the cold sensation (D95, E85). Cold sensations are carried to higher brain centers on a variety of nerves. Cold sensation is mediated by small myelinated A delta fibers (E3, E22, E65) while cold-induced pain by unmyelinated polymodal nociceptors (E78). It is thought that the cold quality of the pain induced by low-temperature stimuli reflects coactivation of cold-specific A delta afferents (E56, E86, E111).

An interesting phenomenon of cold receptors is the "paradoxical cold sensation." With strong heat stimulation (i.e., when the skin is heated above 45°C), some cold receptors begin to fire and the person feels a certain quality of cold (Figure 10.2; see D41 for references). Physiologists are not certain whether a "paradoxical warm sensation" exists (D41, D105), but some (D21, D22) have presented evidence to indicate it may occur during rapid cooling. This sensation may be an explanation for the feeling of warmth that some people get during cryokinetics (see chapter 18).

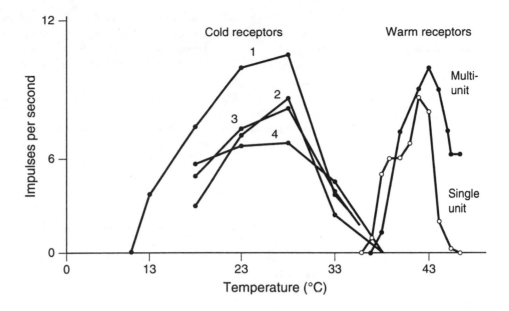

Figure 10.1 Impulse frequency of four cold receptors and two warm receptors in rat skin exposed to various temperatures. Reprinted from Iggo (D49).

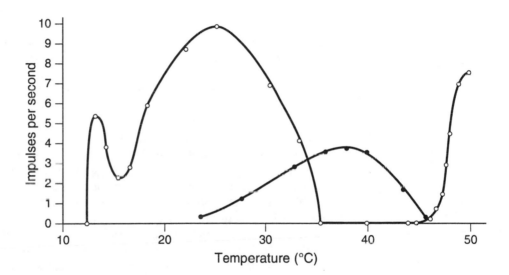

Figure 10.2 Impulse frequency of a single cold fiber (open circle) and a single warm fiber (solid circle) from a cat's tongue exposed to various temperatures. Note the "paradoxical cold" response at temperatures above 45 °C. Reprinted from Zotterman (D106).

Cutaneous Sensations

Cutaneous (skin) sensations are subdued by cooling and show a hierarchical response (D3). In one study, cooling the ulnar nerve (at the elbow) in 2.5°C increments, lasting 6 minutes each, resulted in a loss of sensations (in the hand) in the following order: tickle, cold, first pain, touch, second pain, warmth. The tickle sensation began to disappear when the cooling element was at 2.5°C, which was 5° to 10°C lower than the nerve temperature. The sequence of loss of sensation was the same when cooling was caused much more rapidly. Rapid cooling is accompanied by an intense aching pain, though, apparently caused by stimulation of pain fibers under the cooling element.

There are mixed reports of changes in tactile (two-point) discrimination due to cooling. First, we must separate cooling the body part from cooling the measuring instrument. Cold objects feel heavier than warm ones, and two-point and two-edge discrimination is intensified by cooling the instrument, apparently because of direct thermal stimulation of mechanoreceptors and/or polymodal nociceptor (pain) networks (D95).

Cooling the body part may or may not effect two-point tactile discrimination. Provins and Morton (D86) reported little change in two-point discrimination in the index finger as a result of 20 minutes of cold-water immersion at finger temperatures down to 6°C, but marked impairment at 4°C and complete numbness at 2°C. We reported that two-point discrimination to the bottom of the foot was unchanged following immersing the ankle to 2 to 4 centimeters above the maleolus for 20 minutes in 1°C ice water (E38). Either the bottom of the foot and the finger react differently or our stimulus was not great enough to lower the bottom of the foot to the critical temperature. Or perhaps the few seconds during which our subjects dried their foot and walked to the testing table was enough to warm their feet above the critical temperature. Additional research is needed.

Weeks and Travell (D102) cooled the skin with brief (1- to 3-second) applications of vapo-coolants in an effort to eliminate the pricking pain associated with injections. At skin temperatures above 15°C, 67% of their parents felt pain; between 15° and 12°C, 47% felt pain; between 12° and 10°C no patients felt pain. These results do not imply, however, that the *sensation* of pricking was eliminated.

Conduction Velocity in Sensory Nerves

The velocity of sensory nerve impulse transmission decreases gradually as temperature falls until conduction is totally blocked. In one study, sensory nerve conduction velocity was only 2.5% of normal just prior to being blocked (D81). The decrease in sensory nerve conduction velocity during cold applications has been measured transcutaneously in whole human median (D7, D18, D39, D65), ulnar (D28, D40, D58, D64), sural (D38), and digital (D68) nerves and in cat vagus, saphenous, and cervical nerves (D24, D79–81). The decrease is thought to be linear (to a point), with velocity decreasing 1.4 to 2.6 meters per second per degree and with a Q_{10} ranging from 1.4 to 2.3 for measurements taken at various temperature ranges between 20° and 30°C, which means that activity decreased 43% to 71% as temperature decreased 10°C. (Q_{10} is the ratio of activity of a physiological parameter—conduction velocity in this case—at a given temperature to its activity at a temperature 10°C lower. A Q_{10} of 2.0 means that activity at the higher temperature is double what it is at a temperature 10°C lower.)

Lowitzsch et al. (D64) reported a difference in the Q_{10} when calculated for different temperature ranges. From 35° to 25°C, the Q_{10} was 1.36, but from 30° to 20°C it was 1.44. A similar phenomenon occurred with absolute and relative refractory periods. The authors suggested that 27°C may be a "critical temperature." (*Critical temperature* as used here means a temperature at which the rate of change of a reaction changes. For instance if velocity decreased 2% per degree as the temperature decreased down to 25°C and then decreased 5% per degree as the temperature decreased below 25°C, we would say 25°C was a critical temperature. See D64 for a review of the occurrence of the critical-temperature phenomenon in other mammalian systems.) Paintal (D81) calculated Q_{10} values of 1.6, 2.5, and 4.8 for the temperature ranges 37° to 27°C, 28° to 18°C and 18° to 8°C, respectively, so there may be more than one "critical temperature." Paintal noted that as temperature approached the blocking temperature (i.e., the temperature at which all activity ceased, which was different in different fibers), conduction velocity fell rapidly, causing a sharp deviation in the temperature–conduction velocity curve.

Denny-Brown et al. (D20) reported that nerve conduction was blocked at temperatures below 10°C. Blocking appeared to be time dependent; that is, the longer the duration of cold exposure at a given temperature, the greater the loss of functioning. Motor fibers were affected at higher temperatures than sensory and suffered a greater loss of function at a given temperature than sensory fibers did. Sunderland (I60) reported that different sensory modalities do not fail simultaneously or in a predictable fashion and that function is restored rapidly as recovery from cooling takes place if no tissue death has occurred. Sensory function generally returns before motor function does. Motor function sometimes takes months to recover (see chapter 14).

■ DEEP NERVES ARE LESS VULNERABLE TO COLD

Don't be confused by the fact that nerve conduction ceases at temperatures near 10°C. This would imply that we should never apply a cold pack or use slush buckets colder than 15°C. But the temperatures reported here are actual nerve temperatures, not body surface temperatures. The deeper a nerve is, the less it is cooled by surface applications of cold (see chapter 5). You must be careful when applying cold to superficial nerves, such as at the elbow or the lateral side of the knee, however (see chapter 14).

There is some controversy concerning which fibers are affected by cold first (see D24 and D82 for references). After reviewing the literature on this subject, Paintal (D82) felt that the evidence weighed in favor of the view that cooling blocks conduction in faster-conducting, larger-diameter fibers before slower-conducting, small-diameter fibers. Subsequent research by him (D80) and others (D31), however, has altered this view (D77). The temperature at which conduction was blocked in cat vagal, saphenous, and cervical nerves (all myelinated) was unrelated to respective normal conduction velocities (D80). Conduction of slow and fast fibers of the same nerve filament were blocked at the same temperature: 7.5°C in the vagal, 9.1°C in the normal saphenous, and 16°C in the abnormal (i.e., stretched) saphenous nerves.

It appears that the response of conduction velocity to decreasing temperature in unmyelinated fibers is similar to that of myelinated fibers except that the blocking temperature is lower (D31, D78). In two different experiments, unmyelinated fibers were blocked at 4.7°C (D78) and 2.7°C (D31).

Lee et al. (D58) reported an 18% decrease in ulnar sensory nerve conduction velocity as a result of a small ice pack applied to the thenar eminence for 16 minutes. Conduction velocity decreased throughout the period of application. After the cold pack was removed, sensory nerve conduction velocity increased, but at a slower rate than the decrease during application, and was still depressed 4.8% after 20 minutes of rewarming. Although they did not report the temperature at this time, it can be assumed that it was still depressed (see chapter 5 for temperature responses during rewarming). The authors also reported a difference between males and females; sensory nerve conduction velocity decreased about 10% more (at 16 minutes) in the females.

Although the median sensory nerve conduction velocity between wrist and elbow was less than between elbow and axilla and greater than between fingers and wrist, the effects of cooling were constant in each of these areas (D7).

Sensory Nerve Action Potentials

Sensory nerve action potentials increase in duration with decreasing temperatures (D7, D33, D64, D65, D80). Buchthal and Rosenfalck (D7) measured

Q_{10} values of 2 between 25° and 35°C, and greater than 2 for temperatures below 25°C. Both absolute and relative refractory periods are increased with decreasing temperature (D64, D80). (Absolute refractory period is the time following an action potential when a subsequent action potential cannot be evoked, no matter how great the stimulation of the nerve is. A relative refractory period follows the absolute refractory period; during this time a subsequent action potential can be evoked if the stimulus is great enough— much greater than usual.) Lowitzsch et al. (D64) reported that the absolute refractory period increased from 0.54 millisecond at 35°C to 3.07 milliseconds at 20°C, while the relative refractory period increased from 3.19 milliseconds to 20.09 milliseconds (Figure 10.3). The effect of cold on refractory periods was about twice as great as its effect on sensory nerve conduction velocity, and the rate of change was greater below 27°C than it was above. These changes are thought to be the result of a decrease in the nerve membrane current due to decreasing temperature (D65).

How Does Cooling Decrease Nerve Conduction?

It appears that increased nerve action potential duration following cold application is the result of the lengthened refractory periods. And increasing the duration of nerve action potentials would decrease the number of fibers that could fire in a set time period, thus decreasing the transmission rate. So in summary, cold reduces the nerve membrane current, which lengthens the refractory periods following a stimulus, lengthens the nerve action potential duration, and decreases the rate of impulse transmission. The degree of transmission decrease is directly related to the amount of cooling, which depends on the depth of the nerve and the other factors of conductive cooling (see Chapter 5).

Muscle Spindle and Tendon Organs

It appears that cold acts directly on muscle spindles and tendon organs (D28, D69); however, the response is somewhat complicated and depends on the core temperature (D73), the state of activation of the sensory organ (D69, D70), and the type of organ from which it originates. A roughly linear

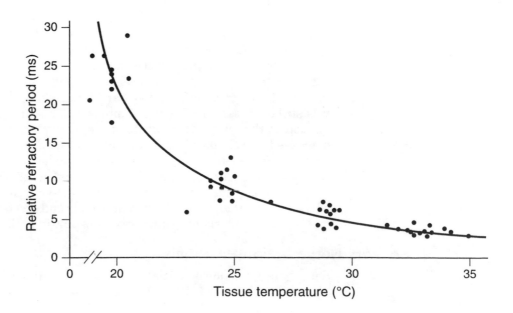

Figure 10.3 Relative refractory period of the ulnar sensory nerve in relation to tissue temperature in 14 healthy subjects.
Reprinted from Lowitzsch et al. (D64).

relationship exists between temperature (38°-28°C) and the rate of discharge in muscle spindles from stretched gastrocnemius (Figure 10.4). Eldred et al. (D28) found that for a 10°C temperature change, afferent discharge from annulospiral endings decreased 56% ± 19%, from flower spray endings the decrease was 42% ± 13%, and from tendon organs, 50%. The slight tension of the spindles when measured masked what later became known as a "cold response" in some slower conducting spindle afferents (D70, D71).

Afferent fibers have been classified according to conducting velocity and origin (D69-71; Table 10.1). Afferents conducting above 70 (or 74) meters per second classified as primary (Type I), while those conducting below 70 (or 65) meters per second are classified as secondary (Type II). In addition, Mense (D69) further differentiated between primary afferents from muscle spindles (Type Ia) and tendon organs (Type Ib). Michalski and Seguin (D70, D71) differentiated between secondary endings that responded to cold in their resting state (CR) and those that did not (NCR). About 65% of the Type II afferents were found to be CR. Mense (D69) had a similar ratio (although he did not call them CR and NCR).

In the resting state, Type I and II-NCR fibers showed no response to cold, whereas Type II-CR fibers increased in activity with cooling down to about

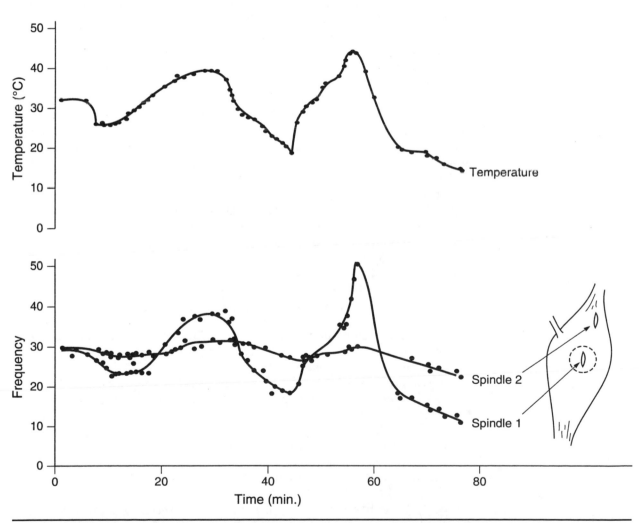

Figure 10.4   Effect of local temperature change on discharge of muscle spindle. Note the difference in response between spindle #1, which was located in the cooled area, and spindle #2, located 2 cm away.
Reprinted from Eldred et al. (D28).

30°C (D70). Further cooling of Type II-CR fibers reversed the response; that is, activity decreased. Chapman (D9) reported the same biphasic response in cat gastrocnemius muscle, even when a synergistic muscle was cooled rather than the involved muscle. When stretched statically more than 6 millimeters, Type II-NCR fibers actively decreased in response at all levels of cooling. Type I and II-NCR fibers also reacted to cold when statically stretched, displaying the same response as Type II-CR afferents. All three types reacted to cold during dynamic stretching (10-millimeter stretch at rates of 10 to 70 millimeters per second). Activity decreased at all rates of stretching. Response was greatest in Type I fibers and least in Type II-NCR fibers.

Golgi tendon organs (Type Ib) do not appear to be as affected by cold as other organs are (D69). Cooling leads to negligible changes in the activity of Type Ib fibers that were active under resting conditions. Perhaps a different effect would be manifest in more active Golgi bodies, but I found no work that investigated this point.

Proprioception

In theory, cold should alter proprioception (sense of body perception and movement), but apparently it doesn't. Cold decreases cutaneous input (D3, D81, D86) and the sensitivity of muscle spindles (D28, D49), both of which are necessary for normal proprioception (D72). However, skilled functional tasks appear to be unaffected by cold (E12, E27, E58, E96). The fear that cold may mask some of the body's protective mechanisms (A30) appears to be unfounded as far as proprioception is concerned.

At present, we must conclude that short-term (20-minute) cold application (immersion or ice pack) has no effect on proprioception. This issue has not been adequately studied, partially because it is difficult to measure proprioception. Of the few studies performed, however, most indicate that cold has no effect on proprioception (E12, E27, E38, E58, E96). The one report (E30) of a decrease in proprioception may have suffered from a flawed design so its results should probably be discounted. They reported loss of balancing ability following immersion of the foot and lower leg (up to the head of the fibula) in a 10°C cold water bath for 15 minutes; but they had no control group and did not allow for warm-up decrement (J15). Studies from which we can infer that short-term cold applications do not alter proprioception are listed here. In each there was no difference between control and cooled body parts, measured on separate days. Subjects were asked to

- stand balanced on one leg ("stork stand") as long as possible after immersing the ankle to 2 to 4 centimeters above the maleolus for 20 minutes in 1°C ice water (E38),
- reproduce ankle joint angles after immersing the ankle and leg to 4 centimeters distal to the knee joint line for 5 or 20 minutes in 4°C ice water (E58),
- reproduce knee joint angles after applying two crushed-ice packs to the knee (medially and laterally) for 20 minutes (E96),
- estimate weight (ankle barognosis) with 1.5 to 5 pounds after immersing the ankle to 4 centimeters above the maleolus for 20 minutes in 1°C ice water (E12), and
- perform agility tests (shuttle run, carioca, cocontraction [J46]) after immersing the ankle 4 centimeters above the maleolus for 20 minutes in 1°C ice water (E27) or applying two crushed-ice packs to the ankle, the calf, or both the ankle and calf for 20 minutes (E48).

■ **WARM UP AFTER YOUR COOL-DOWN**

Even though proprioception and agility appear to be unaffected by cold applications, it is still a good idea to spend a few seconds warming up (loosening up) between a cold application and vigorous activity. Tissue stiffness is increased by the cooling, and this increased stiffness, or decreased elasticity, may cause the tissue to tear rather than stretch when stressed by the activity.

Axioplasmic Transport

Cold slows down axioplasmic transport (flow of nutrients along an axon) in the in vitro cat sciatic nerve (D74, D75). Ochs and Smith (D75) calculated a Q_{10} of 2.0 in the range of 38° to 18°C and a Q_{10} of 2.3 between 38° and 13°C. This change was due to a change in the rate of flow rather than a progressive deterioration over a period of time. A partial failure in transmission occurred at 11°C and completely stopped at temperatures below that. No transmission occurred in 34 nerves cooled to 0° to 10°C for periods of 16 to 46 hours. Since the level of ATP and creatine phosphate remained unchanged during the experiments, the authors concluded that the block was caused by a failure of the nerve to utilize ATP rather than a lack of ATP. They felt that the slowed transport between 38°C and 13°C was due to the reduced utilization of ATP attributable to decreased enzymatic activity within the nerve. The authors speculated that the cold block that occurred below 11°C may have been the result of a disassembly of microtubules; they presented corroborating evidence from others' work (D98) to support this idea. They also reviewed work indicating the absence of transport at 10°C in garfish (D36), at 9°C in goldfish (D34), and down to 4°C in mollusks (D45). But all these are poikilotherms, however, and would be expected to react differently than mammals.

EFFECTS OF COLD ON NEUROMUSCULAR PARAMETERS

Motor Nerve Conduction Velocity

Peripheral motor nerve conduction velocity decreases as tissue temperature is lowered (see D1, D38, and D39 for references). This relationship appears to be virtually linear (A24, D1, D18, D38, D56). A progressive decrease in motor nerve conduction velocity occurred in the median (53.3 meters per second down to 19.1 meters per second) and ulnar (60.3 meters per second down to 24.5 meters per second) nerves during forearm temperature decreases of 29.5°C in the skin, 25.3°C subcutaneously, and 18.1°C intramuscularly (3.5 cm deep) (D1). Halar et al. (D38) demonstrated a linear decrease in human tibial motor nerve conduction velocity with decreases of 2° to 10°C in skin temperature (Figure 10.5).

Although most evidence supports a straight-line relationship, there is evidence of a biphasic decrease in motor nerve conduction velocity similar to that found in sensory nerves, as discussed previously (D81). A more rapid decline in conduction velocity per degree temperature change has been reported in human ulnar nerve below 20°C (D53) and in human peroneal nerve below 24°C to 22°C (D19).

The rates of decrease in motor nerve conduction velocity reported by Abramson et al. (D1) and Halar et al. (D38) are at the low end of the range of

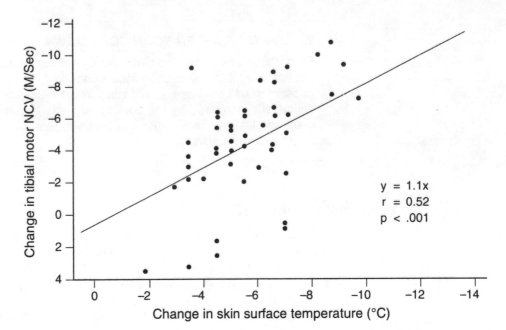

Figure 10.5 Correlation between human tibial motor nerve conduction velocity and skin temperature. Line of best fit determined by regression analysis.
Reprinted from Halar et al. (D38).

values reported in the literature, which range from 1.1 to 1.5 m · sec · °C for skin, and 1.4 to 2.4 m · sec · °C for intramuscular temperatures (D1, D2, D7, D26, D32, D38-D40, D49, D51, D63, D85). Part of this difference is thought to be due to variations in the baseline conduction velocity (D26, D85).

Lee et al. (D58) measured conduction velocity in the ulnar nerve when ice packs were applied to the elbow, where the nerve is very superficial, and when applied over the flexor carpi ulnaris muscle, where the nerve is deep. There was a much greater decrease in motor conduction velocity (30% vs. 17%) when ice was applied to the elbow (Figure 10.6), apparently because the nerve was more superficial at the elbow and therefore cooled more quickly and to a greater degree. Note that motor nerve conduction velocity began to increase shortly after the ice was removed from the elbow, whereas it continued to decrease after ice was removed from the muscle. This change probably was due to the more rapid rewarming of the superficial tissues surrounding the nerve at the elbow. The deeper muscle tissue would remain colder longer.

Along with decreasing motor nerve conduction velocity, the motor nerve threshold to stimulation rises with decreasing temperature (D19, D60, D61, D101). DeJong et al. (D19) reported a constant relationship between temperature and stimulation threshold in human peroneal nerve at temperatures down to 23°C. Below 23°C the threshold rose sharply. At 20°C the maximal output of their stimulator could not elicit a muscle action potential. Li (D60) reported similar results in the rat hind limb, except that the temperatures were 8° to 10°C lower (Figure 10.7).

Firing of Single Motor Units

Firing of single motor units in response to skin cooling appears to vary with the state of excitement of the motor unit (i.e., the activity of the central nervous system) prior to cold application. A nonquantitative study by Clendenin and Szumski (D14) revealed an increase in single motor unit activity in the biceps brachii muscle following a 1- to 2-minute cutaneous ice massage.

A quantitative study by Wolf et al. (D103) revealed that in subjects firing single motor units at the rate of 5.2 hertz, cooling the skin to 10°C tended

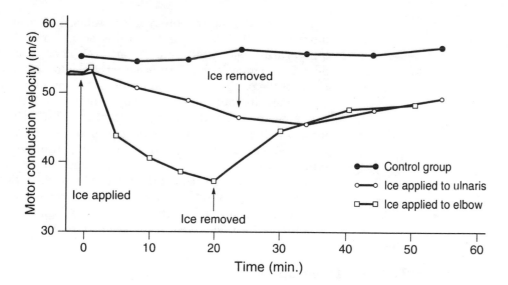

Figure 10.6 Change in ulnar motor nerve conduction during and after ice application to the elbow (squares) and over the flexor capri ulnaris.
Reprinted from Lee et al. (D58).

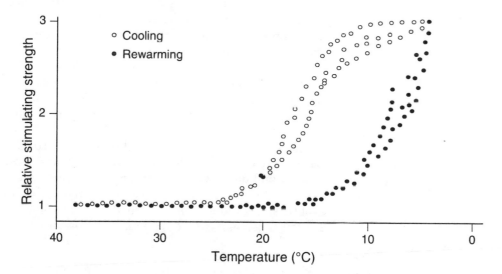

Figure 10.7 Strength of motornerve stimulation required to initiate minimal movement in the rat gracilis anticus muscle during cooling and rewarming.
Note: below 5 °C, no response could be elicited, regardless of the stimulation intensity.
Reprinted from Li (D60).

to decrease the firing during the 1st minute and increase it during the 2nd. These trends were not statistically significant, however. In subjects firing at 0.5 hertz, cooling caused a significant increase in firing during the 1st minute but returned to the precooling level of firing during the 2nd minute. Subjects who were cooled over adjacent muscle groups rather than the one being stimulated did not display noticeable changes, which suggested a specific relationship between the muscle from which the single motor unit was recorded and the site of cold stimulus.

Synaptic Transmission and Muscle Action Potentials

Synaptic transmission is decreased by cooling (D30, D60, D61, D96, D97). Li (D60) reported a blockage of motor nerve transmission at the synapse that occurred in rat obturator nerve at 5°C. There appears to be variability in the temperature at which impulses are blocked at various neuromuscular junctions within the same muscle fiber (D61). A sharp decrease in conduction between the sciatic nerve and the tibialis anterior muscle of dogs which appeared to be presynaptic in nature, occurred at an intramuscular temperature of 28°C (D97). This phenomenon was confirmed by Foldes et al. (D30), who reported that the presynaptic release of acetylcholine decreased by more than 60% at stimulation rates of 0.1 to 50 hertz as neuromuscular temperature decreased from 37° to 17°C. There was, however, a concurrent decrease in muscle cholinesterase activity and a concurrent increase in sensitivity of the postsynaptic membrane factors on neuromuscular transmission.

Latency and duration of the muscle action potential become progressively prolonged as nerve temperature decreases (D19, D60, D61), even though it appears that the resting membrane potential is unchanged until a much lower temperature (D60, D61). There are conflicting reports concerning the effect of cold on amplitude of the muscle action potential (D19, D93). Ricker and Hertel (D93) felt that the increased muscle action potential was due to an effect on the muscle cell membrane and quoted work by others (D5, D35) indicating an increase in the miniature end plate potentials during cooling as support for their hypothesis (see also D61).

Tension Development

The relationships between the variables of duration, frequency of stimulation, and muscle tension are complex (D10). Theoretically, an increased duration of the muscle action potential would result in greater muscle tension development during twitch contractions, if the increase in duration was greater than the decrease in amplitude. The longer duration would allow more time for tension to develop (D46). The duration of the muscle action potential would have no effect on maximal tension during a tetanic contraction, however, since there would be multiple muscle action potentials. But maximal tetanic tension would lessen by a decrease in amplitude in the muscle action potential.

Much research confirms this theory (D6, D10, D15, D30, D46, D57, D90, D100, D101); that is, decreasing temperatures result in increased twitch tension and decreased tetanic tension (Figure 10.8). Foldes et al. (D30), for example, used a rat phrenic nerve–hemidiaphragm preparation that was progressively cooled from 37° to 17°C while being stimulated at 0.1 hertz. Twitch tension, twitch duration, and time of rise to peak tension were all

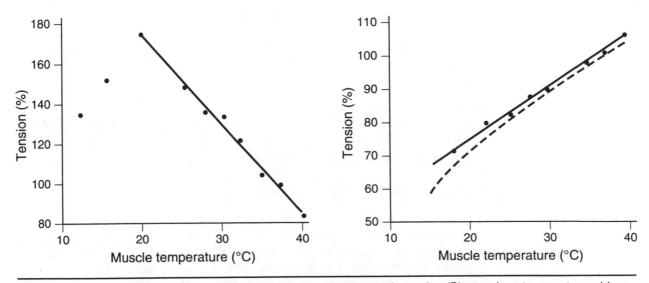

Figure 10.8   Isometric twitch tension (A) and maximal isometric tetanic tension (B) at various temperatures. Lines represent least-square fit to mean values. Line in A excluded values below 20 °C. Solid line in B fitted to values obtained during direct stimulation. Broken line fitted to values obtained during indirect stimulation.
Reprinted from Truong et al. (D100).

potentiated by cooling, increasing 96%, 316%, and 450% respectively during direct stimulation and 70%, 320%, and 515% during indirect stimulation (Figure 10.9). The authors felt these changes were due either to a prolonged association of calcium to troponin or to a decreased rate of formation of the Mg-ATP complex. At tetanic stimulation frequencies (50 hertz), the tension developed was decreased at the lower levels of cooling, for example, 27° to 17°C, by 16% during direct stimulation and 24% during indirect stimulation.

In some studies, however, twitch tension decreased as temperatures fell (D66, F33, D93, D97). In others potentiation of twitch tension in fast-twitch muscles and depression of twitch tension in slow-twitch muscles occurred as temperature went down. The magnitude of the response appears to be species dependent (see Figure 10.10) and may be related to the homogeneity

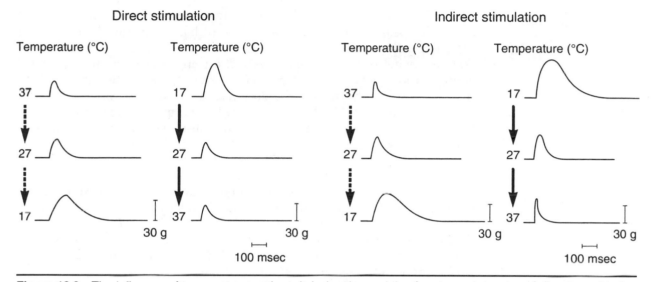

Figure 10.9   The influence of temperature on the twitch duration and the time to peak tension of directly and indirectly stimulated rat phrenic nerve-hemidiaphragm.
Reprinted from Foldes et al. (D30).

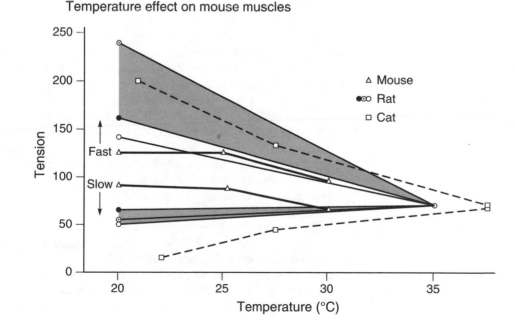

Figure 10.10 Twitch tension variations of fast twitch and slow twitch muscles of the rat, cat, and mouse.
Reprinted from Ranatanga (D90).

of the muscle (D8, D90). For instance, Ranatunga (D90) reported that twitch tension was only slightly potentiated by decreasing temperature in mouse soleus muscle, which contains only about 60% slow-twitch fibers, but depressed by 20% in rat soleus muscle and 40% in mouse soleus muscle, which contain slow-twitch fibers of 80% and 95% to 100%, respectively.

The effect of cold on twitch tension may reverse at lower temperatures (D23, D54, D100). Truong et al. (D100) recorded an increase in twitch tension in the rat triceps surae when the temperature was lowered from 40° to 20°C, but a decrease in twitch tension as the temperature went from 15° to 12°C (Figure 10.8). This is similar to work by Doudoumopoulos and Chatfield (D23), who reported the tension in rat gastrocnemius muscle was greater at 18.0°C and 26.5°C than at either 37.0° or 9.5°C for stimulation frequencies between 15 and 60 hertz. Maximal tension was greater at 18° than at 26.5°C when stimulated between 40 and 60 hertz (tetanic).

Time to peak twitch tension and time to half-relaxation both decrease with decreasing temperature in rat fast-twitch (extensor digitorum longus) and slow-twitch (soleus) muscles (D88). The decrease is linear in the extensor digitorum longus between 35° and 20°C, with Q_{10} values of 2.26 and 2.20, respectively. For the soleus, the decrease is linear from 35° to 25°C (Q_{10} values of 2.79 and 2.59), but appears to have a greater decrease at 20°C. Later research indicated that the time to half-relaxation of twitch tension in both extensor digitorum longus and soleus muscles decreased to a greater degree from 21° to 9°C than it did from 36° to 24°C (D92).

Foldes et al. (D30) interpreted the finding that the influence of cooling was greater on directly stimulated than on indirectly stimulated muscle as indicating that the site of the potentiating effect of cooling is the muscle fiber itself, a conclusion shared by others (D10, D23, D87). They reasoned that since the net effect of cold on neuromuscular transmission was negative, it would partially counteract the beneficial effects of cooling on muscle twitch performance in the indirectly stimulated muscle.

TETANIC TENSION

The level of isometric tetanic tension decreases with decreasing temperature, as do maximum rate of tension development, the time to half-rise of tension, and the time to half-relaxation of tension in rat fast- and slow-twitch skeletal muscle (D92). As with time to half-relaxation of twitch tension, each of these tetanic contraction parameters displays an abrupt change in temperature sensitivity at about 22° to 23°C, indicating an abrupt change in at least one of the underlying contractile processes.

Others have also reported a biphasic response in rat skeletal muscle (D94, D100) and hemidiaphragm (D29) tetanic contractions. Foldes et al. (D29) reported a biphasic response with indirect stimulation of rat triceps surae muscle, but not with direct stimulation (see Figure 10.9). The data of Stephenson and Williams (D94) suggest that the number of cross-bridge interacting sites undergo a considerable decrease at muscle temperatures below 25°C.

The frequency of direct stimulation required for eliciting maximal tetanic tension in Ranatunga's (D88, D92) rat preparations decreased with decreasing temperatures. Duration of impulses was inversely related to temperature. Cooling (from 35° to 20°C) depressed maximum velocity of isotonic shortening (Q_{10} = 1.7) and the maximum rate of rise of isometric tetanic tension (Q_{10} = 1.9) in mouse fast- and slow-twitch muscles (D88, D89). The variations appear to be somewhat less marked than the cooling effects on other isometric parameters (D88).

Isotonic parameters (maximum velocity of shortening, maximum rate of tension development, and force-velocity curve shift) also decrease with decreasing temperatures (D88). A decrease in temperature from 35° to 20°C resulted in a marked reduction in the maximal velocity of shortening (Figure 10.11). Maximal isotonic tension decreased somewhat between 35° and 25°C and then showed a much greater decrease with further cooling to 20°C. The data at 20°C for both the maximal rate of tension development and the maximal velocity of shortening give the impression that these parameters may also have a biphasic temperature dependence. This means that the relationship between velocity of shortening and isotonic force (expressed as a percent of maximal isometric tension at the specific temperature) decreases with decreasing temperature.

Strength Changes Immediately Following Cold Application

The effect of cold applications on maximal isometric contraction is a function of deep-muscle temperature, which is in turn a function of the temperature of the cold modality, how long it is applied, and the depth of the tissue. Coppin et al. (D16) and Johnson and Leider (D50) reported respective handgrip strengths of approximately 60% to 80% of control (contralateral handgrip strength) immediately following forearm immersion for 30 minutes in ice-water baths of 10° to 15°C. Clarke et al. (D13) reported handgrip strength to be unaffected by forearm immersion (30 minutes) in water baths of 18°, 26°, 34°, and 42°C (Figure 10.12). Immersion in baths of lower temperatures, however, led to decreases of approximately 75% at 14°C, 55% at 10°C, and 40% at 2°C.

McGown (D67) reported a significant increase in isometric tension exerted by the knee extensors as a result of a 5-minute ice massage. Her statistical analysis is questionable, however, and interpolation from her graph indicates the increase to be less than 2.5%. Even though the ice was near 0°C, the application was both short-term and intermittent, so the deep-muscle temperature would not have decreased as much as that of the subjects in the research of Clarke et al. did (D13).

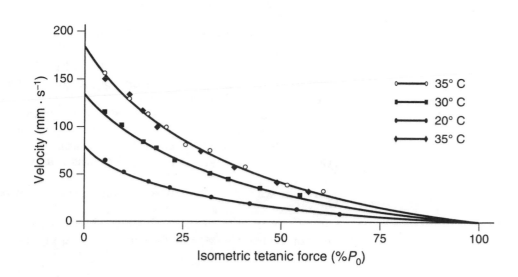

Figure 10.11 Force/velocity relationships at three different temperatures from one extensor digitorum longus muscle. Force is represented as a percentage of maximal isometric titanic tension at that temperature. The sequence in which the data were collected was 35°, 30°, 20° and 35°C (circles with a dot). Reprinted from Ranatanga (D89).

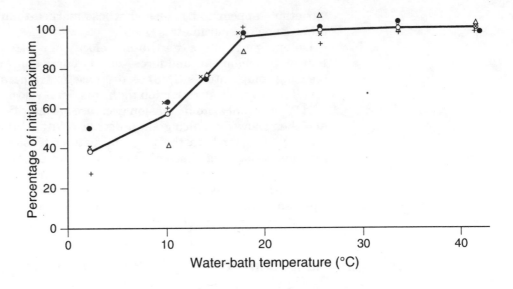

Figure 10.12 Maximal tension (expressed as a percentage of initial maximum tension) recorded after the forearm had been immersed in water at each of seven temperatures for 30 minutes. (Connected open circles represent the mean of four subjects; other symbols represent individual subjects.)
Reprinted from Clarke et al. (D13).

Delayed Strength Changes Following Cold Application

The delayed effect of cold on muscular strength (i.e., during the 3-4 hours following cold application) is unsettled. Johnson and associates (D50, D76) have presented data indicating an increase in strength (isometric tension) in the lower legs and the forearm following 30 minutes of immersion in a 10° to 15°C water bath; the increases ranged from 11% and 19% and occurred from 40 to 183 minutes following immersion. These data have been challenged by Coppin et al. (D16), who reported no increase in strength in the forearm following 30 minutes of immersion. The discrepancy remains unresolved. Muscle power is decreased by massive (half the body) cooling. After immersion up to the waist for 90 minutes in 20°C (68°F) water, subjects' power during a two-legged jump into the air was decreased to 73% of preimmersion levels (D29). This type of cooling is not a common cryotherapeutic technique used in sports. Usually only a single muscle (or muscle group) is cooled; although its temperature is similar to the above. In this experiment, the average decrease in quadriceps muscle temperature (3 cm deep) was 8.5°C (Figure 10.13). Following a 30-minute ice-pack application to the quadriceps, its temperature (2.8 cm deep) decreased (C57). Work is under way in our laboratory to determine the change in force due to cold-pack applications to a single muscle group.

Cote (D17) reported that a 30-minute cold-pack application to the quadriceps had no effect on the peak torque generated in an isokinetic ergometer during knee extension at 0° per second (isometric contraction), 60° per second, 180° per second, or 300° per second, nor on the time required to reach constant velocity. There was no decrease in peak torque during a 30-second fatigue test, but there was a significantly lower power output. Cote speculated that the muscle fiber was inactivated in some way by the cold.

Power was directly related to temperature during rewarming following 90 minutes of immersion up to the waist of human subjects (D29) (Figure 10.13). As mentioned above, this procedure involved cooling the entire lower half of the body, so we must be cautious in applying these results to applications of cold in sports.

Endurance and Fatigue

The duration of submaximal (one third of maximal voluntary contraction) handgrip contractions held to the point of fatigue appears to be longer following 30 minutes of forearm immersion in 18°C water than in water of higher or lower temperatures (Figure 10.14) (D13, D62). Muscle temperature during immersion in the 18°C water was 25° to 29°C (at the time of contraction). By immersing the forearm in hot water then cold, or vice versa, the authors (D13) were able to create a condition in which the subcutaneous and muscular temperatures differed by 30°C. The duration of sustained contractions

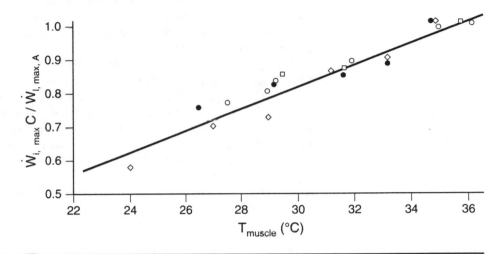

Figure 10.13 Peak power as a function of muscle temperature during rewarming following 90 min of immersion up to the waist in 20°C (68°F) water. Power was computed from ground reaction force during two-legged squat jumps. Four subjects were tested during rewarming; their individual results are represented by circles, squares, and diamonds.
Reprinted from Ferretti et al. (D29).

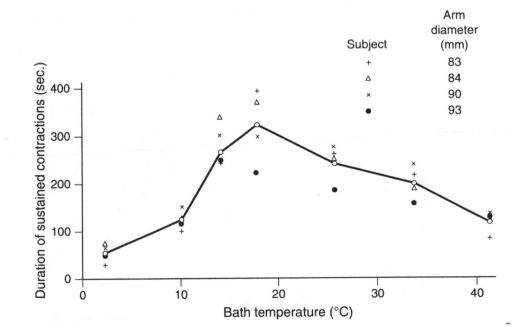

Figure 10.14 Duration of the first of five successive sustained contractions in water at seven temperatures (mean illustrated by connected open circles; other symbols represent individual subjects). Inset shows the diameter of the forearm of each subject, taken 6 cm above the mid-position of the forearm.
Reprinted from Clarke et al. (D13).

was related to muscular rather than subcutaneous temperature. The researcher's felt that at muscular temperatures above 27°C there was an increased rate of metabolism and an earlier accumulation of metabolites. At lower temperatures the cold interfered with neuromuscular transmission, resulting in noncontraction of some of the more superficial muscle fibers.

Clarke and Stelmach (D12) looked at fatigue in another way, measuring tension every 5 seconds during a 2-minute maximal isometric handgrip exercise. Ten minutes of arm immersion in 10°C water prior to the exercise resulted in an 8.3% decrease in initial strength (average tension during the first 30 seconds), but a 5.3% increase in final strength (average tension during the last 30 seconds). Consequently, total work during the entire contraction was unchanged. Similar results during isotonic exercise were reported by Gross (D37).

Recovery from the 2-minute isometric exercise was investigated by measuring handgrip strength each minute during the first 10 minutes following the exercise. Clarke and Stelmach (D12) concluded that recovery was retarded by ice water immersion during the recovery period. These results were probably contaminated, however, because subjects were recovering from different exercise bouts. Control recovery followed control exercise, at normal temperatures, whereas ice water recovery followed exercise influenced by previous ice water immersion. Thus the effects of ice applications during recovery may have been influenced by the application during exercise. Earlier work by Clarke (D11) indicated a slight but nonsignificant decrease in recovery when cold was applied only during the recovery period.

A third way of investigating the effects of cold on fatigue is to measure the duration of sustaining successive submaximal contractions. The duration of quadriceps contractions at two-thirds maximal voluntary contraction with 20-second intervals decreased in excess of 50% between the first and second contractions and then less than 18% between the second and seventh contractions (Figure 10.15). The decrease was greater following immersion in 26°C

Figure 10.15 The relation between water-bath temperature and endurance for successive isometric contractions sustained at 2/3 MVC with intervals of 20 sec between contractions.
Reprinted from Edwards et al. (D27).

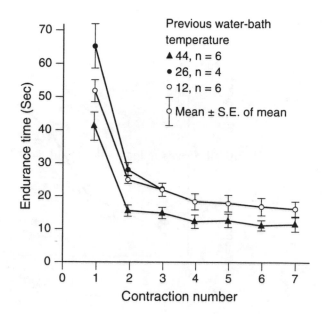

water than in either 12° or 44°C water (D27). Clarke et al. (D13) reported similar results with handgrip contractions at one-third maximal voluntary contraction with 20-minute intervals.

EFFECTS OF COLD ON REFLEXES

At certain levels of central nervous system cooling a hyperresponsiveness occurs, indicating that both the activity of individual structural elements and the patterns of reaction have been modified (D55). For example, monosynaptic and polysynaptic reflexes are increased in magnitude, single stimuli result in repetitive responses, and the numbers of interneurons and motor neurons involved in a reflex are increased, even though the strength of the afferent stimulus and the excitability of the involved neurons are unchanged (see D55 for references). Koizumi et al. (D55) felt that a change in accommodation of spinal neurons could contribute to this hyperresponsive state, and they demonstrated that accommodation was decreased by cooling. They stimulated spinal cord cells with a certain current, varying the time required for the stimulus current to achieve maximum strength. Cells at 33°C would not respond to a current with a rise time of more than 22 milliseconds, but at 25°C a rise time of 54 milliseconds resulted in stimulation.

Cooling a relaxed muscle (medial gastrocnemius) also results in facilitation of the monosynaptic reflex (D71), whereas cooling of a stretched muscle results in its depression (C35). Chapman (D9) reported that cooling the relaxed medial gastrocnemius resulted in facilitation of both phasic and tonic components of the stretch reflex in the lateral (uncooled) gastrocnemius. Facilitation began to increase after a few degrees of cooling, reached a maximum at about 30°C, and began to decrease during cooling down to 24°C. Each of these studies investigated the gastrocnemius-soleus muscles in cats.

Triceps Surae Reflex

Petajan and Watts (D84) demonstrated an increase in half-relaxation time of the triceps surae reflex in humans during and after immersion in 7°C water (Figure 10.16). During cooling the reflex was linear ($Q_{10} = 2.2$). Following 30 minutes of cooling, half-relaxation time continued to increase to a peak at 20 minutes after immersion, then began to decrease very slowly. In 4 subjects studied for an extended period, half-relaxation time averaged 343 milliseconds before immersion and 547 milliseconds 6 hours afterward. Average maximal half-relaxation time was 643 milliseconds. These subjects were relatively inactive throughout testing. Another subject exercised after cooling; his half-relaxation time returned to normal within 2 hours. No mention was made of the level of his exercise.

Petajan and Watts's study (D84) speculated that the conduction velocity of all nerves is lowered by cold, with the velocity of smaller diameter nerve fibers decreasing to a greater degree than that of larger fibers. Desynchronization of activity occurs because of this nonuniform cooling. Cold also causes a decrease in the conduction rate of muscle fibers. The combination of these effects results in decreased maximal tension in the muscle and slowing of relaxation.

Lippold et al. (D63) and Eldred et al. (D28) demonstrated in animal models that muscle spindle afferent activity decreased as muscle temperature decreased. Wolf and Ledbetter (F42) demonstrated in decerebrate cats a decrease in electromyographic activity 1 to 5 seconds after skin cooling began,

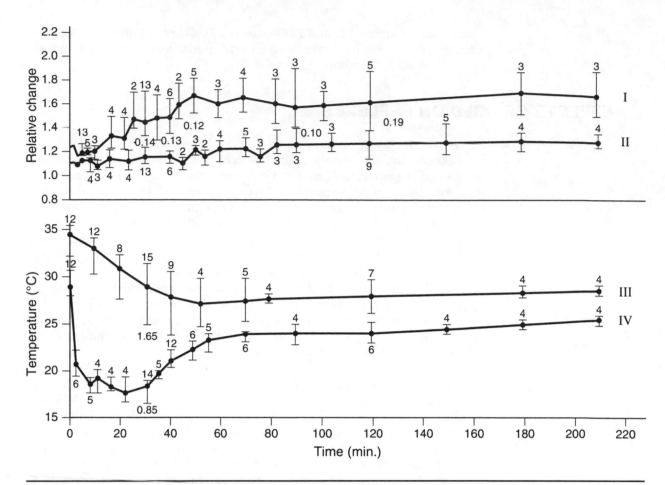

Figure 10.16   Mean changes of the Achilles tendon reflex (ATR) as a result of immersing the calf for 30 min in 7 °C water. Upper two curves represent relative changes in half-relaxation time in the cooled (upper curve) and uncooled contralateral (lower curve) limbs. The bottom two curves represent changes in muscle (upper curve) and skin (lower curve) temperatures.
Reprinted from Petajan and Watts (D84).

and in the absence of appreciable muscle cooling. They postulated a skin–reflex relationship. Tleulin et al. (D99) observed reduced polysynaptic reflex activity with skin cooling in lightly anesthetized cats.

Patellar Tendon Reflex

Miglietta (F35) examined the effect of cold application on the patellar tendon reflex in 10 hemiplegic and quadriplegic patients who had exaggerated deep tendon reflexes. Turkish towels soaked in ice water were applied (changed every 30 seconds) to the quadriceps muscles for 7 minutes. The amplitude of the action potentials elicited by tendon tap reflexes were measured every minute for 2 minutes before cold application, during cold application, and for 5 minutes after cold application. Temperatures decreased from 88°F (31°C) to 66°F (14°C) during cooling and increased to 71.5°F (19°C) after 5 minutes of rewarming. Average reflex amplitude decreased 25% within the 1st minute, decreased an additional 9% by the end of cooling, and increased to a level that was 17% below precooling after 5 minutes of rewarming.

Because of the quickness of the decreased reflex response, Miglietta rejected the idea that it was caused by direct action of the cold on the muscle spindle fibers, muscular tissue, or nervous transmission. Miglietta proposed instead two mechanisms by which the sympathetic nervous system could be responsible for the effect of cold on reflexes. The first was a direct effect based on the work of Hunt (D48), who claimed to have demonstrated that sympathetic stimulation caused significant changes in the threshold of muscle spindle receptors to applied stretch. Spindle afferent discharge decreased or ceased. Hunt's work was accepted by Olson and Stravino (A38), but not by Lehman and de Lateur (A24), who did not reject the Miglietta hypothesis, however. Miglietta's second proposed mechanism was an indirect one suggested by Eldred et al. (D28), who attributed the decreased reflex to sympathetic induced vasoconstriction.

Short-Term Cold Application and Sports Performance

Changes in muscle strength and reflexes have lead some to suggest that athletes would be more prone to injury following cold applications because of a hindered ability to perform (F39). A recent study from our laboratory indicates, however, that agility tests (shuttle run, carioca, and cocontraction E27) are unaffected by ankle immersion (4 centimeters above the maleolus) for 20 minutes in 1°C ice water (E27). Future studies must investigate other performance tests and the effect of knee and large-muscle cooling.

SUMMARY

- The effects of cold on neurological and neuromuscular structures are varied.
- Cold applied to cold receptors increases their activity and thus increases transmission to the central nervous system, whereas cooling the sensory nerve carrying the impulse decreases this transmission.
- Sensory nerve conduction velocity decreases linearly with decreasing temperatures down to a critical temperature of about 27°C. Below this temperature the effects of cold on nerve conduction velocity becomes greater, until a total conduction block occurs.
- It appears that fast- and slow-conducting fibers and myelinated and unmyelinated fibers all react similarly, except that unmyelinated fibers are blocked at a lower temperature than myelinated fibers.
- The effect of cold on muscle spindles is much like its effect on sensory fibers, but is mediated by the state of activity of the spindle fiber.
- Golgi tendon organs do not appear to be as affected by cold as muscle spindles are.
- Motor nerve conduction velocity is decreased by cold, a phenomenon apparently due to an increase in the nerves' threshold to stimulation.
- Synaptic transmission is decreased while latency and duration of the muscle action potential are both prolonged.
- The relationships between muscle tension and the duration and frequency of stimulation are complex. In some muscles, the increased duration of the muscle action potential leads to an increase in the duration and tension of a muscle twitch, but a decrease in tetanic tension. In other muscles (primarily slow-twitch), twitch tension decreases with decreasing temperature. Still others show an increase, then a decrease, in twitch tension as temperature progressively decreases.
- Cold applications result in decreases in isometric tetanic tension, maximum rate of tension development, and the times to half-rise and half-relaxation of tension. This decrease shows an abrupt change at about 22° to 23°C, indicating an abrupt change in at least one of the underlying contractile processes.

- Isotonic parameters (maximum velocity of shortening, maximum rate of tension development, and force-velocity curve shift) also decrease with decreasing temperatures.
- Strength changes in entire muscle groups occur only when the deep muscle is cooled to temperatures below 15° to 18°C (which usually requires at least 20 minutes).
- The effect of cold on fatigue is still an unresolved issue.
- External cooling results in decreased triceps surae and patellar tendon reflexes, whereas certain levels of central nervous system cooling result in increased monosynaptic and polysynaptic reflexes. It appears that these effects are unrelated to the effects of cold on the individual components (sensory input, motor nerve, and muscle twitch) of the reflex.
- Proprioception appears to be unaffected by short-term cold applications.
- Agility appears to be unaffected by cold applications.

11

Pain and Cold Applications

One of the primary reasons for cold applications during both immediate care and rehabilitation of sports injuries is to decrease pain. Yet anyone who has immersed a hand or foot in ice water will tell you that cold *causes* pain— severe pain. Can something that causes such severe pain also relieve it? Yes. Not only can cold reduce pain resulting from musculoskeletal pathologies (E17), but it often does so quite dramatically. Clinical observations leave no doubt that cold applications are effective in reducing many types of pain, but there is also clear experimental evidence of its efficacy (E17). Cold is possibly one of the most effective yet underused physical modalities for relieving pain (E67).

In this chapter, I discuss cold-induced pain, habituation to cold-induced pain, and relief of pain through cryotherapy. An understanding of this material is essential to understanding cryokinetics and other rehabilitation techniques presented in later chapters. Also, read chapter 10 prior to reading this one; it contains the neurological foundation for this chapter.

WHAT IS PAIN?

Explaining how cold affects pain is very difficult. In fact, explaining pain itself is very difficult (E42, E94, E105). But we do know much about pain and its relief. We have all experienced pain and know the joy of pain relief. And many of us know the agony and frustration associated with an ability to relieve pain. The numerous definitions of pain (see box on next page) may help you understand the complexity of the pain experience.

What Is Pain?

- Pain has neither been adequately defined nor objectively measured. Many surgical procedures, drugs, psychological techniques, and physical modalities have been used with varying degrees of success to control pain, but no one method is clearly superior to the others (E94).
- Pain is whatever the experiencing person says it is (E68).
- Pain is an unpleasant sensory and emotional experience associated with actual or potential tissue damage or described in terms of such damage (E10).
- The pain experience varies from individual to individual and is described both in terms of its sensation and the distress or degree of suffering that it causes (E97).
- Although the initial stimuli for pain may occur in the tissues, the pain is not identified or experienced until the higher cortical levels of the brain interpret it as pain and identify its location (E97).
- Pain is multifaceted; it is a label that represents a myriad of different experiences that can be grouped together into four components or qualities: sensory, affective, evaluative, and miscellaneous (E71).

The four qualities or components of pain identified by Melzack and Torgerson (E71) have been amplified and described as follows:

Sensory (or *discriminative*)—pertains to the nature of the noxious stimulation or actual sensation of the pain—that is, the conduction of impulses from sense organs on the periphery to reflex or higher centers (J73). It is often described by words such as *throbbing, stabbing, sharp, stinging, aching,* and *splitting* (E71).

Affective (or *motivational*)—relates to the emotional or autonomic responses associated with the pain. It is influenced by the mental state, personality type, goals, desires, and expectations of the patient (A1). Words that describe the affective qualities of pain include *tiring, sickening, frightening,* and *cruel* (E71).

Evaluative (or *cognitive*)—involves conscious thought processes concerning the pain, such as examining the noxious stimulation, comparing it with past experience, and assigning meaning to the present and to future pain experiences (A1). It is a subjective judgment of the overall intensity of the total pain experience and is described by words such as *mild, intense,* and *excruciating* (E71).

Miscellaneous—refers to combinations of the above and is described by words such as *cold, numb, tight, nagging,* and *penetrating* (E71).

MEASURING PAIN

Most attempts to measure pain in humans have used a questionnaire or one of numerous scales to quantify a person's subjective evaluation of the pain (E9, E11, E15, E32, E33, E83, E95). The five most common instruments, in increasing order of complexity, are discussed next:

- Number scales (see Figure 11.1)
- Verbal rating scales
- Visual analogue scales
- Graphic rating scales (see Figure 11.2)
- The McGill Pain Questionnaire (see Figure 11.3)

Number Scales

Number scales such as the Borg Scale of Perceived Pain (Figure 11.1) are used to quantify pain intensity. These scales consist of a list of numbers, such as from 1 to 10, and associated words to indicate various levels of pain intensity ranging from none to maximal (E11). Patients select the number that they feel best represents their present level of pain.

Verbal Rating Scales

Verbal rating scales use a series of descriptors without numbers. Subjects select the descriptor that best represents their pain experience. Verbal rating scales have been criticized for being insensitive to small changes (E23, E37, E80).

Visual Analogue Scales

Visual analogue scales (Figure 11.2) consist of a line of specific length with the ends of the line labeled with contrasting descriptors, such as *annoying* and *unbearable*, or *dull* and *heavy*. Subjects mark a point between the two extremes that indicates their pain (E95). The distance between the left end of the line and the mark is a measure of the pain. Visual analogue scales are a robust, sensitive, and reproducible means of expressing pain severity (E28, E37, E87).

Graphic Rating Scales

Graphic rating scales are similar to visual analog scales but have descriptors spread across the scale in addition to those at the extremes (Figure 11.2). They are administered and scored in the same manner as visual analogue

Circle the word and/or number which best describes the intensity of your pain.

0	Nothing at all
0.5	Very, very weak (just noticeable)
1	Very weak
2	Weak (light)
3	Moderate
4	Somewhat strong
5	Strong (heavy)
6	
7	Very strong
8	
9	
10	Very, very strong (almost maximal)
*	Maximal

Figure 11.1 Borg scale of perceived pain.
Reprinted from Borg (E11).

Graphic Pain Rating Scale

Name _____   Test session _____

Dull ache	A feeling of discomfort during activity
Slight pain	An awareness of pain without distress
More slight pain	Pain distracts attention during physical exertion
Painful	Pain distracts attention from routine occupation such as writing or reading
Very painful	Pain fills the field of consciousness to the exclusion of other events
Unbearable pain	Comparable to the worst pain you can imagine

No
pain _____ Unbearable
pain

Dull   Slight   More slight   Painful   Very
ache   pain   pain   painful

Figure 11.2   Graphic analogue scale developed after Talig (E75). Subjects mark a point along the 12-cm line between no pain and unbearable pain that represents their level of pain. Pain is quantified by measuring, to the nearest 0.5 cm, the line from the extreme left to the mark made by the subject.
Reprinted from Denegar & Perrin (E23).

scales. Some feel that graphic rating scales are easier to use, improve consistency for each respondent and between respondents (E43), and are a more sensitive measure of pain intensity than visual analog scales (E23).

Verbal rating, visual analogue, and graphic rating scales can be used to measure either pain intensity or the affective quality of pain, depending on the words selected for the scales (E62).

The McGill Pain Questionnaire

The McGill Pain Questionnaire (Figure 11.3) is the most comprehensive and complex pain-measuring instrument. It consists of four parts, as follows.

1. *Pain location* is evaluated by asking patients to circle the location of their pain on a pair of opposite image line drawings (front and back of the body).
2. *What the pain feels like* is the most complex part of the questionnaire. It consists of 20 groupings of three to five associated words, which measure
   - sensory qualities of pain (Groups 1-10),
   - affective qualities of pain (Groups 11-15),
   - evaluative qualities of pain (Group 16), and
   - miscellaneous qualities of pain (Groups 17-20).

   Subjects choose the words that describe their pain. They can choose no more than one word per group, but do not have to choose a word from every group.
3. *How the pain changes with time* is determined by having patients choose one of three groups of words that represent constant, intermittent, or transient pain.
4. *How strong the pain is* (present pain intensity, or PPI) is measured on a five-point numerical scale with the following descriptors: mild, discomforting, distressing, horrible, and excrutiating.

Part 1. Where is your pain? Circle the area of greatest pain.

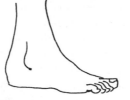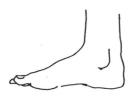

Part 2. Some of the words below describe your *present* pain. Circle only those words that best describe it. Leave out any category that is not suitable. Use only a single word in each appropriate category—the one that best applies.

1	4	8	11	15	18
Flickering	Sharp	Tingling	Tiring	Wretched	Tight
Quivering	Cutting	Itchy	Exhausting	Blinding	Numb
Pulsing	Lacerating	Smarting			Drawing
Throbbing		Stinging	**12**	**16**	Squeezing
Beating	**5**		Sickening	Annoying	Tearing
Pounding	Pinching	**9**	Suffocating	Troublesome	
	Pressing	Dull		Miserable	**19**
2	Gnawing	Sore	**13**	Intense	Cool
Jumping	Cramping	Hurting	Fearful	Unbearable	Cold
Flashing	Crushing	Aching	Frightful		Freezing
Shooting		Heavy	Terrifying	**17**	
	6			Spreading	**20**
3	Tugging	**10**	**14**	Radiating	Nagging
Pricking	Pulling	Tender	Punishing	Penetrating	Nauseating
Boring	Wrenching	Taut	Grueling	Piercing	Agonizing
Drilling		Rasping	Cruel		Dreadful
Stabbing	**7**		Vicious		Torturing
	Hot		Killing		
	Burning				
	Scalding				
	Searing				

Part 3. How did your pain change during the session? Which word or words would you use to describe the pattern of your pain?

31	32	33
Continuous	Rhythmic	Brief
Steady	Periodic	Momentary
Constant	Intermittent	Transient

Figure 11.3 McGill Pain Questionnaire. In Part 2, categories 1 to 10 represent sensory components of pain, categories 11 to 15 represent affective components of pain, category 16 represents pain intensity, and categories 17 to 20 represent combination terms (i.e., involving two or more types of pain).
Reprinted from Melzack (E68).

COLD-INDUCED PAIN

Cold-induced pain has been described by researchers who studied the response of subjects to immersion of the finger (E54), hand (E107), or ankle (E16, E40, E45, E79) in ice-water baths; ice massage to the gastrocnemius (E11); and hand contact with various objects (E35). Also, the cold pressor test (hand immersion in an ice-water bath) has been used extensively as a dependent variable in numerous tests of pain-coping strategies (E61, E88, E89, E108).

Do other types of cold applications, such as crushed-ice packs, cause pain? Except for people with cold hypersensitivity, I don't recall such incidents during my clinical career, nor have I found reports of such in the literature. Is this beacuse other techniques are not as intense as immersion? Or perhaps because crushed-ice packs are usually used during immediate-care procedures when acute pain may be intense enough to gate (overcome) the cold pain? Obviously, this is another area of cryotherapy that needs to be researched.

The immediate sensation from ice-water immersion is cold, but is replaced in 5 to 60 seconds by a deep, aching pain (E54, E107). Hensel (D42) described cold pain as having a dull character, being poorly localized, and radiating intensely into the surrounding areas.

The onset and intensity of pain appear to be related to the temperature of the water bath (Figures 11.4 and 11.5); the lower the temperature, the quicker the onset of the sensation (E107) and the more intense it is (E35, E88, E107). Also, when subjects were asked to write down their sensations each 2 minutes during 20 minutes of ankle immersion, the number of times they mentioned pain was related to the temperature (E80). Within 1 minute after its onset, the pain sensation peaks and either plateaus for a minute or so (Figure 11.6) or begins to decrease (see Figure 11.4). This alteration is followed (in water colder than 12°C) by a sensation of "pins and needles" or "prickling" soon after the peak of the aching pain. The prickling sensation

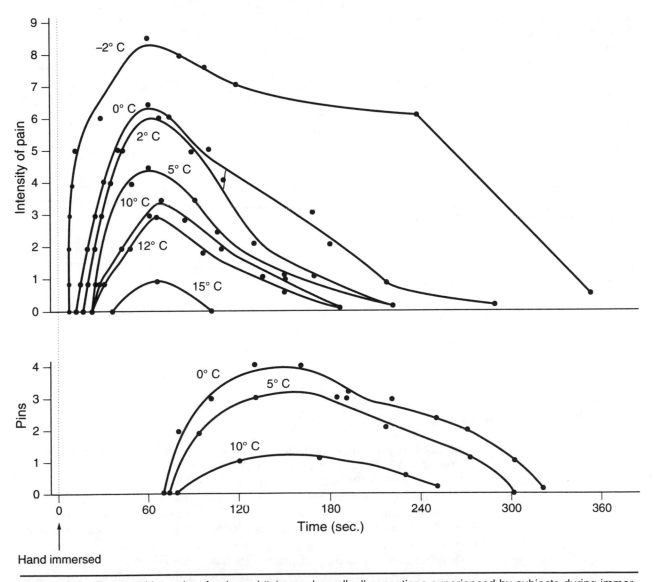

Figure 11.4 Estimated intensity of pain and "pins and needles" sensations experienced by subjects during immersion of the left hand in 15° to –2°C water.
Reprinted from Wolf and Hardy (E107).

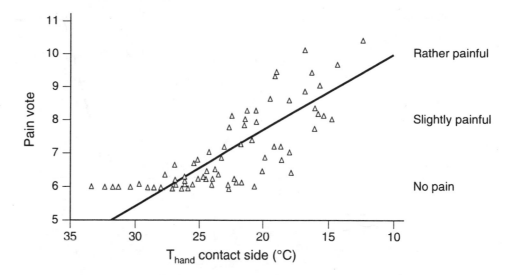

Figure 11.5 There is a direct relationship between subjective pain sensation and actual temperature of the hand. Reprinted from Havenith (E35).

gradually increases in intensity and then abates, lasting 1 to 3 minutes. The intensity of the prickling sensation is also related to the temperature (see Figure 11.4) and is uncomfortable.

Following the prickling sensation, the body part becomes numb. Kunkel (E54) reported that at about the 10th minute pain was mild, the finger felt neither warm nor cold, and tests for both superficial and deep pain indicated the finger was completely numb. Others report different times for the onset of numbness: 1.75 minutes after beginning ice massage to the gastrocnemius (E13) and 17.7 minutes after immersing the ankle in 2°C ice water (C36). This issue definitely needs further investigation.

It is common for people to be unable to perceive numbness, however. I am one of those. During various research projects lasting up to 45 minutes, I have never felt what I could say was numbness. And some athletes being treated with cryokinetics have reacted similarly. Nevertheless, the intensity of pain still varies.

Additional bouts of pain occur in a cyclic fashion if immersion continues. Kunkel (E54) found pain to occur at 3- to 18-minute intervals and to be of variable intensity. In one period of 127 minutes of sustained cooling, 25 separate bouts of pain occurred, but only 7 of the bouts were severe. Like the first pain, the additional bouts of pain were of decreased intensity as the water temperature was raised.

An "after-pain" occurs following removal of the cold modality. It begins a few seconds after removing the body part from the cold and lasts for 1 to 2 minutes (see Figure 11.6). It is a deep, aching, throbbing pain, sometimes with a sensation of warmth (E54).

Progression of Sensations During Ice-Water Immersion

1. Cold
2. Deep, aching pain
3. Pain plateaus or decreases
4. "Pins and needles" sensation
5. "Pins and needles" sensation abates
6. Numbness
7. Bouts of pain at 3- to 18-minute intervals

"After-pain"—a deep, aching, throbbing pain, sometimes with a sensation of warmth—occurs a few seconds after removing the body part from the cold.

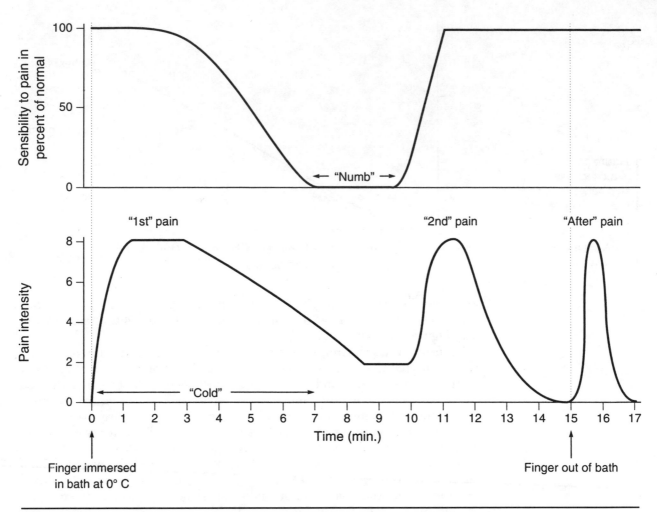

Figure 11.6   Usual course of pain and numbness in a finger immersed in a 0°C water bath. Reprinted from Kunkel (E54).

What Causes Cold-Induced Pain?

Numerous theories have been advanced to explain the cause of cold-induced pain. Kunkel (E54) believed that cold might cause tissue injury that results in a metabolite-mediated excitation of nerve endings or pain fibers. Wolf and Hardy (E107) and Wells (E106) claimed that pain was caused by the increased thermal gradient between superficial- and deep-tissue temperatures. Greenfield and Shepherd (C30) and Abramson et al. (E1) concluded that the pain was due to vasoconstriction of blood vessels. Hensel (D42) also felt that blood vessel spasm contributed to cold pain and explained that it was mediated through nociceptors rather than thermoreceptors.

A closer examination of these authors' work (C30, E1, E106, E107) indicates the possibility of agreement between their results. Greenfield and Shepherd (C30) stated that vasoconstriction was responsible for pain because it lowered the tissue temperature. This relationship would have increased the tissue temperature gradient (E106, E107). And although Abramson et al. (E1) presented evidence that, they felt, indicated that pain was due to vasoconstrictor tone, they may have misinterpreted their data. Their experimental protocol involved placing one hand in an 11° to 14°C water plethysmograph for 140 minutes. From 60 to 100 minutes the body was heated by placing seven Hydrocollator packs over the chest, abdomen, thighs, and one leg and foot. The other leg and foot were immersed in a 52°C paraffin bath, and the entire body was covered with blankets. The authors noted a decrease in blood flow during the first 60 minutes, an increase in blood flow during the bodily heating, and then decreased blood flow following removal of the hot packs. Pain, which was present during the initial period, disappeared during body heating and reappeared after the heating was terminated. Blood flow and pain appeared to be correlated; hence their conclusion. They did not measure temperature, but assumed that the hand in the cold-water bath remained cold throughout the procedure. It seems doubtful that it did, however. With almost total body heating, the head, hand, and lungs would have been the only heat sinks for dissipating the excess heat. Heat probably was transferred to the cooled hand through the vascular system and conducted into the water. Thus, had they measured the temperature of the hand, they may have found a correlation between pain and the temperature of the hand, as have others (E53).

Temperature, or Rate of Change of Temperature?

It appears that the temperature at which pain occurs depends on the rate of change of the temperature; that is, the faster the cutaneous temperature is decreased, the lower the pain threshold temperature (E21, E35, I37, I64). This is probably due to methodological artifacts, however. In one study, rates of cooling of 0.5°, 1.3°, 2.0°, and 2.8°C per second were investigated (E21). Subjects were asked to indicate, by pressing switches, when they first felt pain and when the pain became intolerable. The mean pain threshold was about 11.8°C for cooling at 0.5°C per second and decreased linearly to a mean of about 7.8°C for cooling at 2.8°C per second. The author suggested that this difference was an artifact, however, due to the time lag between the subject's pain sensation and their motor response to the pain (E21). This doesn't mean that subjects responded more slowly in some situations, but only that the temperature decreased more during the time the subjects were responding. Another explanation for the inverse relationship between pain temperature and rate of cooling is that with faster cooling of the skin the deeper tissues (site of the pain receptors) do not cool as fast (E35). Thus, by the time the deep tissues are cooled enough that the pain receptors are stimulated, the surface temperature is lower.

Pain Threshold Temperature

The pain threshold of 11.8°C observed by Croze and Duclaux (E21) is lower than that observed by Wolf and Hardy, 18°C (E107). The difference is probably due to methodology. Croze and Duclaux were cooling hands with a device that decreased in temperature at a constant rate, whereas Wolf and Hardy immersed body parts in water baths of constant temperatures. Even though Wolf and Hardy's subjects experienced pain at 18°C, the sensation occurred after 60 seconds of immersion. A direct relationship existed between water temperature and the time between immersion and sensation of pain; the lower the temperature, the quicker pain was sensed.

If the rate of cooling is too slow, however, pain does not occur. Wolf and Hardy (E107) immersed subjects' hands in 20°C water, a temperature at which no pain was felt, and then lowered the temperature to 0°C in successive steps over a period of more than 60 minutes. The subjects felt no pain, but did report a "pins and needles" sensation. The slower the cooling, the less marked the sensation was. The authors' interpretation of this pattern was that with slow cooling, the tissue temperature gradient was never great enough to elicit pain. After observing an increase in pain sensation both during skin cooling and as it rewarmed after being cooled, LeBlanc (A22) also concluded that pain was due more to a change in the thermal gradient than to absolute temperature.

Tolerating Cold Temperature

Croze and Duclaux's (E21) subjects reported temperatures below 7.8°C to be intolerable. What was their definition of tolerable? Obviously, the subjects were expecting the cold to become intolerable at some point since they were instructed to indicate that point. In our clinic, we routinely treat sprained ankles by immersing them in a "slush bucket" of ice water that is 0° to 1°C. Research protocols using this method have resulted in surface temperatures of 2° to 7°C for the finger, ankle, and forearm that have been maintained for 20 to 45 minutes (C36, C42-C45, E79).

COPING WITH AND ADAPTING TO COLD-INDUCED PAIN

First, why worry about coping with cold pain? If it causes so much pain, just avoid the pain by not using cold. This is a bad option, for two reasons. First, this option eliminates one of the greatest rehabilitative techniques for acute joint sprains. Second, in my own clinical observations I've found that most people adapt to the cold in the first or second session and so have little problem with pain after that. It is uncommon for one of our athletes even to mention pain after the first immersion. The key is to help them get through the first cold-immersion session.

Coping With the First Ice-Water Immersion Session

Coping strategies do not alter the pain sensation or its intensity, they just help patients tolerate the pain (E6, E112). Several studies have found that the more highly susceptible people are to hypnosis, the more they respond to coping procedures (E74, E76). Moods also seem to affect pain tolerance (E112). One the other hand, adaptation actually decreases the intensity of the pain (E2, E16, E51, E61, E93).

Research on basic pain mechanisms, using the cold pressor test to induce pain (E61, E88, E89, E105, E108, E109), provide some valuable tips in dealing with cold pain during therapy. Perceived control is a basic mediating variable for both acute and chronic pain (E105, E108). You achieve this by actively involving the patient in the treatment (E105). I always give patients a choice as to whether or not to use the treatment—without really giving them a choice. For instance, prior to cryokinetics I'll say, "By using cryokinetics we can rehabilitate your ankle in 4 or 5 days; other types of therapy usually take 3 weeks or a month [implying that there is really only one choice]. But this first ice immersion session will be very, very painful. You'll soon adapt to the pain, though, and it will go away. Within 2 or 3 days you'll be plopping your foot into the ice water and won't even know it is cold, like Craig and Bob over there. What do you think? Do you want to endure 15 or 20 minutes of ice pain and be rehabilitated in days, or should we go for the month-long, less painful treatment?" Since most people want quick resolution of their injury, they will choose what you were going to use anyway, but by allowing them to choose, you give them control. This is very important in helping them cope with the pain.

Talking about the pain beforehand is important, but what you say about its intensity may not be. We randomly assigned more than 90 varsity athletes into four groups (E91). Each group received one of the following explanations about the pain they would feel during ankle immersion for 20 minutes in a 1°C ice-water bath: (a) pain will be very intense, (b) pain will be moderate, (c) pain will be mild, or (d) no explanation. The three groups receiving an explanation reported less pain than the group receiving no explanation, but there was no difference in reported pain among the first three groups.

What you ask patients to think about during ice-water immersion can affect their tolerance time to a cold pressor test (E108). Four groups of college students immersed their forearms in 1°C water for 5 seconds, removed their arms from the water, read a typed page of instructions, and then immersed their forearms in the ice water again for as long as they could. Their tolerance time and type of instructions were as follows:

Time (in seconds)	Instructions
69	Combined ineffective strategies: Count backward by 3's from 1,000; become aware of your sensations; imagine a blank wall; imagine you're attending a lecture.
139	No instructions
198	Pleasant imagery: Keep thinking of pleasant things and move from one to another.
285	Combined effective strategies: Concentrate on other things; imagine the sensations as unusual rather than painful; imagine that your hand is wax or rubber; imagine that your hand feels dull and insensitive.

Clear, straightforward oral directions were more helpful than written ones in decreasing pain sensation during a cold pressor test, although tolerance time did not increase (E109). Presumably this was because it allowed the instruction giver to impart encouragement, even though the words were identical for both groups.

■ *HELPING INDIVIDUALS COPE WITH COLD-INDUCED PAIN*
- Actively involve the patients in their treatment. Discuss with them the pros (quick resolution of injury) and cons (pain).
- Talk with the patient about the potential pain before beginning treatment.
- Explain that they will adapt to the pain after the first treatment.
- Ask the patient to do any one or more of the following during treatment: concentrate on other things, imagine sensations as unusual rather than painful, imagine that your body part is wax or rubber, imagine that your body part feels dull and insensitive.

Adaptation to Cold Pain

Most people readily adapt to ice-water immersion (E2, E16, E51, E92). During cryokinetics (see chapter 18), the first ice immersion session seems intolerable, and often your salesmanship is taxed in keeping the patient in the water. If the patient endures 15 to 20 minutes of immersion, though, subsequent immersion is much more tolerable. In fact, it is not uncommon in my clinical experience to hear patients utter a sigh of relief upon immersing their body part for the second time because the pain is so greatly reduced.

Adams and Smith (E2) reported that pain in fingers immersed in an ice-water bath for 20 minutes four times per day diminished and finally disappeared completely, but they did not mention the time course of this adaptation. Strempel (E92) exposed subjects to a cold pressor test (hand immersed in 4°C water for 1 minute) seven times a day for 21 consecutive days. He observed a very distinct subjective adaptation to the pain from one exposure to another. In a later study, Strempel (E93) exposed subjects to the cold pressor test once each day for 21 consecutive days. Both objective and subjective evaluation of the pain intensity indicated an adaptation. Adaptation has also been demonstrated in hands immersed in 4°C water for 2.5 minutes twice a day for 19 days (E62) and in ankles immersed intermittently in 1°C water for 40 minutes daily for 8 days—simulated cryokinetics (Figure 11.7).

Adaptation is specific to the body part treated (E2, E16, E60, E61, E107), water temperature (E16, E106), and activity during adaptation (E61). For instance, if a person immerses one ankle for a number of sessions and then immerses the other ankle, the pain in the second ankle is usually as intense as it had been in the first ankle during the first session (see Figure 11.7). Thus, even though one ankle had adapted to the ice water, the second one has to go through its own adaptation, although this second adaptation is usually faster than the first (E16).

Wolf and Hardy (E107) reported that adaptation was partially specific to the temperature of the water. That is, if a body part was immersed in water of a certain temperature, reimmersion in water at the same or a higher

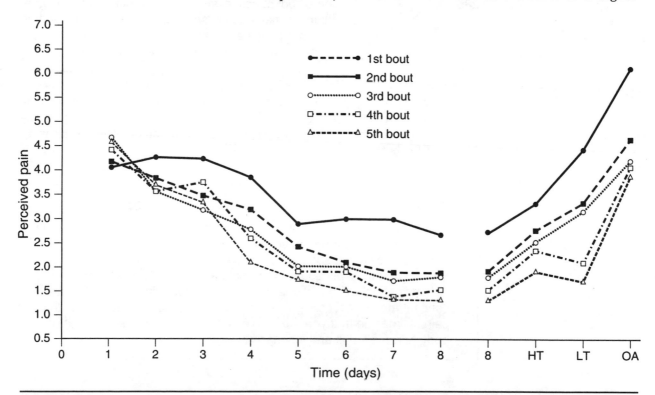

Figure 11.7 Perceived pain intensity during the five bouts of 10 days of simulated cryokinetics in normal subjects. Subjects underwent 8 days of cryokinetics with either 1 °C or 5 °C water (data combined). On days 9 and 10, treatments were to the opposite (left) ankle (OA) or to the right ankle at the opposite temperature (HT = higher temperature, habituated at 1 °C, then tested at 5 °C; LT = lower temperature, habituated at 5 °C, then tested at 1 °C). Scores during HT, LT, and OA indicate that the habituation during the first 8 days was specific to the body part treated.
Reprinted from Carmen and Knight (E16).

temperature did not evoke pain. Reimmersion in a lower temperature bath, however, resulted in the cycle of pain as usual, although its onset was a little delayed and its intensity reduced. We confirmed these conclusions, except our subjects who went to a higher temperature (1° to 5°C) had as much pain as those who went from 5° to 1°C (see Figure 11.7).

A fascinating study in this area was performed by LeBlanc and Potvin (E61). They had 16 male subjects immerse the left hand in 4°C water for 2.5 minutes twice a day for 19 days. Half the group performed mental arithmetic during immersion, the other half just immersed. The researchers pretested and post-tested all subjects' left hands with a cold pressor test, an arithmetic test, and a combined cold pressor and arithmetic test and also posttested them with the cold pressor test using the right hand. They demonstrated habituation (i.e., subjects could tolerate cold water longer), which was specific to the left hand as well as to the activity during immersion. That is, subjects who performed the arithmetic activity during immersion showed no habituation when tested with either the plain cold pressor or arithmetic tests, and those who immersed their hands without performing mental arithmetic showed no habituation when tested with either the plain arithmetic or the combined tests. Retesting 1 month later indicated that the habituation was gone.

There is much that we don't understand about habituation to cold-water immersion. This is illustrated by comparing the work of Ingersoll and Mangus (E40) with a study from our laboratory (E14). They reported no habituation among students who immersed their ankles in 1°C ice water for 21 minutes per day for 7 days (Figure 11.8). Subjects were in semi-isolation, could speak to no one, and were told to concentrate on the pain experience while filling out the McGill Pain Questionnaire every 3 minutes. Contrast this with the habituation that occurred under the somewhat similar circumstances illustrated in Figure 11.7. Both studies involved general students, ankles in a slush bucket, and the McGill Pain Questionnaire. Differences were that we talked to our subjects before and during the sessions to help them cope with the pain, tested them in groups of 5 to 10, encouraged them to socialize with one another, and immersed them 5 times daily (40 minutes total: 20 minutes initially and 4 times for 5 minutes interspersed with 3 minutes of exercise) as opposed to once daily for 21 minutes by Ingersoll and Mangus (E40). Which of these differences accounted for the habituation? We need further research.

Physiological or Psychological Adaptation?

The specificity of adaptation indicates that it is physiological rather than psychological. However, the quicker adaptation the second time indicates that a psychological component exists. Perhaps the second adaptation is much more tolerable because the person has gone through the adaptation previously and knows from experience the temporary nature of the pain. Another way of saying this is that more than one component of pain adapts. Clearly evaluative pain adapts, and probably affective pain does also. Does the sensory component adapt? And what about the cold sensation itself? According to LaBlanc and Potvin (E61), habituation applies to cold pain and not to the cold sensation itself.

Central and Local Adaptation

Cold adaptation results in central as well as local changes. Rats placed in a 2°C room for 6 hours per day for 20 days adapted so that brain norepinephrine turnover, uptake, and endogenous levels were all increased (E8).

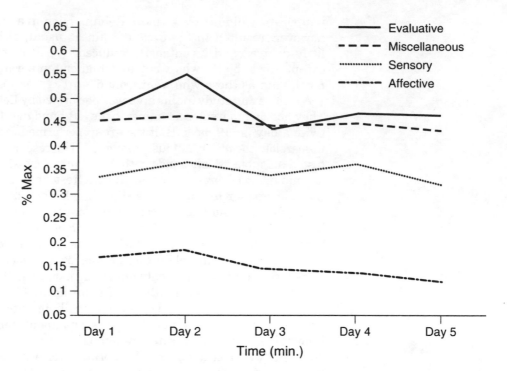

Figure 11.8 Little change occurred in any of the four areas of pain assessed by the McGill Pain Scale during 5 days of 21-minute immersion per day. Subjects were isolated during immersion and were instructed to concentrate on the pain. Reprinted from Ingersoll and Magus (E40).

LeBlanc et al. (E60) reported a decreased sympathetic response and an increased parasympathetic response, which, he explained, reduces the strain of cold exposure on the cardiovascular system, improves the peripheral circulation, and alleviates some of the disturbing psychological effects of this stress. The adapted person is then able to function more efficiently in the cold while being somewhat protected against cold injury.

USING COLD TO RELIEVE MUSCULOSKELETAL PAIN

The major reason for cryotherapy during rehabilitation is to relieve residual pain so that active exercise can begin more quickly and be more vigorous. One of the consequences of injury is neural inhibition of the neuromuscular system, which is manifest as a decrease in physical functions such as range of motion and muscular strength (see Figure 3.17, page 33). Pain-free, graded physical activity will overcome the neural inhibitions and restore normal function.

Although we cannot give a definitive explanation for how superficial cold decreases musculoskeletal pain, there is no question that it does. Here we define some pain relief terms and discuss theories and techniques of using cold to relieve pain originating from acute musculoskeletal injury.

Analgesia vs. Anesthesia

There are two general types of pain relief: analgesia and anesthesia. *Analgesia* derives from Greek roots meaning "without pain," *anesthesia* from the Greek for "without feeling" (J73). Both terms refer to a decrease in pain, but *anesthesia* additionally refers to a partial or total loss of other sensations (temperature, touch, etc.) as well (J73).

Irrespective of its Greek roots, *analgesia* does not mean total loss of pain. Rather it is defined as the absence of a normal sense of pain (J73).

Some have felt that local cold applications reduce pain through an anesthetic effect. Recent research, however, indicates that two-point discrimination and topognosis are unaffected by the short term (20-minute) cold applications (E38) usually used to relieve pain during cryokinetics. Thus, since some sensations are unaffected by the cold, cold-induced pain relief would have to be due to analgesia rather than anesthesia.

Hyperalgesia means excessive sensitivity to pain. The opposite, lessened sensitivity, is *hypoalgesia* (or *hypalgesia*). Ingersoll and Mangus (E40) recommended using hypalgesia rather than analgesia to refer to the pain relief caused by ice-water immersion, because such immersion results in decreased pain rather than total relief of pain. But based on the above definitions, either term is appropriate for describing the decreased pain of ice immersion.

HOW DOES COLD RELIEVE PAIN?

Unfortunately, we don't yet have a definite answer to the question of how cold relieves or reduces pain. Many theories have been proposed to explain the pain-relieving effects of cold:

- Cold decreases nervous transmission in pain fibers (A14, A15, A19, A30, A38, A39, A43, B18).
- Cold decreases excitability of free nerve endings (A15, A30).
- Cold reduces metabolism in tissue to relieve the deleterious effects of ischemia (B24).
- Cold causes asynchronous transmission in pain fibers (D13).
- Cold raises the pain threshold (A15, A30, A38, A40, E51).
- Cold acts as a counterirritant (A31, E24, E25, E72, E98).
- Cold causes a release of endorphins (B35).
- Cold inhibits spinal neurons (E45).

Some of these theories relate to vapo-coolant application, others to local hypothermia.

How Do Vapo-coolants Relieve Pain?

Klaus (E51) suggested that ethyl chloride spray raises the pain threshold, but later stated there was no adequate scientific explanation for the fact that surface anesthesia could lessen pain in deep structures (E50). Others (A28, E24, E25, E73, E99, E100) have attributed the success of vapo-coolants to counterirritation. This was explained by Ellis (E25), who claimed that the area of the central nervous system that received pain impulses was bombarded with such a barrage of cold impulses that the pain impulses were swamped and obliterated. Mennell (E73) went into more detail, explaining that the cold sensory impulses would arrive at the central nervous system faster than slower moving pain impulses and thereby make the central nervous system refractory to the pain impulses. Although he did not mention it, Mennell was explaining the essence of the gate control theory of Melzack and Wall (E72), which states that intense sensory stimulation can "close the gate" to, or block, transmissions at the spinal cord.

Counterirritation

Historically, *counterirritation*—relieving pain in one place by irritating another place—has been one of the most important methods available to the medical community for pain control. Gammon and Starr (E28) studied the effectiveness of a number of different counterirritants in relieving induced pain in human subjects, animals, and clinical patients. Hot-water bottles, ice packs, vibration, tactile sensation, electric muscle stimulation, and static electricity were all employed as counterirritants. The authors concluded that irrespective of the type of pain or counterirritant, temporary relief of pain occurred both after application and removal of the counterirritant. Intermittent application was more effective than continuous application. Neither circulatory changes nor pain fiber transmission changes were responsible for the pain relief. The authors concluded that a central sensory depression or inhibition was responsible for the decreased pain.

Travell and Rinzler (E101) measured the effects of 1-minute applications of ethyl chloride and ice-water immersion (12° to 20°C) on muscular endurance during ischemia. Ethyl chloride markedly reduced pain and resulted in greatly increased muscular activity. These effects were not evident during the cold-water applications, although the water may not have been cold enough.

Parsons and Goetzl (E81) studied the counterirritant effects of cold applied to the leg in reducing pain that has been induced in subjects using electrical stimulation of a tooth filling. A second application of ethyl chloride to the leg elevated the pain threshold in the tooth for over 2 hours. They felt that it was the pain induced by the ethyl chloride, rather than tissue cooling, that was responsible for the analgesia.

Pain Relief With Local Hypothermia

Lehman and de Lateur (A24) concluded that cold relieved pain by both direct and indirect effects. An elevation of the pain threshold occurs as a direct effect of decreased temperature of nerve fibers and receptors. Also, pain is indirectly relieved by removing the cause of pain (i.e., relieving conditions such as muscle spasm, spasticity, and swelling). Later in their review, however, the authors stated that cold could relieve pain through counterirritation, which they felt could be accounted for by the gate control theory (E72). Further evidence in favor of the gate control theory was supplied by Kamui (E45), who demonstrated that thermal stimuli may inhibit spinal cord neurons in the rat and cat, and Arendt-Nelson and Gotiebsen (E44), who reported that laser-induced pain was lowest when evoked from the dermatome to which cold was concurrently applied.

Raether (B35) mentioned work had been done at McGill University that indicated that ice applications stimulated endorphin release, thereby decreasing pain, but he did not elaborate.

A number of authors have written that cold relieves pain by blocking nervous transmissions of pain receptors or pain fibers (A15, A19, A31, A43, B18, E13). Stangel (E90) challenged this interpretation, explaining that although therapeutic applications of cold cause a decrease in nervous transmission, they do not cause a complete block. Intramuscular temperatures plateau at about 25°C (D84), but small fibers that carry pain continue to conduct at temperatures down to 0°C (A13). Stangel reasoned, therefore, that pain relief was due to counterirritation and not nerve blockade.

One would infer from Stangel's argument that she feels that pain must be totally blocked. Is it possible that, as a direct result of lowering tissue temperatures, the pain threshold is raised, thus partially blocking pain? Must we look only at ways of totally blocking pain? Discovering the answer to this question has great clinical significance.

Travell (E99) and Mennell (E73) both emphasized that the effectiveness of vapo-coolant sprays was compromised if the muscle mass was cooled. Counterirritants work better if applied intermittently. If pain is relieved only by counterirritation, and not by a direct effect, continuous applications of ice bags or immersion would be less effective in situations in which the chief aim was to control pain. More experimental work must be done in this area.

Cryoanalgesia

A relatively new technique known as cryoanalgesia, in which nerves are actually destroyed by freezing, needs to be mentioned briefly. Cryoanalgesia is a surgical technique that uses devices much colder than the ones used in sports medicine and physical therapy. I mention it here so that you will not confuse it with local cryotherapy.

Cryoanalgesia involves a cryosurgical probe whose tip is cooled to −60°C by circulating nitrous oxide gas (E7, E62, E64). The probe is applied to nerves for 1 minute, causing them to freeze. The nerve is allowed to thaw out and is then refrozen by application of the probe for another minute. Among 64 patients with pain from assorted pathology, cryoanalgesia produced pain relief for a median of 11 days (range 0 to 224 days) (E64). Comparisons among posthoracotomy patients treated with and without cryoanalgesia indicate less of a demand for postoperative analgesic medication among the cryoanalgesic group (E31, E44, E85).

Don't confuse cryoanalgesia with cold-induced pain relief.

PAIN REDUCTION WITH CRYOTHERAPY: CLINICAL USES

Cold applications have been used in a number of situations to relieve pain. Some of these are mentioned below and discussed in more detail in other chapters.

Rehabilitation

During rehabilitation of joint sprains, cold applications lessen pain so that active exercise can be initiated (see chapter 18). It is a common clinical impression that ice-water immersion is preferable to cold-pack application, but to my knowledge this point has not been adequately studied.

Cold is more effective than heat in lessening pain (E17, E66), but heat may be equally or more effective in decreasing dull aches. For example, athletes who sprain an ankle and delay getting professional help for a week or so usually progress through cryokinetics very quickly and are able to practice at near normal levels, but still have dull aching pain. My experience is that these athletes get more pain relief with heat applications than cold. The same is true with general aches and pains that athletes feel the morning after a vigorous game.

■ **WHEN TO USE COLD AND HEAT FOR REHABILITATION**
- Treat specific injuries with cold packs, but general aches and pain with a warm whirlpool or hot tub.
- In a subacute injury, if pain prevents normal range of motion or gait, use ice to facilitate exercise. If range of motion and gait are normal, use heat applications to relieve the dull aches.

Surgery

The effectiveness of cold in lessening surgical pain has been debated for years (see chapter 8). Allen and associates (H1, H13) used immersion and ice packs to provide total aesthesia for high risk amputee patients. Applications ranging from 1 hour for thin tissue to 5 hours for thicker tissue provided enough anesthesia that nothing else was required. In addition, the amount of pain medication needed postsurgically was reduced. Others (E20, H10, H38, H61) reported decreased need for pain medication with cryotherapy following surgery (see Table 8.1, p. 100).

Allen and associates (H1, H13) felt that immersion was superior to ice packs, which confirms our observations. Mennell (E72) preferred ice massage to ice packs for treating painful trigger points.

A majority of dental patients experienced at least 50% pain relief with massage of the *hoku* acupressure point (L14) of the ipsilateral hand with ice until the web space became numb or for 7 minutes (E69).

Induced Pain and Muscle Soreness

The effects of cryotherapy on experimentally induced muscle soreness have produced mixed results in experimental studies. Four studies (B6, D25, E23, E31) indicate that cryotherapy is effective in lessening pain associated with induced muscle soreness when 20 to 30 minutes of ice immersion is used; two studies (E35, E90) found that 15 minutes of ice massage is not effective in decreasing pain. The most obvious reasons for this difference are either the mode or length of application. (Besides the obvious time difference of 15 vs. 20 to 30 minutes, any single area received an intermittent application with ice massage as it passes back and forth). Other possible factors include the type of induced soreness and the fitness level of the subjects.

Carbajal and Nelson (B6) and Kato (E46) induced soreness in the arms of physical education students by having them pitch baseballs for speed and accuracy. Immediately after pitching, the subjects received some type of therapeutic intervention. Three days later the process was repeated. When subjects were treated with ice immersion for 20 minutes in 1° to 2°C water (B6, E46), or ice immersion (20 minutes) and static stretching (E46) immediately following pitching, their subsequent pitching performance improved. The authors attributed this to a decrease in pain. There was no statistical difference in Kato's study between ice immersion alone and combined ice immersion and static stretching.

Yackzan et al. (E110) induced pain in the elbow flexor muscles through eccentric contractions on an NK table. Subjects received 15 minutes of ice massage to the arm either immediately after exercise, 24 hours later, or 48 hours later. They were tested for pain and range of motion at 24, 48, and 72 hours following exercise. Neither pain (delayed muscle soreness) nor range of motion benefited from the ice massage treatment.

A fourth study that is somewhat related concerned the effects of ice immersion (15 minutes in 11° to 12°C water) and static stretching on muscle tension following induced muscle soreness of the triceps surae muscle group (D75). Electromyographic measurements 48 hours following exercise and treatment revealed decreased muscular tension in muscles treated by either ice immersion or static stretching, but no difference between the two treatments. But in a similar study (F29) subjects treated with cold packs and stretching relaxed more than those treated with hot packs and stretching. And myofascial pain and disfunction of the masticatory system were relieved more by cold packs and stretching than by reflex inhibition or nonintervention controls (E14).

Deneger and Perrin (E23) used eccentric elbow flexion to induce soreness into the nondominant arm of 40 female students. After 48 hours they applied crushed-ice packs and compression for 20 minutes. Pain decreased, and range of motion increased more in groups that were treated with cold, transcutaneous electrical nerve stimulation (TENS), and combined cold and TENS than in sham TENS and control. Isokinetic flexion and extension were not different between any groups.

Isabell et al. (E41) induced soreness in 22 male and female physical education students with concentric and eccentric elbow curls. They massaged the subjects with ice for 15 minutes at 0, 2, 4, 6, 24, 48, 72, and 96 hours following exercise. Pain, range of motion, isokinetic flexion, and isokinetic extension were no different between groups who were treated with ice, exercise, ice and exercise, or control.

Electrical Stimulation of Muscle and Nerves

A 2-minute ice massage to the quadriceps muscle prior to electrical stimulation increased the maximal voluntary contraction that the electrical stimulation elicited (E75). Since electrical stimulation was applied according to subjects' pain tolerance levels, the increased intensity of muscle stimulation with cold indicates that the cold application decreased pain in the subjects (healthy college-aged females). But since only the single 2-minute ice massage protocol was studied, we do not know if this is the optimal ice protocol to promote electrical stimulation. In a similar study, TENS applied for 10 minutes was also associated with an increase in electrically induced quadriceps torque (E104).

Ice massage was as effective as TENS in relieving chronic low back pain (E70). Patients who had habituated to TENS no longer obtained the desired pain relief. In such cases, ice massage provided pain relief. After a few sessions of ice massage, TENS was effective again.

Ethyl Chloride Spray

Kraus (E51, E52) has been credited with introducing the technique of relieving pain and muscle spasm by spraying the area with liquid ethyl chloride (E98). It's "surprising efficacy in [relieving] skeletal muscle spasm and other painful states" has been confirmed by a number of investigators (see E98 for references). However, the treatment apparently fell into disuse by the early 1960s. Ellis (E24, E25) believed that this discontinuance was due to the exquisite pain experienced by the patient as the skin thawed following freezing with ethyl chloride.

There appears to be a renewed interest in this technique, but with fluoromethane instead of ethyl chloride (E34, E78, E103). Fluoromethane is an inert gas that is not explosive, flammable, highly toxic, or a general anesthetic like ethyl chloride (E73). Also, it will not freeze the skin as ethyl chloride does (E73, E78). But it may not be environmentally safe.

Kraus (E50, E51) felt that the key to rehabilitation of musculoskeletal injuries was mobilization of the injured body part. Motion is often not possible, however, either because pain and muscle spasm are too intense or because the motion aggravates pain and muscle spasm. He felt that ethyl chloride was the most effective and easily applied physical modality to break the pain-spasm cycle and thereby allow active motion.

Travell (E99) used ethyl chloride for treating chronic conditions. She felt that any number of causes (including trauma, ischemia, fatigue, arthritis, and hysteria) could cause trigger points—localized areas of deep hypersensitivity—to develop in myofascial structures (E99, E102). Trigger points bombard the central nervous system with impulses, resulting in referred pain. Whenever a trigger point is stimulated by pressure, needling, extreme heat or cold, or motion that stretches the myofascial area, pain is elicited. Trigger points continue long after their precipitating cause has vanished and therefore can maintain pain cycles indefinitely. These pain cycles can often be permanently relieved by any one of a number of procedures applied directly to the trigger point, including ethyl chloride spray, procaine infiltration, dry needling, and sustained heavy pressure.

Note that all the authors cited here emphasized that the involved area must be stretched after spraying with ethyl chloride. The interruption of painful stimuli is not enough; the input of normal impulses must be fully reinstated (E29).

Halkovich et al. (E34) demonstrated that a combination of fluoromethane spray and static stretching is more effective in increasing hip flexion than static stretching alone in normal subjects. The fact that the technique was successful in subjects who were not suffering clinical pain indicates that vapo-coolant sprays must act in some way other than, or in addition to, relieving pain.

■ *EXERCISE WITH COOLING*

Exercise must be combined with cooling when you are attempting to relieve painful myofascia, trigger points, or muscle spasm.

SUMMARY

- Although pain has not been adequately defined nor objectively measured, we do know much about the interaction between cold and pain.
- Cold applications are capable of both causing pain and decreasing or eliminating pain, but when one or the other occurs is not certain.
- Cold-induced pain usually occurs during cold immersion, a technique employed during injury rehabilitation. Most people adapt to this pain, though, so it is not a serious threat to the clinical use of cold.

- There are many proven techniques to help people cope with cold-induced pain while adapting to it, such as concentrating on other things, discussing the adaptation, or thinking of the sensation as unusual rather than painful.
- The mechanism through which pain is decreased by cold has not yet been determined. Counterirritation or gating is part of the effect. Whether there is a direct effect due to decreased temperature in pain receptors and pain fibers remains to be determined.
- One way cold applications reduce pain is by reversing the pain-spasm-pain cycle, which occurs as a result of injury. Cold acts to reduce both pain and muscle spasm, as explained in the following chapter.

12

Reduction of Muscle Spasm With Cold Therapy

The clinical literature abounds with references to the efficacy of cold in reducing spasticity, increasing relaxation, leading to earlier mobilization, and promoting increased range of motion. (See chapter 1.) Figure 12.1 presents the commonly accepted relationships among these effects. These relationships apply to reversible muscle spasm secondary to acute musculoskeletal trauma (i.e., sprains, strains, and contusions), however, and not necessarily to all types of spasm or spasticity (F19, F22).

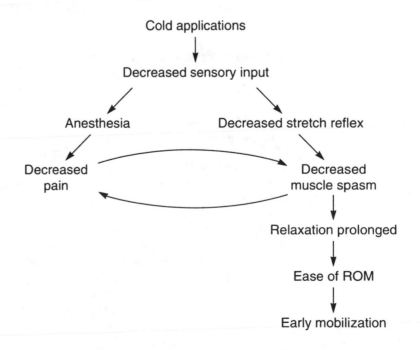

Figure 12.1 Commonly accepted relationship of cold application to pain, spasm, and mobilization (see text for exceptions).
Reprinted from Knight (A19).

Muscle spasm is any involuntary movement or muscular contraction (J73). It may be temporary in nature (i.e., lasting from a few seconds to a few days), or more permanent (i.e., lasting for months, years, or a lifetime). Permanent spasm can be constant (called tonus), or can alternate between muscle contraction and relaxation (called clonus). When muscle spasms are strong and painful they are called cramps. When they are caused by an upper neural lesion (an injury to the nerves of the central nervous system, the condition is known as spasticity (J73).

Spasm occurs because a constant stream of impulses bombard a muscle's motor nerve. These impulses come from one of two sources: the higher centers of the central nervous system, in which case the spasm is called alpha-mediated; or the muscle spindle, which is known as gamma-mediated. Gamma-mediated spasm is always temporary.

CLINICAL STUDIES

Using cold to reduce muscle spasm appears to have been introduced by Meade and Knott (see F27, F12). Their technique involved cold applications followed by passive and active exercise (F17, F18, F28, F30, F31). They speculated that the mechanism involved cold analgesia of peripheral sensory end organs that changed the balance of facilitatory-inhibitory influences playing on the anterior horn cell. Thus, resistance to stretching the muscle would be decreased.

Clinical research using ice massage (B10, B16, B25), cold packs (F2, F5, F20, F21, F38), Turkish towels dipped in ice water (F5, F8, F13, F16, F27), and cold-water immersion (D68, F2, F4, F26, F27, F32, F42) has demonstrated that cold applications do decrease muscle spasm due to multiple sclerosis (F2, F4, F5, F31, F34), cerebral vascular disease (F31, F46), spinal cord disorders (F3, F16, F20, F31, F32, F34), acute poliomyelitis (F5), acute musculoskeletal conditions (B10, B16, F11, F18, F25, F38), and delayed onset muscle soreness (DOMS; F29).

Cold applications cannot, however, be looked upon as a panacea for spasm relief. Although many authors have reported marked decrease in spasticity and clonus (see F34) after cold applications, some have also reported that 25% to 35% of their patients found no relief (F2, F4, F5, F21). Knutsson (F21) even reported that spasticity increased in some patients as a result of cold applications. Miglietta (F34) reported decreased clonus with cold-water immersions in all 15 (hemiplegic, quadriplegic, or multiple sclerosis) patients. Although the duration of each bout of clonus was unchanged, the frequency and amplitude of bouts was decreased. The longevity of the effects varies; some patients found relief for up to 24 hours (F31), some for 12 hours (F2, F34); but for some relief was not as long lasting. Boynton et al. (F4) reported that even though some of their patients found no change in level of ambulation, the patients did report feeling more relaxed. In a study of 117 patients with low back pain, Landen (E57) reported that hot packs and flexion exercise were more effective in acute cases (those with onset of less than 48 hours), whereas cold packs and flexion exercise were more effective in chronic cases (those with onset of 14 days or more).

Miglietta (E33) studied surface and deep temperature changes, changes in triceps-surae duration of twitch contraction, half-relaxation time, and clonus relief in 40 spastic patients (30 with hemiplegia, 5 with paraplegia, and 5 with multiple sclerosis) following leg immersion in 7°C water for 10, 20, and 30 minutes. Clonus frequency decreased and half-relaxation time increased progressively with increasing duration of cold exposure, but the two variables were not correlated. There was no relationship between clonus presence, absence, or return and the duration of the twitch contraction. In some patients, clonus was abolished before any change occurred in twitch contraction; in the 5 patients in which clonus was unchanged, average half-relaxation time was almost as long as in the entire population. Miglietta concluded that clonus relief was due to a direct effect of cold on muscle spindle excitability.

Knutsson (F19) believed that the variable effects of cold on spasm may be due in part to a bimodal action and in part to differences in types of spasm. This assumption was based on a number of observations: Local cooling depresses muscle spindle sensitivity and therefore gamma-mediated spasm (F22, F24); alpha-motoneurons, however, become facilitated (E23, F44), so alpha-mediated spasticity will either be unresponsive to cold (F21, F22) or increased by it (F21, F45).

MECHANISM OF SPASM RELIEF

Relieving muscle spasm with cryotherapy is another area where technique leads theory. Efforts to provide a theoretical explanation for clinical success have lead to three hypotheses: (a) decreased sensory input, (b) a reflex mechanism, and (c) breaking of the pain-spasm-pain cycle. Each will be discussed.

Figure 12.1 summarizes the common explanation for the role of cold in decreasing muscle spasm, namely, that cold applications cause decreased sensory input, which leads to reduced muscle spasm (A11, A16, A18, A39). A closer look at the evidence, however, suggests this may not be the case. The quickness with which cold causes reflex responses to decrease (F25, F51); the fact that cooling a skin flap without cooling the muscle causes a decrease in the tonic stretch reflexes of the underlying muscle (F50, chapter 11); and the work of Hunt (D48), who demonstrated that sympathetic stimu lation causes a significant decrease in muscle spindle afferent discharge during stretching, indicate that decreased muscle spasm during cryotherapy may be due to a reflex mechanism rather than the direct effect of decreasing the sensory input. Further research must be conducted before a definitive explanation can be given.

Clinicians must also recognize that cold applications increase stiffness within muscle and associated connective tissue (see chapter 13). In a patient who is suffering gamma-spasticity, the net result of cold applications will be an increase in range of motion because the decrease in spasticity will be much greater than the increase in tissue stiffness. In a normal person, however, or in a person suffering alpha-spasticity, the net effect of cold applications will be to temporarily decrease range of motion.

Pain-Spasm-Pain Cycle

Kraus (E49) and others (C16, E5, E102) have explained that cold decreases spasm by breaking the *pain-spasm-pain cycle*. In this cycle, pain originating anywhere in the sensory-motor chain leads to reflex muscular spasm and locking of joints (E49). Compression from the muscle spasm results in additional pain, and vicious cycle ensues. An excitatory state is created in which pain is provoked by trivial stimuli (E5). Once the cycle begins, it is easily perpetuated and often continues after the initial painful stimulus has ceased (E5, E15). Elimination of the pain at any point in the chain results in the breaking of the chain and allows the muscle to relax (E49, E82). The excitatory state must then be reduced. Cold applications are very effective for doing this, if combined with graded exercise.

Peppard (personal communication), using the terminology of the gate control theory (E72), explains this as "resetting of central biasing." In simplistic terms, central bias refers to impulses that higher centers are constantly sending to the body to establish the resting state of the body. Pain and injury cause this central bias to change and, in some cases, cause muscle spasm. Often the pain-spasm-pain cycle becomes so firmly established that pain relief by itself does not reset central biasing; it must be combined with graded exercise. The cryostretch technique (chapter 19) is an example of this combination. Kraus (E49) stated that cold application without exercise does as much good as surgery with anesthesia but no cutting.

SUMMARY

- Muscle spasm is any involuntary movement or muscular contraction (J73). It may be temporary or permanent (tonic or clonic) and may be alpha- or gamma-mediated. Gamma-mediated spasm is always temporary.
- Strong and painful spasms are called cramps.
- Techniques of relieving muscle spasm with cryotherapy are much more established than the theoretical rationale behind their success.
- The three most common explanations for decreasing muscle spasm include (a) decreased sensory input, (b) a reflex mechanism, and (c) breaking of the pain-spasm-pain cycle.
- The decreased sensory input theory stems from the decrease in conduction velocity of sensory and motor nerves caused by cooling and the subsequent decrease in motor activity.
- The reflex theory is based on several facts: (a) Many motor nerves are too deep to be directly cooled by the time the cold effects its reflexes, (b) motor activity decreases after cooling a skin flap, (c) motor spindle activity decreases after cooling, and (d) muscle spindle discharge decreases by sympathetic stimulation.
- Decreasing spasm often requires both cryotherapy and active graded exercise (such as cryostretch), which together reset central biasing.

13

Tissue and Joint Stiffness

Cooling normal muscle, connective tissue, and joints causes them to become more stiff (or less elastic) and resistant to movement. Thus subsequent activity feels awkward and unnatural. Fine motor tasks are hindered, but gross motor skills are not. Also, very sudden or explosive activity could result in tissue tearing. Muscle stiffness occurs secondary to injury and exhaustive exercise; both heat and cold applications are used to relieve thse symptoms.

CONNECTIVE TISSUE

Connective tissue stiffness increases and its extensibility decreases as temperature decreases (A13, F14, F27, F48, F49, J45). Apparently the mechanisms for this have not yet been studied, but the ramifications are clear.

Attempts to forcibly extend cooled tissues may result in tears in connective tissue. Although combined cooling and stretching is effective for decreasing muscle spasm (see chapter 18), it is detrimental for lengthening connective tissue. Even mild stretching, if the tissue is extended to near its maximal length, will cause cooled tissue to tear (J66). Connective tissue must be warmed before it is stretched (see "Stretching Connective Tissue" in chapter 21).

MUSCLE STIFFNESS

There are two causes of muscle stiffness, one is mechanical and the other is neurological. Muscle spasm is neurological in origin; a constant low grade muscle contraction, mediated through the nervous system, and involving both gamma and alpha motor neurons. Cold applications help decrease gamma spasm but have little affect on alpha spasm (see chapter 12).

Mechanical muscle stiffness results from increased muscle fiber viscosity as muscle temperature decreases (C18, F2, F10, F32, F36, F37). Muscle stiffness impaires manual dexterity (F37), but doesn't seem to affect whole body agility (E27, E48).

JOINT STIFFNESS

Joint stiffness increases with decreasing temperatures (A24, A27, D16, F1, F10, F13, F14, F32, F47-49). This is due to a number of concomitant and complex changes, including impaired function of muscles that surround the joint, decreased connective tissue elasticity, and increased viscosity of synovial fluid in the joint (F15).

At normal temperature, the joint capsule connective tissue and muscles are the major factors in joint stiffness in the intact wrist of a cat, which is similar to the human metacarpophalangeal joint (F15). The joint capsule accounts for 47% of the total midrange joint stiffness, muscles for 41%, tendons for 10%, and skin for 2%. Tendons accounted for a greater percent of the total during motion at the extremes of the range of motion. Synovial fluid viscosity has little effect on joint stiffness at normothermia; in either the cat or human (F15).

Synovial fluid viscosity increases during joint cooling (A13, A27, C9, F10, F13, F14, F26, F47). Hunter et al. (F13) observed that as joint temperature decreased, resistance to movement increased and the maximal speed at which the joint could be moved was decreased. They attributed both of these effects to increased viscosity of the synovial fluid. Wright and Johns (F52), on the other hand, reported that elastic stiffness was increased throughout a large part of flexion range of motion during and following cold applications to the hands of normal subjects. Others (F15) claim muscle and joint tissues are inseparably involved in joint stiffness. Further research is needed to determine the relative contribution of increased synovial fluid viscosity to joint stiffness.

MANUAL DEXTERITY

Both finger and hand dexterity decrease with cooling (C18, F8-F10, F13, F37), and are caused by impairment of both extrinsic and intrinsic hand muscles. This decrease is due to local cooling of the arm and hand, and is independent of the core temp (A13, F9, F13).

LeBlanc (F26) measured performance of two tasks involving different degrees of finger dexterity following three different cooling situations: finger only immersed, hand and finger immersed, arm only immersed. The simple task performance decreased approximately 19%, 9%, and 2% after cooling of the forearm, hand, and finger, respectively; the more complex task decreased 16%, 25%, and 18%, respectively.

Fox (F8) measured grip strength and a standardized typing task before and after 30 minutes of immersion at nine different temperatures between 10° and 42°C. The time required to complete the typing task began to increase at temperatures below 34°C, with the greatest changes between 22° and 14°C. Grip strength did not decrease until the 22° to 18°C increment. Licht (A27) interpreted these data as meaning that the loss of dexterity was due to factors other than a loss of muscle power. He may be right, but note that the rate of loss in typing performance became greater as muscle power decreased.

MANUAL PERFORMANCE

Cold causes reduced dexterity and reduced sensitivity (E26, F29, F40, F43, I38), which together act to decrease manual performance. The reduction in sensitivity and/or manual performance seems to occur most clearly between 15°C and 20°C (F29, F40, F43, I38) and coincides with the sensations of slightly painful and uncomfortably cool (E35). Cold's influence on sensitivity is moderated by sensory integration of input from all parts of the body, and to heat input from the unexposed parts to the exposed parts caused by blood flow and heat conduction (E26).

CRYOTHERAPY DURING SPORTS ACTIVITIES

Cryotherapeutic treatments immediately prior to or during sports activities have been discouraged because of the possible detrimental effects of decreased temperature on the performance and because of fear that the activity would tear the cooled tissue. Since manual dexterity is decreased by cooling (C18, F8-10, F13), it is reasonable to assume that fine motor sports skills such as shooting a basketball and batting a baseball would be adversely affected by muscle or joint cooling. In the absence of specific evidence on this point, clinicians should follow the assumption.

The effect of cooling on gross motor skills is unsettled. It is logical to assume that increased muscle and joint stiffness would adversely affect gross motor skills. In addition, strength is decreased by cooling the muscles; there are reports of decreased isometric force production (D13, D16, D50, F32), decreased isokinetic force production (F39, H42), no change in isokinetic force production (D17), and decreased ground reaction force during a two legged jump (F7) with cooled muscles. And it requires more force to produce passive movement in a cooled cat joint (F14). On the other hand, ankle (E27, E48) and calf (E48) cooling have no effect on timed agility tests (shuttle run, carioca, cocontraction). Perhaps the body compensates for decreased force production with increased motor unit recruitment (F13). Neural activation in single motor units increases with cooling (D14, D103, F32). Further research is needed to sort out this puzzling situation.

In uninjured subjects, heat applications, mild activity, and a combination of heat applications and mild activity are more effective than cold applications in increasing range of motion in the wrist, elbow, and ankle (F41). There is no difference, however, in their effects on knee flexibility.

MUSCLE AND JOINT STIFFNESS AS A SYMPTOM

Muscle and joint stiffness occur secondary to injury and exhaustive exercise. Research on induced muscle soreness indicates that ice immersion leads to decreased muscle tension (as measured by EMG; D24) and increased physical performance (throwing a baseball; B7, E46) while ice massage has no effect on pain and range of motion (E50; see chapter 12).

My clinical impression is that general body soreness, secondary to exhaustive exercise responds well to ice applications immediately after the activity and warm baths and mild exercise the next day.

SUMMARY

- Connective tissue and muscle stiffness increased and their extensibility decreases as temperature decreases.
- Attempts to forcibly extend cooled tissues may result in tears in connective tissue.
- Connective tissue must be warmed before it is stretched (see "Stretching Connective Tissue" in chapter 21).
- Muscle stiffness increases when cooled because of increased muscle fiber viscosity. This results in impaired manual dexterity but has no effect on whole body agility.
- Don't confuse muscle stiffness with muscle spasm. Muscle stiffness is mechanical in origin, spasm is neurological in origin.
- Joint stiffness increases with decreasing temperatures due to numerous changes, including increased synovial fluid viscosity in the joint, and increased muscle and decreased connective tissue stiffness.
- Both finger and hand dexterity decrease with cooling, and are caused by impairment of both extrinsic and intrinsic hand muscles.
- Although there is no direct evidence on the point, it is reasonable to assume that fine motor sports skills would be adversely affected by muscle or joint cooling.
- The effect of cooling on gross motor skills is unsettled. Force is decreased but agility activities are not.
- A combination of heat applications and mild activity are best for treating general body stiffness due to exhaustive exercise.
- Ice immersion leads to decreased muscle tension (as measured by EMG) and increased physical performance (throwing a baseball) following induced muscle soreness.
- Treat general body soreness, secondary to exhaustive exercise, with ice applications immediately after the activity and warm baths and mild exercise the next day.

14

Problems, Precautions, and Contraindications in Cold Therapy

Cryotherapy, like other methods of physical therapy, is not without problems. Although problems are rare (A22, B27, H36), they do occur. On the other hand, fear of problems (such as frostbite and neuropathy) causes some clinicians to be too conservative in their use of cryotherapy, with the result that their patients do not receive its full benefits. Also, fear of possible problems from cryotherapy has resulted in a number of contraindications and precautions such as "Do not apply ice packs directly to the skin." Most of these, however, are purely theoretical and lack any scientific basis (B24).

This chapter includes discussions of the pathophysiology relating to many problems that occur during cryotherapy and culminates with a list of contraindications and precautions to the therapeutic application of cold. My intent is to provide you with the necessary information concerning the problems associated with cryotherapy so that you can make proper decisions concerning when and how to use cryotherapy. You should be neither so liberal that you cause a patient injury, nor so conservative that your patients receive less than maximal benefits from cryotherapy. (Concerning the theoretical background on cold-induced pain, see chapter 11.)

This chapter begins with a discussion of frostbite and associated tissue damage, including mechanisms, temperature–time interactions that cause frostbite, tissue damage that occurs at temperatures above freezing, and how and why frostbite might occur during sports medicine cryotherapy. I discuss frostbite first because it is the most talked about problem with cryotherapy.

The chapter deals next with how pressure, such as from elastic wraps, combined with cryotherapy occasionally results in transient (reversible) nerve palsy. This is a very minor problem, but nevertheless most cases can be avoided.

Some people are hypersensitive or allergic to cold. The various manifestations of cold hypersensitivity and how to deal with it are briefly discussed.

Vasospastic disorders are conditions in which the blood vessels of the extremities do not dilate properly; Raynaud's disease, livedo reticularis, and acrocyanosis are examples.

The last sections of the chapter include lists of specific contraindications and precautions to therapeutic application of cold.

FROSTBITE AND RELATED CONDITIONS

Many clinicians fear frostbite from direct application of ice packs to the skin and therefore advocate placing a towel between the ice packs and the skin. (See chapter 7 for references and further discussion.) This policy is overly conservative. Short-term (≤ 1-hour) applications of ice packs will not cause frostbite. There is evidence, however, that either a long-term (24- to 72-hour) continuous application of ice packs (H2, I51) or an application of some cold-gel packs (unpublished observations) can result in frostbite.

What Is Frostbite?

Frostbite is the localized freezing of tissue (I45, J73); some classify frostbite as either superficial or deep, depending on the depth to which tissues are frozen (I35). (Some clinicians consider frostnip—prefreezing symptoms—as a form of frostbite because some nonfreezing cold injuries result in the same tissue damage, signs, and symptoms as freezing injury does [I37].) One classification of cold injury uses the burn classification system (Table 14.1)—that is, the depth of tissue involved (G67, J79).

Frostnip

Frostnip, also called incipient (or beginning) frostbite (I1, J56), is characterized by the symptoms that occur prior to the freezing of the skin. It usually occurs in the face, hands, and cheeks and comes on slowly in persons exposed to extreme temperatures, such as those active in the out-of-doors during severe winter weather. Frostnip causes the skin to blanch and is characterized by a tingling or burning sensation (I64), which eventually turns to numbness (I1). Frostnip can easily be reversed by warming the affected body part (I62).

Table 14.1 Classification of Cold Injuries According to Degree of Tissue Damage				
Classification	**First degree**	**Second degree**	**Third degree**	**Fourth degree**
Tissue damage	Erythema and swelling	Blister formation, but with intact appendages	Damage to skin and subcutaneous tissue (also called full thickness)	Muscle and bone involvement with loss of a body part
Examples (other types)	Frostnip Chilblains Immersion/ trench foot Urticaria	Superficial frostbite	Deep frostbite	Deep frostbite

Superficial Frostbite

Superficial frostbite is the freezing of skin and subcutaneous tissues (I1, I62) and usually results when frostnip is left untreated. The skin can tolerate being frozen for 4 to 7 minutes without experiencing injury other than slight peeling of the superficial epithelial skin layer, as occurs after a light sunburn (I25, I64). Longer freezing, however, causes problems once the skin is rewarmed.

Blue or purple spots or streaks appear in the skin rewarmed after freezing for longer than 7 minutes. Initially the area is numb, but this gives way to a stinging or burning sensation and to severe itching (H1, I62), which may last for several weeks (I62). The area becomes swollen. Blisters may form and ulcerate (Figure 14.1) but usually dry up and become hard and black within 2 weeks (I62, J73). Whether or not blisters form, the skin peels. The area will remain red and tender, be extremely sensitive to cold, and perspire abnormally for months or years after (I62). There is usually no permanent loss of tissue.

Deep Frostbite

Deep frostbite involves frozen blood vessels and muscle in addition to frozen skin and subcutaneous tissues. The symptoms are much like those of superficial frostbite, only more severe. The blisters are larger and the entire foot or hand may be swollen. In addition to the aching and throbbing, shooting pains are experienced (I62). In extreme cases, when tissue is not rewarmed quickly enough, permanent loss of muscle tissue occurs; the skin does not become red and blistered after thawing, but turns grey and remains cold (I62). In about 2 weeks it turns black. The rest of the limb becomes either black, dry, and shriveled (up to the line of demarcation with good flesh) or wet, soft, and inflamed, and extremely painful. More tissue will be lost in the latter case than in the former (I62).

Immersion Foot and Trench Foot

Immersion foot results from prolonged exposure (days or weeks) to cold or cold water in ambient temperatures above freezing (I35). Mild cases result

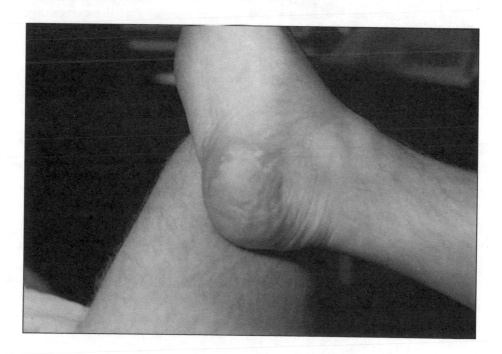

Figure 14.1 Superficial frostbite on the heel of a student following a 30-minute application of an Ice Down™ pack. The blister formed overnight, was protected, reabsorbed, and peeled 10 to 14 days later.

in edema, hyperemia, and transitory anesthesia. There usually is no permanent damage from mild immersion foot. Following severe cases, however, patients experience years of pain, numbness, and muscular weakness. Gangrene can, but usually does not, occur (I34, I45).

Trench foot is the same as immersion foot, except it occurs as a result of prolonged exposure to damp conditions (as opposed to water) such as those experienced by soldiers in foxholes (I35, I59).

Chilblain

Chilblain (or perniosis) is an inflammatory condition of the feet, toes, fingers, or ears caused by mild frostbite (J73) or above-freezing temperatures (I45). The involved skin becomes reddish purple and swollen and in persistent cases may smart, burn, or itch, especially during rewarming. Using the above classification, chilblain would probably include some cases of frostnip and the milder cases of superficial frostbite. Chilblains usually resolve in 1 to 3 weeks (I45) and do not result in permanent damage.

Mechanism of Frostbite

A combination of factors, listed next, interact to cause tissue damage during frostbite (I1). The first two factors are direct effects of and occur during freezing; the third is an indirect effect that follows freezing and thawing (I1, I19, I39, I52).

1. Direct cellular damage due to ice crystallization
2. Intracellular molecular damage due to dehydration of cells as water moves out of the cell to form extracellular ice crystals
3. Vascular damage

Ice crystals many times the size of individual cells develop in the intracellular spaces during tissue freezing (I34). Although some credit this occurrence as the cause of injury (I47-49), Meryman (I36) claimed that irreversible injury does not occur as long as the percentage of water frozen out of the cell does not exceed a critical amount. The critical factor in freezing injury is related to tissue cell dehydration, but the exact mechanism is still debated (G95, I1, I8, I14, I19, I34, I47, I48).

Vascular damage and microcirculatory failure occur within minutes after thawing of frozen tissue (I4, I16, I22, I39). Mundth (I39) described the sequence of events following thawing as follows:

1. Blood flow is reestablished within seconds after thawing.
2. Numerous white emboli (platelet clumps) appear in the blood stream within minutes.
3. Red cells aggregate; thus, few red cells circulate through the capillaries.
4. Platelets aggregate to form white thrombi at the venular bifurcations.
5. Circulating platelet emboli adhere to the thrombi.
6. The thrombi occlude vessels, often totally within 10 minutes.
7. Complete stasis (no blood flow) occurs.
8. The packed red cells lose their morphological identity, giving the vessel an appearance of being packed with a homogenous pink material.
9. Nearly complete thrombosis of all precapillary arterioles, capillaries and postcapillary venules occurs within 1 hour. Blood flow is slow and irregular through the larger arterioles and venules (see also I4 and I63).

It is failure of the local circulation that is responsible for tissue loss (I28, I29, I55). With no circulation, the tissue becomes hypoxic and dies. Normal wound healing follows (I4).

Frostbite Temperature

At what temperature does tissue damage occur? There appears to be a great deal of confusion on this point (A27, E55, I16) because temperature is not the only factor involved (I14, I19). The length of application, body part involved, method of cooling, humidity, external compression, and skin pigmentation all play a role. The amount of heat loss is more important than the length of application and temperature (I19), although heat loss is related to both these factors (see chapter 5).

Lewis and Love (I30) could not freeze forearm skin at skin temperatures above –2.2°C using a metal bar. In many of their experiments supercooling occurred, during which the skin did not freeze even though its temperature was much lower than freezing. During one 4.5-minute application, the skin cooled to –17.1°C without freezing; in another case an arm was supercooled to –4.5°C with a cold air current and remained at that temperature for over 30 minutes without freezing. When the skin is cooled by contact with a cold object it freezes at higher temperatures than when it is cooled by exposure to cold air (E35), since contact results in greater heat loss (I19).

Kreyberg (I27) stated that mammalian tissue could freeze solid and then thaw out without gross damage; however, if cooled to somewhere between –10° and –20°C, tissue would always be destroyed. A literature review by Gage (I16) indicated that –20°C is lethal for cells and is therefore the ideal temperature for cryosurgical tissue destruction. The author indicated, however, that in some cases –20°C was not adequate to cause tissue destruction. Wilson and Goldman (I64) demonstrated that the fingers very often did not freeze when exposed to air temperatures of –10° to –15°C for periods of 45 to 60 minutes. They concluded that due to supercooling and cold-induced vasodilation (CIVD) during the supercooled state, there is no well-defined value of the wind-chill index below which freezing routinely occurs. Further research by these authors (I37, I64) confirmed these results and led them to conclude that the factors that determine whether freezing or supercooling occurs at a given temperature remained to be discovered.

There is an inverse relationship between intensity of cold and duration of exposure (I9). The longer the cold is applied, the higher the temperature that causes frostbite. Fuhrman (I15) found that temperature and time of exposure were also determining factors in the extent to which oxygen consumption was impaired in rat tissues rewarmed after being cooled.

Black people are more susceptible to frostbite than whites. In guinea pigs, pigmented skin is damaged more by cold than nonpigmented skin (I50).

Establishing a specific temperature at which frostbite occurs is also complicated because different cells freeze at different temperatures (see I16 for references). During a single experiment with rabbits the duration of exposure required for freezing varied markedly from one animal to another, from one hind foot to another in the same animal, and from toe to toe on the same foot (I29).

Nonfreezing-Cold Damage

Tissues do not have to freeze to undergo damage similar to that which occurs with frostbite. Individually caged mice kept at 3° to 10°C for periods of over 7 days developed gangrene in their ears (I29). These injuries developed in five stages:

1. Generalized vasoconstriction, beginning within minutes after exposure, led to vascular insufficiency, which began to develop after a few hours.
2. Venular dilation occured after 1 day of exposure (segmental arteriolar spasm persisted).
3. Segmental venular leakage, which appeared after 2 to 4 days, was usually most prominent at the sites where venular dilation was maximal.
4. Venular-capillary erythrostasis, which usually began after 3 days, led to subsequent necrosis of the vessels in which it occurred.
5. Arteriolar-venular shunting: After 6 to 8 days, the venous portions of the shunting channels began to undergo necrosis. The spread of necrosis correlated with the spread of microcirculatory insufficiency, which was not correlated to the areas of greatest exposure to the cold.

Proulx (I51) reported a case of what he called "Southern California frostbite" in a man who had treated a broken great toe with continuous applications of ice packs for 3 days. The toe was swollen, with purplish discoloration and vesicle formation. Sensation was intact. Healing was uneventful and complete. Edholm et al. (I11) reported redness and swelling in the forearm of a subject 20 hours after the forearm was immersed in a −1.0° to 9°C water bath for 1 hour. Two other subjects suffered the same symptoms after 40 minutes of immersion in 6°C water. On previous days these subjects had been subjected to immersion of 18°, 12°, and 9°C water baths. An additional 3 subjects suffered no ill effects following this regimen, even after a further immersion of 3°C. The authors felt the degree of injury was minor and was not chilblain or frostbite. It may have been urticaria (see later in this chapter).

The minor injury reported by Edholm et al. (I11) is in contrast to research from our laboratory. In one study (C43), 12 subjects suffered no ill effects following 45 minutes of immersion in water at 15°, 10°, 5°, and 1°C (in a randomized order on separate days). During other research, single bouts of immersion in 0° to 2°C water for 35 to 45 minutes did not result in injury to the ankle (C42, C44, C45), finger (D42, D45), or forearm (C44, C45, C60). The lowest average skin temperature obtained during this work was 2.8°C, in the finger (D45). It appears, therefore, that the critical factor in causing tissue damage during cryotherapy as used in sports and physical medicine is the length of application.

Frostbite and Sports Medicine

Most of the current cryotherapy techniques are probably not cold enough to cause tissue damage unless they are used continuously for 1 hour or more or are combined with pressure. Be extremely careful, however, with gel packs from a freezer. These are much colder than crushed-ice packs prepared from an ice machine and can cause superficial frostbite if applied under an elastic wrap.

What to Do if Frostbite Occurs

If frostbite occurs from your application of cold packs, it will probably be superficial. There will probably be nothing more than a red spot or a welt when you remove the cold pack, but a blister will develop within a few hours. Do not massage the skin (I46, J73). Often the damage is not as great as it seems to be. Do not complicate matters by using overly aggressive treatment such as popping the blister or scrubbing the wound (I21, I45, J79). Instead, follow these procedures:

■ *WHAT TO DO WHEN FROSTBITE OCCURS*

If the blister is intact: Place a large sterile gauze pad over it and secure it with an elastic wrap, snug but not tight. Alter the activity of the patient sufficiently to protect the blister from being ripped open. The pressure from the bandage will cause the fluid in the blister to be reabsorbed, and the skin over the tissue will keep the tissue from drying out and dying. In time new skin will grow under the blister and the old skin will shrivel and peel off. Allow this to occur naturally.

If the blister pops: Keep the skin in place and cover it with salve and a bandage. Do not scrub the wound; seemingly necrotic skin often heals normally (I21, I45, J79). Keep the area covered 24 hours a day with the salve or new skin so that it does not dry out.

■ *WHAT NOT TO DO IF FROSTBITE OCCURS*

Do not pop a cold blister or debrile or scrub the wound. Such activities are overly aggressive and will add to the injury. Cover the area with an elastic wrap and the blister will reabsorb.

PRESSURE-RELATED NERVE PALSY

There are five reports of nerve palsy in athletes using cryotherapy, including the initial report by Drez et al. in 1981 (I6, I20, I32, I46). (Two additional reports have appeared [I2, I7] but they were duplicate publication of a previous report [I32].) These reports comprise 14 cases of nerve palsy (Table 14.2). Ten cases involved the lateral fibular head, and in six the ice pack was held on with an elastic wrap. There was no recurrence in four of the five reported by Drez et al. (I10) when application position was changed. All 14 patients recovered completely, some within 1 to 3 hours, others after 6 or 7 months.

How much did compression have to do with these instances of palsy? At first Drez et al. (I10) thought that compression of the nerve with an elastic bandage was the cause, but they discredited this theory upon noticing that reapplication of the ice pack after the symptoms had disappeared caused recurrence of the symptoms.

Although I do not necessarily disagree with the conclusion that ice was the cause of the palsy, research from our laboratory causes me to question it. In a study on the effects of various lengths of ice-pack application (10 to 60 minutes), a subject suffered nerve palsy during a session in which ice was applied to the lateral ankle for 10 minutes (H47). An elastic wrap was applied to the ankle for 190 minutes (during the 10-minute ice-pack application and for 180 minutes after application). We concluded that pressure was the cause of the palsy because the subject completed—without recurrent ill effects—three additional sessions during the next week in which ice packs were applied for 45, 20, and 30 minutes.

Others have also reported palsy occurring because of pressure (I9). It is hypothesized to result from decreased blood flow, and therefore ischemia,

Table 14.2   Summary of Nerve Palsy Cases Reported in the Literature

Authors	Athlete	Injury	Duration of application	Other therapy	Immediate symptoms	Subsequent symptoms	Time to resolution
Drez et al. (1981)	26 y FB	L knee	?	?	Weak toe extensor and dorsiflexor muscles	Drop foot	36 hours
	15 y FB	B knee	IB-2 hr	Elastic wrap	No dorsiflexion	Axonomosis of peroneal nerve	19 months
	31 y FB	L knee	20 to 30 min	?	Weak toe extensor and dorsiflexor muscles		3 days
	26 y FB	Knee	?	?		No problems with ice on inner side of elbow	4 days
	16 yr bb	Elbow	?	?			
Parker et al. (1983)	15 yr FB	Knee	IB-2 hr	?	Anesthesia over anteriolateral tibial muscle and dorsum of foot	Decreased nerve conduction, superficial and deep peroneal nerve	5 weeks
Collins et al. (1986)	26 y thin	L Knee	IB-1 hr twice	None	Drop foot	Same	
Green et al. (1989)	18 y college FB	L knee	IB-20 min	Elastic wrap	Heaviness in lower leg Common peroneal nerve axon damage	No dorsiflex or evert foot	7 months +
Malone et al. (1992)	22 y FB	1 knee	IB-30	Elastic wrap			6 months
	24 y BB	1 knee	IB-30/60	Elastic wrap			6 months
		hip	IB-30/60	Elastic wrap			6 months
	21 y T	ASIS	IB-15/20	None			4 days
	20 y FB	Shoulder	IM-10	None			14-21 days
	21 y FB	1 knee	IB-30	Elastic wrap			1 hour
Bassett et al. (1992)	Same as Malone et al.						
Covington/ Bassett (1993)	Same as Malone et al.						

to the nerve (I12). Lee and Warren (H36) felt that many cold injuries occurred because of pressure-induced ischemia, particularly when combined with cold-pack application. Perhaps cold-induced vasoconstriction (J74) aggravates the pressure-induced ischemia. On the other hand, the decreased metabolism of the nerve due to cold application may allow it to endure a greater length of pressure-induced ischemia. More information is needed before definite conclusions about the effects of cold on palsy can be made.

Possible mechanisms for nerve palsy include direct injury to the nodal membrane, endoneural edema, ischemia, suspension of axioplasmic transport, or a combination of these (I42). Sunderland (I60) concluded the following with regard to cold and nerve palsy:

- Motor functions succumb before and to a greater degree than sensory functions.
- Different sensory modalities do not fail simultaneously or in a predictable fashion.
- Function is restored rapidly as recovery from cooling takes place if no necrosis has occurred. Sensory function generally returns before motor function.
- There are individual differences in resistance of nerves to cold injury.
- Nerves can tolerate cooling to 10°C (50°F).
- Cold can disturb function at temperatures above freezing, with total motor and sensory functional loss occurring between 0° and 5°C (32° and 41°F).

Incidence of Nerve Palsy

Although cold does contribute to nerve palsy, the problems must be put into perspective. A rough, very conservative estimate is that problems occur in less than 0.001% of the instances in which cold packs are used; there are few treatments in medicine that enjoy such a low failure rate. This estimate is based on the number of plastic bags we purchase for ice packs each year times estimates of the number of college and professional teams that do likewise, and on the reported number of cases of nerve palsy, as follows:

3,000 ice packs/year × 300 teams (100 professional + 200 college) = 900,000 applications/year

10 injuries/year ÷ 900,000 applications = 0.0011% incident rate

This estimate is very conservative for the following reasons:

- The number of ice packs per year is a gross underestimation of the actual number of cold treatments. This number does not include the treatments when an ice pack is used repeatedly or when commercial, refreezable cold packs or ice immersion is used.
- There are many more than 300 professional and college teams. But since I don't know how many use fewer ice packs than we do, I want to be conservative. Those who use more than we do will make the incident rate even lower.
- Since there has been a total of only 11 instances of nerve palsy among college and professional athletes reported in the past 12 years, my estimate of 10 per year seems overly conservative. If indeed, less than 10 occur per year, the incident rate would be even less.
- This analysis does not include the thousands of high schools that apply cold packs to their athletes.

Some of the recommendations for cold-induced nerve palsy by the authors are extreme:

UNCALLED-FOR RECOMMENDATIONS

- Limiting ice applications to 20 minutes (I2, I6, I7) or 20 to 30 minutes (I10, I21, I34). For most injuries, this will not provide adequate time to cool the injured tissues. Ice applications are of little value if they do not cool the deep injured tissues. The notion that the maximal benefits of cold are achieved in 20 minutes is totally unsubstantiated.
- Never applying any kind of ice, except ice massage, directly to the skin (I7). Just the opposite is true: Failure to apply ice packs directly to the skin will result in less-than-optimal cooling (see Figure 7.4, p. 95). The advice is correct for cold-gel packs because they are cooled to many degrees below freezing (I6), and also for application over superficial nerves (ulnar at elbow and peroneal at knee).
- Avoiding compression when applying ice (I2, I7). On the contrary, it is imperative to include compression for immediate care of musculoskeletal injuries (chapter 7).

COLD HYPERSENSITIVITY

There are many forms of cold hypersensitivity, sometimes referred to as allergic reactions, in humans (I18, I23, I56, I58). These have been grouped into four categories based on their major signs (I23, I56):

- *Cold urticaria*—hives; caused by the release of histamine and other mediators during rewarming that follows localized cooling (I45)
- *Cold hemoglobinuria*—free hemoglobin in the urine; occurs when red blood cells break down in the vessels so quickly that not all of the hemoglobin can combine with blood proteins.
- *Purpura*—hemorrhage into skin and mucous membranes; a sign (among several) reflecting the presence of cryoglobulins, abnormal proteins in the blood that form a gel at low temperatures (J73)
- *Cold erythema*—redness; a nonallergic, congenital, abnormal response to cooling characterized by severe pain, muscular spasms, sweating, and an axon reflex erythema, without urticaria.

The most common, cold urticaria, is discussed in more detail in the next section.

Cold Urticaria

Cold is just one of several causes of urticaria (I45, I61). Causes are internal (e.g., ingested drugs or foods or inhaled pollen) and external (e.g., skin contact, pressure from clothes, and heat) (I61). Cold urticaria occurs most frequently in young adults; 90% of cases are idiopathic (i.e., occur spontaneously without apparent cause) (I40). It sometimes occurs in combination with other urticarias, such as heat- or exercise-induced urticarias—that is, when cold is used following vigorous exercise. The response is associated with the breakdown of skin mast cells (connective tissue cells), tissue degranulation (change to a less complex form), and the release of histamine and other mediators, such as prostaglandins and platelet factors (I24, I33, I43). The signs and symptoms associated with cold urticaria are illustrated in Table 14.3.

Table 14.3   Signs and Symptoms of Cold Hypersensitivity Syndromes

Reflecting	Skin	Respiratory	Gastrointestinal	General	Eye	Blood	Other
Histamine release*	Erythema Itching Urticaria Sweating Facial flush	Hoarseness (laryngeal edema) Sneezing Dyspnea Caught Chest Pain	Dysphagia Gastric hyperacidity Abdominal pain Diarrhea Vomiting	Malaise Headache	Puffiness of eyelids	Passive transfer in idiopathic type only Cold-sensitive basophils	*Vascular:* Shock (cold anaphylaxis) Syncope Hypotension Tachycardia Extrasystoles
Cold hemolysins and agglutinins†	Cold urticaria Ulcers Raynaud's phenomenon Acrocyanosis	—	—	Maslaise Chills Fever	—	Anemia STS: Biologic false positives Cold hemolysins§ Cold agglutinins	*Renal:* Paroxysmal cold hemoglobinuria
Cryoglobulins‡	Erythema Itching Purpura Cold urticaria (unusual) Raynaud's phenomenon (atypical) Ulceration Necrosis	Dyspnea	Stomatitis Melena Gingival bleeding	Chills Fever	Decrease in visual acuity Blindness Conjunctival hemorrhages	Anemia Fibrinogenopenia No passive transfer# Sedimentation rate elevated Cryoglobulin inclusion cell Cryoglobulins•	*Ear and Nose:* Deafness Epistaxis

*Presents as classical (essential) cold urticaria. Pathogenesis: effects of histamine on capillary vasculature and smoooth muscle throughout body. †May present as paroxysmal hemoglobinuria. Associated, e.g., with syphilis, atypical pneumonia, infectious mononucleosis, hemolytic anemia. ‡May present as purpura. Associated, e.g., with multiple myeloma, leukemia, kala-azar, malignancy, lupus erythematosus. Pathogenesis: occlusive vascular effects of cryoprotein precipitate. §Donath-Landsteiner test. #Except with cryoprotein. •Precipitate in chilled serum. Modified from Juhlin and Shelley (123).

Urticaria can be induced by cold applications of 3 to 10 minutes (I24, I45). Wheals (2 to 4 millimeters high) develop within minutes of rewarming, but are transient and disappear within 30 to 120 minutes of rewarming (I24, I61).

The standard treatment for urticaria is to avoid the precipitating conditions (I13, I24, I45, I61), but that is not always a desirable choice, especially for an athlete with an injury (I13, I24, I61). Drug (antihistamine) therapy is generally effective (I24), although the wheal may not be totally blocked (I44). Subcutaneous epinephrine and intramuscular diphenhydramine (Benadryl) administrations are often helpful (I61), although some clinicians prefer cyproheptadine (I17, I57).

Repeated cold applications can result in a tolerance to cold, characterized by a progressively diminishing response to the cold (I13, I24). It appears the tolerance is due to depletion of the antigen that triggers mast cell degradation (I24). We have had two athletes at Indiana State who decided that urticaria was less of a problem than not using ice; they soon had only a minor response.

■ ICE CUBE TEST FOR URTICARIA

The ice cube test is a simple diagnostic tool for cold urticaria (I21). Massage the skin with an ice cube for at least 3 minutes. Erythemia (redness) will occur within 5 minutes after massage. If the erythemia is replaced after 5 to 10 minutes by a wheal that covers the area treated, the test is positive and the patient suffers from urticaria. In unaffected persons the erythemia will last for approximately 5 minutes and then the skin will appear normal.

Treating People Who Have Cold Hypersensitivity

Cold hypersensitivity is frequently overlooked because its symptoms are relatively mild (I18) and because cold causes intense pain in nonhypersensitive people during their first treatment or two. It sometimes is difficult to know during the initial numbing period of cryokinetics whether the pain a person feels is due to hypersensitivity or is just the normal pain experienced by an unadapted person. Suspect hypersensitivity if the subject has a severe emotional response along with the pain (such as crying) or if the pain does not decrease during subsequent immersions (i.e., adaptation does not occur) (see chapter 11). If you suspect a person is hypersensitive to cold, you can test for hypersensitivity by applying a small ice cube to the skin for a few minutes, as noted in the technique tip above (H36). An adverse reaction indicates hypersensitivity.

Be careful when using cryotherapy to treat a person who suffers from cold hypersensitivity. Let the patient make the choice. If the symptoms are too intense, you will have to choose an alternative method. Peppard (B32) has been successful using transcutaneous electrical nerve stimulation (TENS) and exercise to treat acute ankle injuries in cold-hypersensitive patients. He uses a program similar to cryokinetics, but with TENS for analgesia rather than cold applications.

VASOSPASTIC DISORDERS

Vasospastic disorders are conditions in which the vessels of the extremities do not dilate properly. A person who suffers from a vasospastic disorder should never be treated with any form of cryotherapy. The extreme arterial spasm (additional vasoconstriction) caused by cryotherapy would very likely lead to ischemic necrosis. Fortunately, most people who suffer from one of these diseases know it, are aware of the problems that even mild cold exposure causes, and will not allow themselves to be subjected to cryotherapy. However, you must be aware of the symptoms associated with vasospastic disorders in the event that a person with an undiagnosed disorder comes under your care.

Raynaud's Phenomenon

↓ Blood Flow + excessive vasoconstriction (can completely close vessels)

Raynaud's phenomenon refers to local functional changes in the peripheral circulation, such as decreased finger blood flow and excessive vasoconstriction in response to sympathetic nervous stimulation (I54). If the phenomenon is caused by Raynaud's Disease, it is known as Primary Raynaud's Phenomenon; if caused by anything else, it is called Secondary Raynaud's Phenomenon.

Small arteries and arterioles in the extremities constrict, resulting in pallor (J73) and/or cyanosis—a slightly bluish, grayish, slatelike, or dark purple discoloration (J73)—of the skin, followed by hyperemia and redness (I5). Vasoconstriction may be great enough to cause complete closure of the vessels (I41). Numbness, tingling, and burning may also occur during the attack (J73). The exact cause of and specific pathophysiology of Raynaud's phenomenon remain a mystery (I3).

Raynaud's disease is a condition affecting predominantly young women in which mild exposure to cold, such as repeatedly putting the hands into a refrigerator or freezer (I58), or an emotional upset results in *Primary Raynaud's phenomenon* (J73). There are apparently no other contributing conditions.

Secondary Raynaud's phenomenon—the term applied when the condition is caused by anything other than Raynaud's disease—is associated with a number of disease processes. Trauma due to surgery or related to occupation, such as typing or operating a pneumatic hammer, can precipitate secondary Raynaud's phenomenon. It can also result from neurogenic lesions, such as carpal tunnel syndrome, occlusive arterial disease, cold sensitivity disease, and rheumatoid arthritis (see I5 and I57 for additional information and references).

Livedo Reticularis

Livedo reticularis is a semipermanent bluish mottling of the skin of the hands and legs that is aggravated by exposure to cold (E63, I45). Some patients also experience feelings of coldness, numbness, dull aching, and paresthesia (I5, I58). The symptoms result from a narrowing of the arterioles with dilation of the capillaries and venules. Like Raynaud's phenomenon, it too can be either primary or secondary to other disease processes.

Acrocyanosis

Acrocyanosis is painless and persistent coldness and cyanosis of the distal parts of the extremities (I45, I58). Its etiology and pathophysiology are both obscure, but like livedo reticularis, it appears to involve a narrowing of the arterioles with dilation of the capillaries and venules. Acrocyanosis is a primary entity and is the least common and most innocuous of the vasospastic disorders.

COLD-INDUCED PAIN

Cold-induced pain sometimes keeps athletes from using cryotherapy, especially ice-water immersion. We must, therefore, acknowledge pain in this chapter on problems. But there is no need to repeat the information of chapters 11 and 20 here.

CONTRAINDICATIONS

Contraindications are situations in which a given treatment is not advisable. The following are contraindications to cryotherapy:

1. Do not apply any type of cryotherapy directly to the skin for longer than 1 hour continuously; it may cause frostbite.
2. A chilled gel pack should not be applied under a compression bandage; it may cause frostbite.
3. Never apply cryotherapy of any type to persons who suffer any of the following conditions:
   - Raynaud's or one of the other vasospastic diseases
   - Cold hypersensitivity
   - Cardiac disorder
   - Compromised local circulation

PRECAUTIONS

Even when all contraindications to cryotherapy for a given patient have been ruled out, a number of precautions must always be taken to prevent serious injury:

■ *PRECAUTIONS WHEN ADMINISTERING CRYOTHERAPY*

- Do not apply any type of cryotherapy to the skin for longer than 1 hour continuously; this may cause frostbite.
- Be very careful when applying a cold-gel pack directly to the skin for longer than 5 to 10 minutes.
- Do not apply cold-gel packs under a compression bandage; frostbite might result.
- Be very careful when the patient is performing exercises that cause pain following cold applications. Additional injury may occur.
- Be very careful when using cryotherapy for treating persons who
  - have certain rheumatoid conditions,
  - are paralyzed or in a coma,
  - have coronary artery disease, or
  - have certain hypertensive diseases.
- Be very careful when applying an elastic wrap over a cold pack, especially in thin people and to body parts where the major nerves are superficial, such as the elbow or knee. Do not apply the wrap too tightly.

SUMMARY

- Do not apply any type of cryotherapy directly to the skin for longer than 1 hour or a cold-gel pack for any length of time under an elastic wrap.
- Contrary to some stated opinions, frostbite apparently does not occur from short-term (30- to 40-minute) ice-pack applications directly to the skin.
- Frostbite represents part of a continuum of tissue injury to cold. This continuum includes frostnip, superficial frostbite, and deep frostbite.
- Although problems resulting from cryotherapy are rare, cryotherapy should not be used on persons with Raynaud's or other vasospastic diseases, cold hypersensitivity, cardiac disorders, or compromised local circulation.
- Be cautious when using cryotherapy on persons who are paralyzed or in a coma or have coronary artery, rheumatoid, or hypertensive diseases.

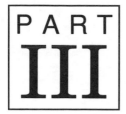

PART

III

Clinical Techniques Involving Cryotherapy

The most common—and some of the not-so-common—cryotherapeutic techniques are presented in the chapters in this part. Chapter 15 introduces the proper application of various cryotherapy modalities. Subsequent chapters cover rest, ice, compression, elevation, and stabilization (RICES) for immediate care of injuries; cryokinetics for acute joint-sprain rehabilitation; cryostretch for acute muscle-strain rehabilitation; presurgical and postsurgical applications; techniques for relieving pain, such as menstrual cramps and headaches; and other miscellaneous techniques, including blister control, medicated ice for abrasions, and stretching connective tissue contractures.

The rationale underlying the techniques is briefly summarized, but the emphasis is on how, not why, to apply the techniques. You may want to review Part II for the detailed pathophysiological and theoretical basis of the techniques. For your reference, summary statements in most of the chapters of Part III include references to the theory chapters in which the concept is discussed in detail. Each chapter in Part III is heavily illustrated to enhance the written description of the techniques.

15

Methods of Cold Application

There are numerous techniques for applying cold to (or, actually, withdrawing heat from) the body. In this chapter I describe the most popular methods and comment on their usefulness. Except for a few gimmicks, such as using a package of frozen peas as an ice pack (B49), most methods are variations of the following.

ICE PACKS

Ice packs are containers of crushed, shaved, or chipped ice that are applied to the body. Containers include towels, plastic bags (Figure 15.1), and ice caps. Plastic bags are more economical than ice caps and less messy than towels, which cannot hold the water from the melting ice. Ice packs cool the body more than commercial packs (C48, C54) and last longer outside of a freezer unit (C48). Thus, they can be prepared ahead of time and carried onto a field or court during practice without losing their effectiveness.

A plastic bag that holds a gallon of liquid or more is preferred unless an injury is very small and contained, such as a sprained finger or bruised eye.

Use the following procedure to apply an ice pack:

1. Place the ice in the bag.
2. Remove excess air by squeezing or by sucking with your mouth (Figure 15.2).
3. Tie a knot in the top of the bag.
4. Place the ice pack directly on the skin and secure it. (Pillows or elastic wraps are most commonly used to hold ice bags in place.)

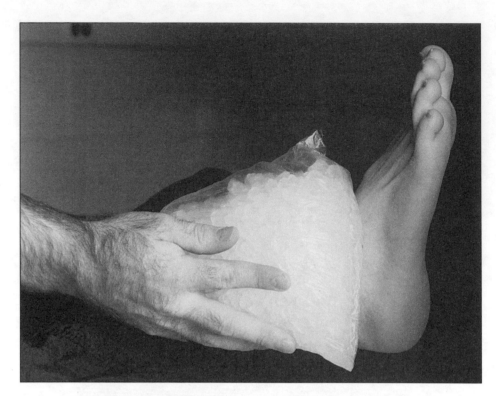

Figure 15.1 Ice pack containing about three pounds of crushed ice in a plastic bag. Note the knot in the bag. Air was evacuated before the knot was tied.

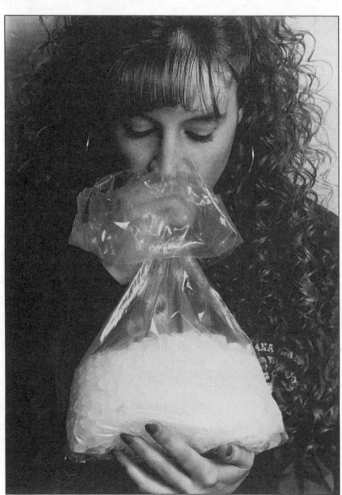

Figure 15.2 Remove as much air as possible from crushed-ice packs. An easy way to do so is to gather the open end of the plastic bag in one hand, place the opening to your mouth, and suck the air out. Then twist the bag and tie a knot in the end of it.

COLD-GEL PACKS

In commercially prepared cold-gel packs, a gelatinous substance is enclosed in a vinyl cover (Figure 15.3). The packs contain water, an antifreeze (such as salt) to keep them from freezing (so they stay flexible) and gelatin or shredded paper to give the pack substance. The packs are chilled in a freezer unit and then applied to the body. Cold-gel packs are much less messy than ice packs; they can be used over and over again as long as the vinyl bag remains intact and they are chilled for at least 2 or 3 hours between applications. They are convenient for use in a general training room or clinic, but three facts weigh against using them for immediate care of acute injuries:

- Because cold-gel packs do not freeze solid and therefore do not have the heat-absorbing capacity of ice (chapter 5), they do not cool the body as much as ice packs do.
- Because they immediately begin to warm when taken out of a freezer unit (C48), they cannot effectively be taken on the court or field and held in ready for later use.
- They are potentially more dangerous than ice packs when combined with compression because they may cause frostbite.

Be cautious when using cold-gel packs. Because they are normally chilled to far below 0°C, they may cause frostbite if used improperly (H71). Do not apply a cold-gel pack for longer than 30 minutes at a time, and, depending on the type of cold-gel pack and the temperature to which it is cooled, layer a damp cloth between the pack and the skin.

Blue Ice™ packs, which are no longer marketed, were made with a gel formula that apparently cooled more than other types of cold packs. These packs were too cold to apply directly to the skin; three cases of superficial frostbite occurred in our own research laboratory, one with Blue Ice and two with Ice Down™ packs (whose gel came from the Blue Ice Company). In all three cases the cold packs were applied directly to the skin and held in place with compression. I strongly discourage applying elastic wraps over cold-gel packs.

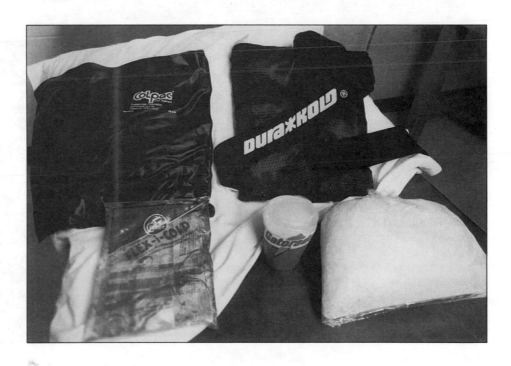

Figure 15.3 Chattanooga ColPaCs (upper left) and Craner Flex-i-Cold (lower left) are gel packs. They are shown here with a Dura*Kold pack (upper right), crushed-ice pack (lower right), and a partially used 12-oz ice cube (center).

ARTIFICIAL ICE CUBE PACKS

Another type of commercial ice pack is one made from "artificial ice cubes" (Figure 15.4). Developed to keep produce cool during shipping, artificial ice cubes consist of sheets of vinyl bubbles (1 by 1.5 inches in size) filled with water and glycerine. Frozen sheets of these ice cubes are placed around boxes of produce in trucks and train cars.

The Dura*Kold Corporation was the first to use artificial ice cubes in cold packs for therapeutic use. Their packs consist of two layers of the cubes inside of a nylon envelope (Figure 15.5). Elastic straps with Velcro are sewn at each end to the nylon and are used to attach the pack to the body. Although they are not as effective as ice in cooling the body, Dura*Kold packs share some of the advantages of both ice and cold-gel packs while avoiding some of the disadvantages of both:

- They are not as messy as ice.
- The water in them freezes solid and so have a greater capacity to withdraw heat than cold packs do, but they are still flexible because of the joints between the bubbles.
- Their application can be delayed after they are removed from the freezer without losing effectiveness. Thus, they can be taken on the court or field or sent home with an athlete for later use. (Our research [C48] involved a 20-minute delay without insulation of the packs. They will last longer than this, especially if stored in an insulated cooler.)
- They are safer to use than cold-gel packs because they have a nylon cover that protects the skin against accidental long-term application.
- They are better as a take-home device than ice packs because they can be refrozen and used again. (A refrozen ice pack is a solid mass that must be broken up before it can be reapplied.)
- The icc in the packs stays evenly distributed, even when the pack is applied in a dependent position, such as the shoulder. When a crushed-ice pack is applied in dependent position, the ice falls to the bottom of the pack.

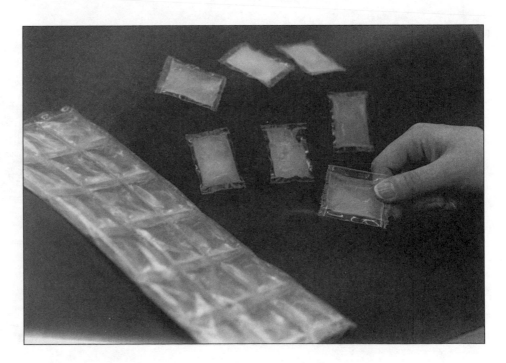

Figure 15.4 Sheets of vinyl bubbles (lower left) are filled with water to form "artificial ice cubes" and are the basis of Dura*Kold packs. The individual bubbles on the upper right were cut from a larger sheet.

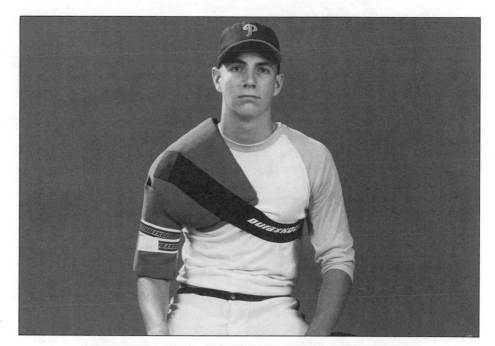

Figure 15.5 Dura*-Kold packs are made from two layers of artificial ice cubes (see Figure 15.4) in nylon covers. Elastic straps with Velcro closures are attached to the nylon covers.

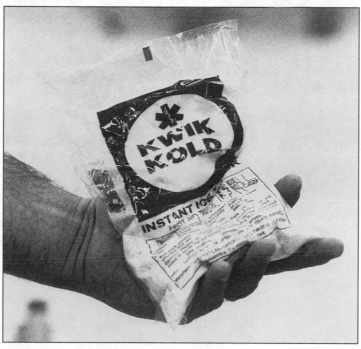

Figure 15.6 A chemical pack does not decrease temperature nearly as much as ice packs do. There is also a possibility of chemical burn if the outer vinyl pack is punctured. Avoid using these if possible.

CHEMICAL COLD PACKS

Chemical cold packs consist of two chemical substances, one in a small vinyl bag within a larger bag (Figure 15.6). Squeezing the pack until the smaller bag ruptures and its fluid spills into the larger bag causes a chemical reaction between the two substances that lowers the temperature of the combined mixture. These cold packs cannot be reused. Although chemical cold packs are convenient for emergency use, they are not suitable substitutes for ice packs or cold-gel packs. They do not adequately lower the body temperature (C54, C76), and the fluid occasionally leaks out, causing a chemical burn. I do not recommend them, unless there is absolutely no other choice.

ICE IMMERSION

Ice immersion is perhaps a misnomer, for it is actually immersion of a body part (such as the ankle) in an ice water bath, sometimes called a "slush bucket" (Figure 15.7). Any container big enough to hold the body part can be used. The container is filled with ice and water, and the body part is simply immersed in it. Ice immersion is the preferred technique for cooling feet, ankles, hands, arms, and elbows during cryokinetics. It is rather difficult to use for other body parts, however, since too much extraneous tissue has to be chilled. (For instance, when treating the back with ice immersion, the legs must also be immersed. Nevertheless, many therapists do use immersion for the lower back.)

Ice immersion should not be used during immediate-care procedures. You have to sacrifice either compression or maximal cooling, both of which are essential. If you apply an elastic wrap for compression prior to immersion, the wrap insulates the body part, reducing cooling. If you leave the wrap off to get maximal cooling, you do not get compression.

The optimal temperature for ice immersion is not yet known. Some therapists use 2° to 4°C (33° to 36°F); others use 10° to 15°C (49° to 59°F). The latter is preferred for lower back immersion, because of the large amount of tissue cooled. My clinical impression is that the lower temperature is better for cryokinetics. It seems to cause quicker and more complete hypalgesia and therefore allows more complete exercise.

COLD WHIRLPOOLS

The cold whirlpool is essentially ice immersion. It has two advantages in cryotherapy: It is large enough to allow immersion of larger body parts (e.g., the knee and lower back), and it combines cold water with the massage

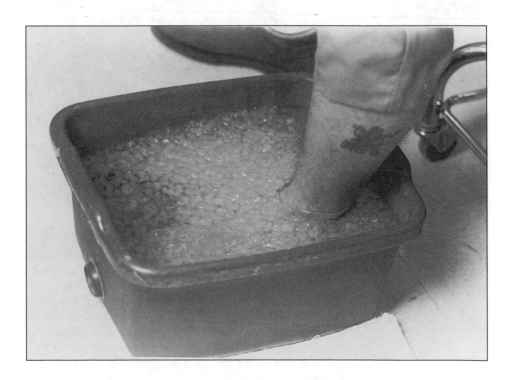

Figure 15.7 Immersion of the ankle in an ice-water bath, or "slush bucket," in preparation for therapeutic exercises. The temperature of the water is about 1°C and remains there as long as there is ice in the water, and it is kept stirred.

action of the whirlpool agitator. However, I do not advocate cold whirlpools for the following reasons

- Too often this treatment is used to the exclusion of anything else. For efficient rehabilitation, exercise must follow cold applications (see chapter 9).
- A whirlpool is larger than needed for lower leg or arm immersion and requires too much ice to cool the large volume of water.
- Immersion of more than a single extremity is too painful for most people.

ICE MASSAGE

Ice massage is exactly what its name implies: massage with a cube of ice. The ice cubes are usually prepared in 150- to 300-milliliter (5- to 10-ounce) cups. Each cube is then big enough to last through an entire treatment. To protect your fingers while massaging with ice, you can do one of the following:

- Put a tongue depressor in the cup prior to freezing. The ice cube then has a handle (Figure 15.8). This is the preferred method.
- Leave the ice in the cup and tear the edges away as the ice is used (Figure 15.9).
- Wrap a towel around the top of the ice cube and massage with the exposed sides.

Rub the ice cube back and forth in a motion parallel to the underlying muscle fiber. Each stroke should extend the length of the treatment area and, in terms of width, should overlap about half the area covered by the previous stroke. The physiological response to ice massage may be affected by two factors that are unique when compared with other forms of cryotherapy. First the application is phasic. As the area is massaged, the ice is in contact with a specific area of the tissue only briefly; then the tissue is exposed to atmospheric temperature. This is a disadvantage when your goal

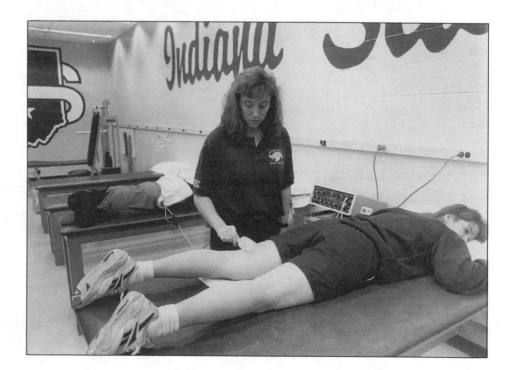

Figure 15.8 Ice massage with a popsicle made with a tongue depressor in a 12-oz cup of water.

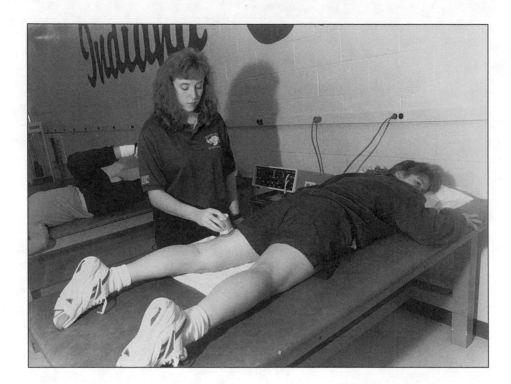

Figure 15.9 Ice massage with a tear-away cup. Some athletic trainers wrap a small towel around the ice cube to prevent their fingers from getting so cold.

is to decrease the tissue temperature. Second, the massage action of the ice cube stimulates mechanoreceptors more completely than other forms of cryotherapy. Presumably, this is the reason ice massage results in quicker numbness than ice or cold packs.

Ice massage is a very effective means of achieving numbness in muscles prior to cryostretch and as part of cryokinetics in joints such as the knee, hip, and shoulder, which are not easily immersed.

COLD MACHINES

There are a variety of appliances that provide cryotherapy. These consist of a reservoir that holds ice and water or a unit that chills a fluid (water or Freon). The chilled fluid is then circulated through pads that are applied to the body.

Cryo Cuff

The Cryo Cuff is a combination cold and compression device developed by the Aircast Corporation (Figure 15.10). It consists of a double-walled nylon sleeve connected to a 1-gallon thermos jug. The thermos is filled with ice and water, some of which flows into the sleeve. Raising the jug causes more water to flow into the cuff, increasing the pressure; the higher the jug is raised, the greater the pressure in the cuff. The water in the cuff can be rechilled by lowering the jug to drain the cuff, mixing the warmer cuff water with colder jug water, and raising the jug to refill the cuff.

The Cryo Cuff is used both following surgery and for immediate care of acute injuries. Its greatest advantages are its portability, ease of use, and cost (less than $100). Its greatest disadvantage is that the user must remember to keep rechilling the water in the cuff.

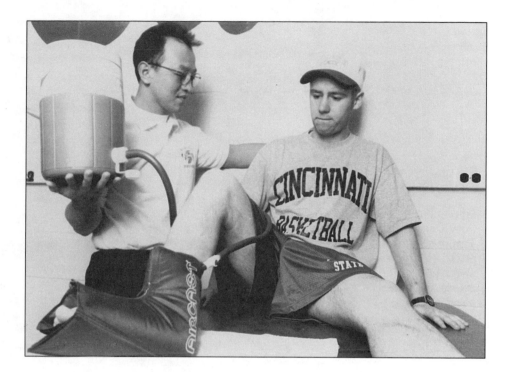

Figure 15.10 The Cryo Cuff provides both cold and compression. It is applied over the limb and then inflated with ice water from the jug. The higher the jug is lifted, the greater the pressure in the Cryo Cuff.

Polar Care Cooler

Polar Care also has a low-cost (about $200), portable, easy-to-operate unit. It consists of a cooler, a pump, and several pads of different sizes and shapes for different parts of the body (Figure 15.11). The low-voltage submersible pump has an in-line thermometer and flow control valve. The pump connects to a pad through insulated double hoses with self-sealing couplings. The pump is submersed into any appropriate-sized container of ice and water; an 11-quart insulated polyurethane reservoir is available with the device. The pads can be placed under or over a surgical dressing, although the benefits are much greater if placed under it (E20; see Figure 8.1, p. 102).

The device was originally developed for postsurgical use, but is now being used for more general cryotherapeutic applications. It maintains a constant temperature more easily than the Cryo Cuff does, but is not as portable. It operates in essentially the same manner as the Icy/Hot type of machines (discussed next), but is much less expensive.

Icy/Hot Machine

The Icy/Hot machine was the first cryotherapy machine developed exclusively for postsurgical use. There are now a variety of machines on the market by other manufacturers. All chill and circulate water through small vinyl pads that are placed over the incision and surrounding area. The size and expense of these machines prohibit their use outside of a hospital.

Cryomatic

No longer available, the Cryomatic (Chattanooga Corporation) is a refrigeration unit that circulates Freon through coils in a pad (Figure 15.12). The pad is wrapped around a limb or placed over the back or abdomen. The user may select any temperature between –6° and 27°C. Sensing devices keep

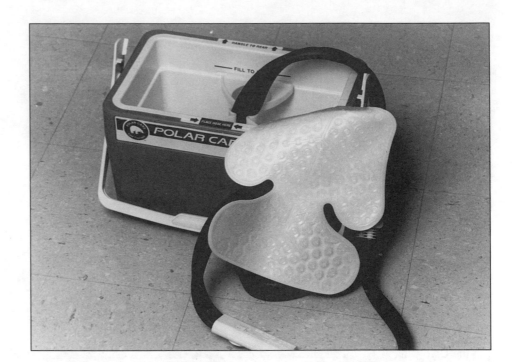

Figure 15.11 The Polar Care unit consists of an insulated, plastic 40-gal cooler, pump, hoses, and a bladder. The cooler holds ice water, which is circulated through the bladder by the pump.

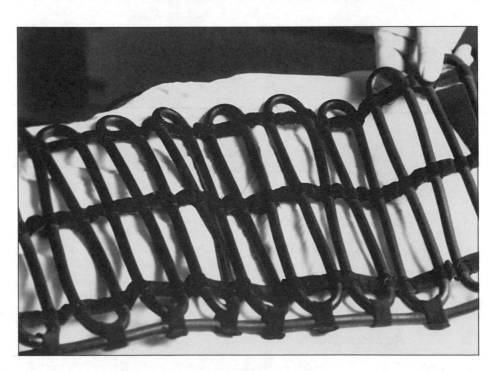

Figure 15.12 Freon is circulated through the coils of a Cryomatic pad.

the temperature close to the selected temperature. The Cryomatic had great promise. It was used at many race tracks for treating musculoskeletal disorders in thoroughbred race horses. Unpublished reports by orthopedic physicians using it before and after surgery and by physiatrists treating spastic paraparesis were encouraging. But the market never developed and the manufacturer discontinued the device.

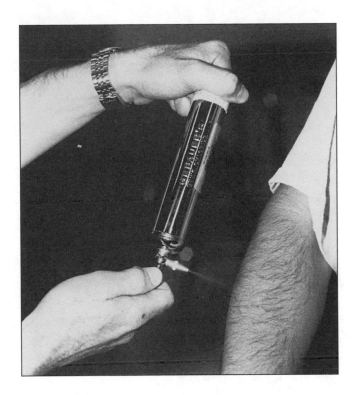

Figure 15.13 Ethyl chloride, sprayed on the skin, evaporates very quickly and cools the skin. But the effect is short lived, and does not involve deeper tissue cooling.

VAPO-COOLANT SPRAY

Liquid ethyl chloride and fluoromethane evaporate very quickly when applied to the body, removing heat from the skin in the process. Because they evaporate so quickly, their effects are very superficial. Fluoromethane is preferred; ethyl chloride is flammable and can freeze the skin hard (B18, B31, B47, E77).

The superficial effects of vapo-coolant sprays limit their use to techniques that rely on stimulating the sympathetic nervous system to treat pain and muscle spasm. Vapo-coolant sprays should never be used when the goal is to decrease the temperature of underlying tissues.

Use the following procedure to apply vapo-coolant sprays:

1. Hold the container about 30 centimeters (1 foot) from the body and deliver a moderately fine jet spray at an angle to the body.
2. Spray the body part in a sweeping motion at the rate of about 10 centimeters per second (Figure 15.13).
3. Sweep in a single direction (B35) and proceed in a rhythmic fashion until the entire injury area has been covered twice.
4. Take care not to frost the skin.

VAPO-COOLANT CUFFS

Cryomatic cuffs are double-layered nylon sleeves that fit over selected body parts, such as the ankle. Vapo-coolants are sprayed into the envelope between the layers, thus providing both cold and compression. I know of no evaluation of the degree of temperature decrease or compression provided by these devices. They have apparently been marketed more to emergency response personnel than to sports medicine personnel.

16

Initial Care of Acute Injuries: The RICES Technique

The combination of rest, ice, compression, elevation, and stabilization (RICES) is without question the appropriate treatment for immediate care of acute injuries (Figure 16.1). When used properly, the RICES treatment regimen reduces the total amount of tissue damage, reduces limb swelling, reduces pain, and results in much quicker rehabilitation (e.g., days as opposed to weeks).

Summary of Rationale for RICES

See chapters 3 and 5–7 for a complete discussion of the research base for RICES.

EFFECTS

- Ice applications lower metabolism in the injured tissue, which decreases the need for oxygen. This inhibits secondary hypoxic injury in cells within the injured tissue that escaped primary traumatic injury.
- Ice limits swelling by decreasing total injury. Less total injury means less free protein in the tissue. Thus, there is less tissue oncotic pressure and lower capillary filtration pressure. Lower capillary filtration pressure means less edema.
- Both compression and elevation contribute to swelling control by decreasing capillary filtration pressure.
- Stabilization allows musculature around the injury to relax, which, along with ice, aids in limiting the pain-spasm-pain cycle.

ADVANTAGES

- The total amount of injured tissue is decreased; thus, less healing is needed.
- Swelling is decreased, resulting in less pain.
- Ice is relatively inexpensive.

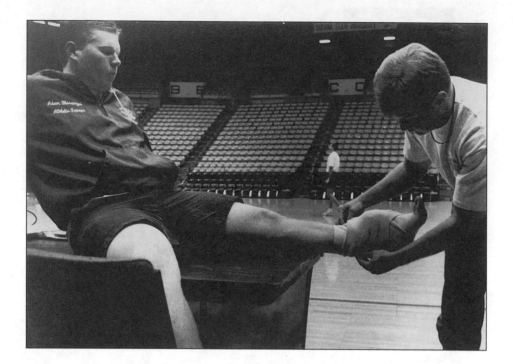

Figure 16.1 Apply an ice pack and wrap to an acute injury (sprained ankle in this case) as quickly after the injury as possible (within the first 10 min). After securing the wrap, elevate the injury above the heart.

DISADVANTAGES

- Effectiveness of cold diminishes with time. Its full effects are achieved only if it is applied within 5 to 10 minutes following the injury; it is probably of little benefit when the initial application is 8 to 24 hours following injury.

INDICATIONS

- Immediate care of acute injuries

CONTRAINDICATIONS

- Do not use with a person who is hypersensitive to cold.

PRECAUTIONS

- Do not apply ice packs directly to the skin for more than 30 to 60 minutes at a time.
- Cold packs that have been refrigerated at −17°C or below should not be applied directly to the skin.

Equipment Needed

- Ice pack
- 15-centimeter (6-inch) elastic wrap
- Pillow(s) to elevate the injured limb
- Brace or splinting material to stabilize the injured joint

Preapplication Procedures

- Evaluate injury before applying RICES. You must know what the injury is.

- Check contraindications: Ask the injured person if he or she is hypersensitive to cold.
- Prepare the patient physically by removing shoes, clothing, bandages, etc., as needed.
- Position the patient so that he or she is comfortable and so that the injury can be elevated.
- Prepare the patient psychologically. Reassure him or her. Injured people are often depressed because of pain and being frustrated that they were injured.

Application Procedures

WHEN DO YOU BEGIN?
Begin as soon as possible after the injury—within minutes. The longer you wait, the less effective will be the procedure.

PROCEDURE

1. Place the ice pack on the skin directly over the injury and shape or mold it to the general contour of the body part (Figure 16.2).
   a. Apply within 10 minutes after the injury occurs.
   b. Chilled commercial packs may be too cold initially. Do not apply them directly to the skin.
   c. Chemical packs do not get nearly as cold as ice packs and may cause skin problems if they leak.
2. Secure the ice pack with a 15 centimeter (6-inch) elastic wrap (see Figure 16.1).
   a. Apply the wrap snugly, but not too tightly (stretch it to about 75% of its length).
   b. The wrap must cover the entire injured area, even areas that the ice pack does not cover.
   c. The elastic wrap must be on constantly for the first 20 to 24 hours

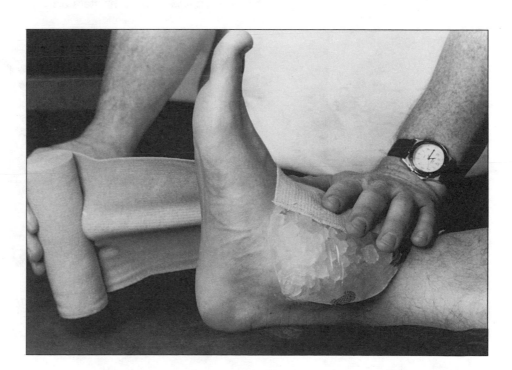

Figure 16.2 Crushed-ice pack applied directly to the skin and shaped to the contour of the body part.

after the injury (except for the few seconds it takes to remove or reapply the ice pack).

3. Elevate the injured part 15 to 25 centimeters (6–10 inches) above the level of the heart.

4. Stabilize.
   a. The goal is to allow the surrounding musculature to relax completely.
   b. Use a sling for upper extremity injuries if muscle guarding occurs.
   c. Use a brace for lower extremity injuries if muscle guarding occurs.

5. After 30 to 45 minutes, remove the ice pack, replace the elastic wrap, and continue elevation (Figure 16.3).

6. The patient may take a quick shower if necessary, but the body part must be wrapped during the shower (Figure 16.4). Reapply the ice pack as in Step 2 immediately after the shower or after the patient gets home.

7. Reapply the ice pack, as above, every 2 hours until the patient goes to bed.

8. The elastic wrap should be worn throughout the night.

9. Use crutches for lower extremity and abdominal injuries if walking causes any pain or limping (Figure 16.5). Use a swing gate.

DURATION OF APPLICATION

- Apply ice packs intermittently, 30 to 40 minutes on, 60 to 90 minutes off, for most injuries.
   a. For most joints, 30 minutes is adequate; more fleshy areas require 40 minutes.
   b. Treat fingers and toes for 20 to 30 minutes on, 40 to 60 minutes off.
   c. If the injured body part must be in a dependent position for longer than 10 minutes (such as while showering or while the athlete is on the way home), do so immediately after cold-pack application

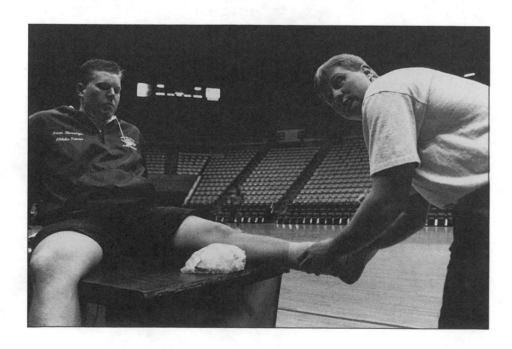

Figure 16.3
Reapply an elastic wrap to the body part after removing a cold pack. An injured body part should be constantly compressed, except for the minute or so that it takes to apply or remove a cold pack.

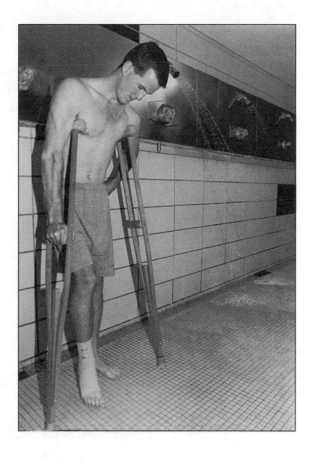

Figure 16.4 An athlete with a sprained ankle preparing to shower. Note that the ankle is wrapped and the athlete is using crutches. The shower should be a quick one, and the ankle should then be elevated as quickly as possible. Apply a dry wrap following the shower.

and apply a cold pack immediately after the activity that required a dependent position. Then begin the normal on-off procedure.

- Apply compression and elevation continuously.

FREQUENCY OF APPLICATION

- *Rest*—until body part can function without pain.
- *Ice*—intermittently for the first 12 to 24 hours following injury.
- *Elevation*—as much as possible during the first 24 hours postinjury.
- *Compression*—constantly until swelling is gone.
- *Stabilization*—until body part can function without pain.

Postapplication Procedures

- Make an appointment for the athlete to return for treatment the next day.
- Instruct the patient to follow the procedure exactly as outlined. Emphasize that noncompliance will complicate the injury and result in delays of 1 to 3 weeks in resolving the injury. Written instructions such as those in Table 16.1 are often helpful. Tell the patient to do the following:

1. Reapply an ice pack as soon as he or she gets home. This is done by removing the elastic wrap, applying the ice pack to the skin, and reapplying the wrap.

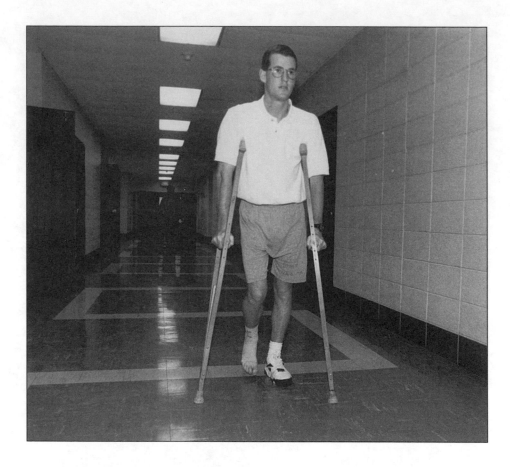

Figure 16.5 An athlete with a lower extremity injury should use crutches as long as walking causes pain or is done so with an abnormal gait.

2. Elevate the injury above the heart.
3. After 30 minutes, remove the ice pack, reapply the wrap, and elevate the injury again.
4. Repeat Steps 1 to 3 every 1 to 1-1/2 hours until bedtime.
5. Remove ice pack at bedtime.
6. Keep elastic wrap on injury overnight.
7. Repeat Steps 1 to 3 first thing in the morning.
8. Keep elastic wrap on until appointment.

- Instruct the patient concerning what level of activity he or she can participate in.
- If the injury involves the upper extremity, place the involved arm in a sling.
- Place the patient on crutches if the injury involves the lower extremity. Instruct the patient to do three things:

  1. Use a "three-point gait" with the crutches (i.e., move both crutches and the injured leg simultaneously [Figure 16.5]).
  2. Attempt to walk with a normal gait, using the crutches to support the injured limb. At times this means putting 90% to 100% of the body weight on the crutches, at others as little as 5% to 10%.
  3. Use the injured limb as much as possible without causing pain or limping.

- Continue these measures as long as pain is present when the measures are not used.
- Record treatment (and injury if not already recorded).

Table 16.1 Extended Immediate Care Procedures
Indiana State University Sports Medicine

Your activities during the next 12-72 hours are critical to the resolution of your injury. Failure to follow the following procedures may delay your return to full sport participation by as much as two weeks. Help us to help you by doing the following:

Before leaving the training room make sure you have:

1. Had an initial 30- to 40-minute application of ice, compression, and elevation.
2. Had a second evaluation of the injury.
3. Showered.
4. An elastic wrap applied to the injured area.
5. Been fitted for a sling (if shoulder or arm injury) or crutches (if lower extremity injury).
6. Received instructions in proper use of the sling or crutches (if fitted with them).

After you get to your dorm/apartment/home

1. Apply an ice or cold pack to the injury for 30 minutes at the times circled below. To do this, remove the elastic wrap, put the ice pack directly over the injury, and reapply the ice pack. The wrap should be snug, but not real tight (remove about 3/4 of the stretch).

    1:00   2:00   3:00   4:00   5:00   6:00   7:00   8:00   9:00   10:00   11:00   12:00

2. After each 30-minute ice-pack application, remove the ice pack and reapply the elastic wrap (snugly, as above). Following the last ice-pack application, wear the elastic wrap through the night until you return for treatment tomorrow.
3. Keep the injured part above the level of your heart as much as possible (constantly if possible) until you go to bed tonight.
4. Tomorrow, report to:

    The Student Health Center at _____ am/pm

    The Rehabilitation Clinic at _____ am/pm

    _____ at _____ am/pm

    _____ at _____ am/pm

5. This form filled out by _____

Key Points for Applying RICES

Apply RICES to acute injuries in the order described by the acronym RICES: rest, ice, compression, elevation, and stabilization.

- Rest the injured body part by limiting the athlete's activity.
- Apply the ice pack directly to the skin of the injured body part as soon as possible after you evaluate the injury (within 10 minutes after the injury).
- Secure the ice pack with a 15-centimeter elastic wrap applied over the ice pack and around the body part with firm pressure. Stretch the wrap to about 75% of its length during application.
- Elevate the injured body part with any device that holds it above the level of the heart.
- Stabilize the injury with a sling or brace.
- Use crutches until the athlete can walk without pain or further injury (if the injury involves the lower extremity).

17

Cryokinetics in Rehabilitation of Joint Sprains

Sprains = ligaments
Strains = mm. tendons

Cryokinetics is a systematic combination of cold applications to numb the injured body part and graded, progressive, active exercise (B23). It is the most effective form of cryotherapy for rehabilitation of ligament sprains. The technique is especially effective for ankle sprains, but can be used for any acute musculoskeletal joint injury. Cryokinetics allows rehabilitation to begin much sooner than traditional thermotherapy and can reduce rehabilitation time by days or even weeks (H4).

Although cryokinetics is especially effective for treating acute joint sprains, it is not the best treatment for acute muscle strains. Muscle strains should be passively stretched in the early stages of rehabilitation. The cryo-stretch technique (explained in chapter 18) combines cold and passive stretching. It should be used during the early phases of muscle strain rehabilitation and followed by cryokinetics.

Pain-free exercise is the key to cryokinetics (B23, C46). Cold applications serve only to diminish pain so that active exercise is possible. Unlike procaine injections, cold does not remove the pain-sensing mechanism; rather it removes residual pain (such as pain due to damaged tissue and pressure from the swelling on nerves). If the exercise during cryokinetics becomes so vigorous that further damage may result, the body responds with a pain sensation. Thus, cryokinetics has a built-in safety valve: Pain during cold-induced numbness indicates that the exercise is too vigorous and that the level of activity must be lowered.

Five exercise bouts, with cold-induced numbness in between, should be performed during each treatment session. Two or three treatment sessions per day is common among athletes who want to return to play quickly.

217

Summary of Rationale for Cryokinetics

See chapters 4, 9, 10, and 11 for more in-depth details on cryokinetics.

EFFECTS

- Cold decreases pain.
- Exercise increases blood flow.
- Exercise reestablishes neuromuscular functioning.

ADVANTAGES

- Cryokinetics allows exercise much sooner than normally would be the case.
- Cryokinetics retards muscular atrophy and neural inhibitions.
- Cryokinetics reduces swelling dramatically through muscular "milking action."
- Ice is relatively inexpensive; exercise is free.
- You can progress at the patient's speed.

DISADVANTAGES

- Ice is very painful during the initial ice immersion (a person usually adapts to this, though, so subsequent treatments of the body part are not so painful).
- Melting ice can be messy.

INDICATIONS

- Ankle sprains (cryokinetics is more effective on ankle sprains than on any other body part. Cryokinetics is more effective on ankle sprains than any other form of treatment of the ankle.)
- Finger sprains
- Shoulder sprains
- Other joint sprains

CONTRAINDICATIONS

- Do not perform any exercise or activity that causes pain.
- Do not use ice on a person who is hypersensitive to cold.

PRECAUTIONS

- Pain must be used as a guideline. The patient should not consciously or willfully attempt to overcome pain (see "Psychological Preparation" later in the chapter).
- With lower extremity injuries, patients may limp if not frequently reminded to refrain from limping. This could lead to overuse injuries in other muscles.
- There may be an increase in pain 4 to 8 hours after treatment.

Equipment Needed

- Slush bucket or ice packs
- Toe cap (if treating the foot or ankle)—helpful, but not necessary
- Towel

Preapplication Procedures

PSYCHOLOGICAL PREPARATION

The initial numbing during the first treatment session is usually difficult for the patient; he or she experiences intense pain before the body part numbs. The body part adapts to this pain, however, so that subsequent ice applications are not nearly as intense. Be sure to prepare the patient for the initial intense pain and make certain that he or she understands that it is only temporary and will not occur during subsequent cold applications and that the benefits of the treatment, primarily decreased disability time, greatly outweigh the temporary discomfort. Patients who are not prepared for the intensity of the initial cold pain sometimes refuse to continue the treatment.

The preapplication procedures are as follows:

1. Enlist the patient as a partner in the treatment.
    a. Explain the three types of pain he or she will experience and the role of each in the treatment:

    Residual pain—caused by the injury (damaged tissue and swelling). This pain prevents the patient from exercising. It will be neutralized by the numbness from the ice water.

    Cold pain—caused by the ice water until the patient adapts to it. This pain is merely a nuisance; it serves no useful purpose.

    Reinjury pain—caused if the patient stresses the tissues to the point of reinjuring them. Such pain will not be covered up by the numbness. This is the safety valve, so the patient should respect it and respond to it. Reduce the intensity of the patient's activity when he or she feels this pain.

    b. Patients should not feel any pain during exercise. If they do, either return to the ice bucket to renumb the body part or reduce the exercise intensity.
    c. Make sure that patients understand that recovery will be hindered if they ignore pain during exercise—that even though you are going to be aggressive and push them to the limits of pain, they must not go beyond this limit.
    d. I often tell patients that the effectiveness of the treatment depends on how well we work together—that my ability to help them depends on my knowing what activities cause pain. I tell them, "You yourself must let me know when it hurts; *I'm* not the one feeling the pain."

2. Explain to patients the sensations they will experience.

    Pain—very intense during the first application, slight during subsequent treatments
    Ache or numbing
    Numbness—relative anesthesia

3. Explain that the ice will be very painful during the first application, but that the advantages of the treatment are worth the discomfort.

Application Procedures

1. Numb the body part.
    a. Use ice immersion, ice massage, or cold-pack application.
    b. Numbing generally takes 12 to 20 minutes (C36).
    c. Numbing lasts 2 to 3 minutes, during which time the patient performs exercise (Step 2).
    d. The patient's sensation is more significant than the time of application of the cold modality. When the patient reports numbness, begin exercising (F18). Continued cold application wastes time. Some patients (10%–20% in my experience) cannot perceive numbness, even after 40 minutes of ice immersion in some cases. If the patient does not report numbness after 20 minutes (5 minutes when renumbing), assume that pain is sufficiently decreased and proceed with the exercise phase of the treatment.
    e. Help patients adapt to cold pain. Patients may become discouraged with the pain if you leave them alone to think about it. Avoid this by talking to patients continuously during the initial immersion. Any topic that will take their mind off the cold is appropriate.
    f. Use a toe cap (Figure 17.1) when treating sprained ankles. It will spare the patient much pain if worn during immersion (B45, E79), since most of the pain during ankle immersion is in the toes. The toe cap keeps the toes warm and therefore relatively pain-free, but has no effect on the uncovered portions of the ankle (E79).
    g. Remember, numbing serves no purpose other than to allow the body part to actively exercise.
2. Exercise the numbed body part.
    a. All exercise should be
       • active (performed by the patient),
       • progressive (increasing in both intensity and complexity), and
       • pain-free.
    b. Exercise should last 2 to 3 minutes, the duration of the numbness. As the numbness begins to wear off, reapply the cold modality. (It will only take 3 to 5 minutes to renumb the area.)
    c. Exercise must be performed without pain and in a normal, rhythmic, coordinated fashion.

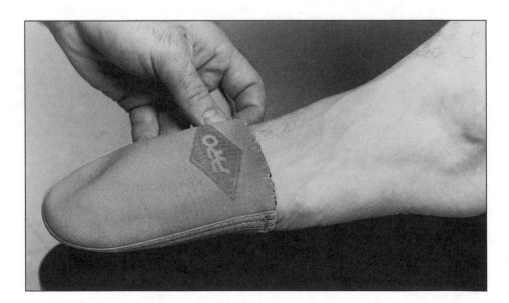

Figure 17.1 Toe cap over toes decreases pain during ice-water immersion.

d. Begin with simple range-of-motion activities and progress through full-sport activity. Constantly encourage the athlete to progress to the next level of activity (as long as all exercise is performed properly). With some injuries, progression through full-sport activity will take place in a single treatment session, while with others it may take weeks.

e. Neither the time spent performing an activity nor the number of repetitions is important. The key to cryokinetics is the ability to perform exercise of increasing difficulty properly and without pain.

EXAMPLE OF AN EXERCISE PROGRESSION FOR AN ANKLE SPRAIN

Use similar progressions for other joints. Design an exercise progression that begins with range-of-motion exercise and successively becomes more difficult until full-sport activity is achieved.

1. Non–weight-bearing range of motion (Figure 17.2)

   Plantar flex, dorsiflex, invert, evert, and circumduct (point toes to ground, towards nose, to right, to left, and move in a circle) the ankle to the limits of motion or pain. Exercises such as writing the alphabet with the big toe or picking up marbles with the toes have been suggested (H34, J50). These are all right, but not necessary; they do nothing more than require the patient to go through an active range of motion. Move on to the next step when full pain-free range of motion is achieved.

   If full range of motion is not achieved within 2 or 3 exercise bouts, use biofeedback by providing specific range-of-motion goals for the patient to achieve. Establish these goals with your hands and ask the patient to touch your hand with his or her toes (Figure 17.2). As the goal becomes easier to reach, move your hand(s) to require more range of motion.

Figure 17.2 Non–weight-bearing active range of motion is usually the initial form of exercise during cryokinetics. Most often these exercises are performed by the patient while seated next to the slush bucket, and are completed within one or two bouts. If, however, a reasonable amount of range of motion does not return quickly, it is helpful to use some biofeedback by giving the patient goals to work toward, as shown.

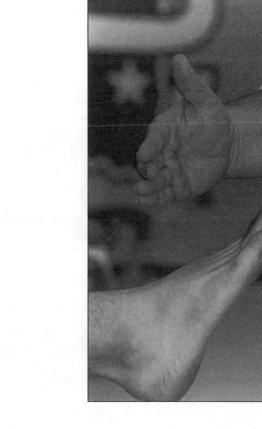

2. Weight-bearing (Figure 17.3)
   Have the patient stand with most of the weight on the uninjured leg. Have him or her slowly shift the weight back and forth between the uninjured and injured legs, while progressively bearing more weight on the injured leg. When the full body weight can be borne by the injured leg, have the patient progress to the next step.

3. Weight-bearing range of motion
   With weight on both legs, plantar flex and dorsiflex the ankle. Do this by alternately crouching and then raising up on the toes (Figure 17.4). If dorsiflexion is difficult or extremely limited, perform heel cord stretching exercises (Figure 17.5) as part of each subsequent treatment session (J50).

4. Walking
   Have the patient begin with short (heel-to-toe) steps straight ahead. The patient then gradually lengthens the steps (Figure 17.6) and walks in gentle arcs or large circles, then progresses to making sharper cuts on turns.
   Do not allow patients to limp, which they will often do unconsciously. Merely telling patients not to limp will not eliminate limping. You must constantly supervise walking (and subsequent running) patterns, looking for limping or any other unnatural gait. If patients limp, work with them until the limping is eliminated. If there is pain when a patient is forced to walk without a limp, he or she is not ready for this level of activity and should return to an earlier level (short-step walking or weight-bearing range of motion). Sometimes limping is caused by the obvious—having one shoe on and one off. Be sure that both shoes are off before beginning to walk.

5. Strengthening the ankle musculature
   Have the patient perform inversion, eversion, and dorsiflexion exercises on an ankle machine (Figure 17.7) or with a weighted boot, using the daily adjustable progressive resistive exercise (DAPRE) technique (J37, J38). Plantar flexion exercises on a weight machine are not necessary. Walking and normal toe raises are adequate to develop

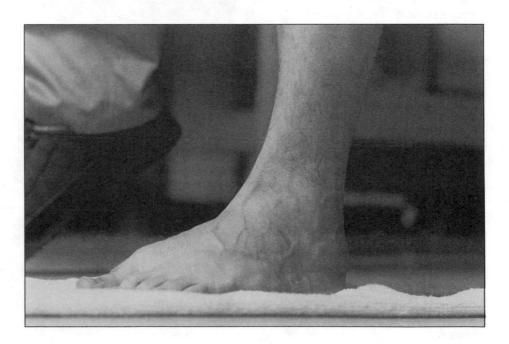

Figure 17.3 Stand on both feet and gradually shift weight back-and-forth, increasing the amount of weight borne by the injured ankle.

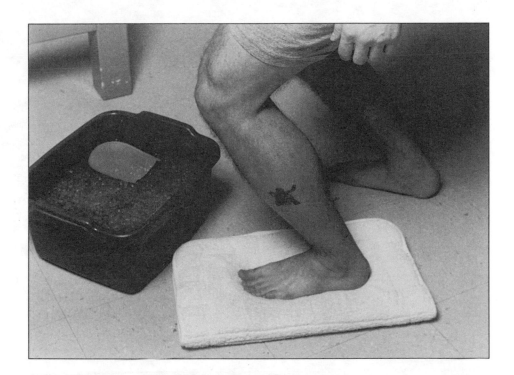

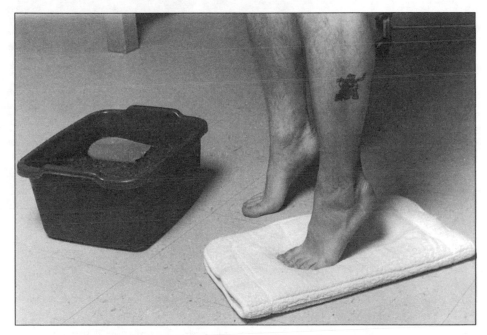

Figure 17.4 Plantar flex and dorsiflex the ankle by crouching (top) and then raising up on the toes (bottom).

plantar flexion strength. Perform these weight-training exercises once daily, after one of the cryokinetic sessions. It is not necessary to apply cold prior to or during weight training.

6. Jogging

Have the patient begin jogging straight ahead and progress to jogging in a lazy-S or figure-eight pattern, then in a sharp-Z pattern.

A hallway is a convenient location for jogging. The patient can begin the lazy-S pattern jogging with large sweeps from side to side of the hallway (Figure 17.8). Gradually the S is tightened until the pattern is a sharp Z.

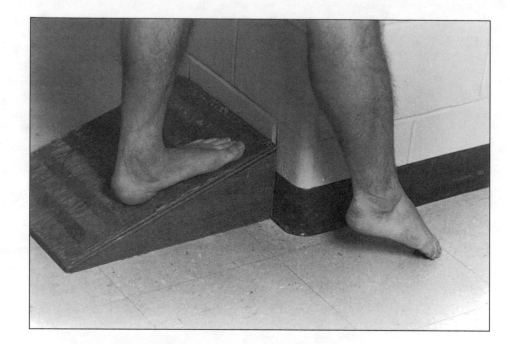

Figure 17.5 Stretching the heel cords; necessary if normal dorsiflexion is reduced. (Note that the left leg is out of position to show the injury.)

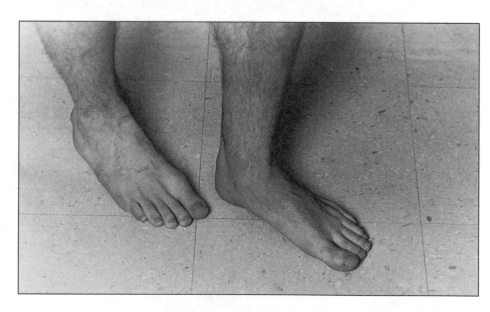

Figure 17.6 Walk first with short steps (often less than 10 inches long). Make sure the patient doesn't limp. Gradually lengthen the steps, as tolerated, until the patient is taking long steps.

7. Hopping and Jumping

   The four-square program (J78) provides excellent guidelines for progressing through hopping and jumping (Figure 17.9). Make a large + on the floor with adhesive tape. Tell the athlete to jump from quadrant to quadrant in the following progression, as tolerated: both feet ahead and back, side to side, then diagonally (Figure 17.10); one foot (injured) ahead and back, side to side, then diagonally. Progress also from short, shallow hops to long, high hops.

   After the athlete has mastered the four-square program have him or her hop on the injured foot back-and-forth across a crack or imaginary line in the floor while progressing forward across the room (Figure 17.11).

8. Sprints

   Begin with 5- to 10-yard (5.5- to 10.9-meter) straight-ahead sprints. Start and stop slowly at first and gradually progress to

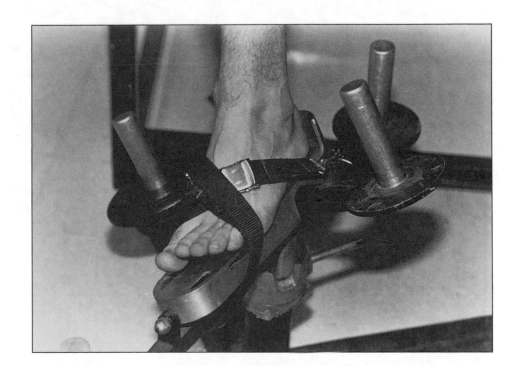

Figure 17.7 Strengthening the ankle musculature. This is a necessary, although often overlooked, aspect of ankle rehabilitation.

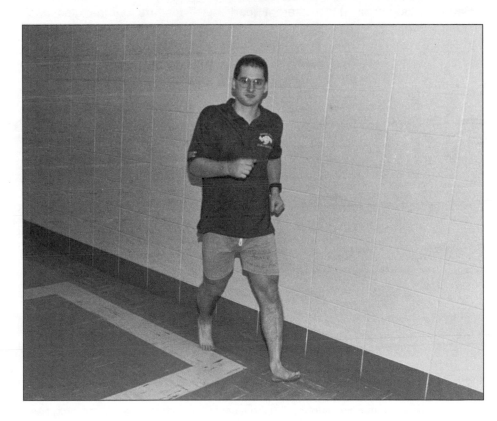

Figure 17.8 Jogging in an S pattern. As the athlete can accomplish this without pain or limping, the pattern is gradually condensed until it is a Z pattern. At this point the athlete is planting and cutting.

Side to side: Hop laterally between two quadrants

Front to back: Hop forward and backward between two quadrants

Four Square: Hop from square to square in a circular pattern. Sets are performed clockwise and counterclockwise

Triangles: Hop within three different quadrants. There are four triangles, each requiring a different diagonal hop.

Crisscross: Hop in an X pattern.

Straight-line hop: Hop forward and then backward along a 15- to 20- foot line.

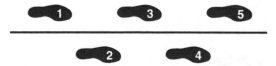

Line zigzag: Hop from side to side across a 15- to 20- foot line while moving forward and then backward.

Figure 17.9 The seven basic hopping patterns in the four-square ankle rehabilitation program, arranged in order of increasing difficulty. First, place a cross on the floor with two 3-ft pieces of adhesive tape to use as a guideline. The arrow denotes the direction the athlete faces. Start with number 1, and progress consecutively.

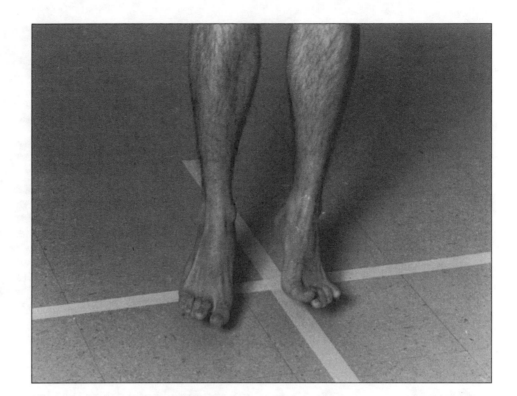

Figure 17.10 Diagonal hopping is part of the four-square exercises used during ankle rehabilitation. Begin hopping on both legs, and then progress to hopping on the injured leg only.

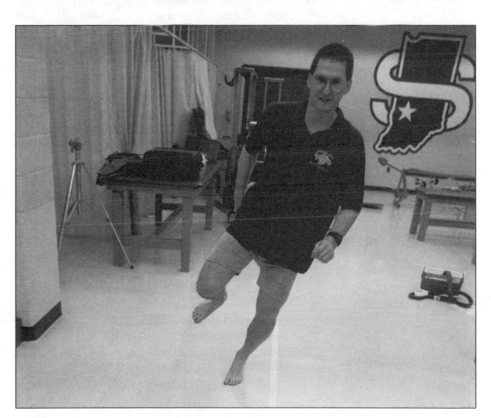

Figure 17.11 Hop back-and-forth across a line.

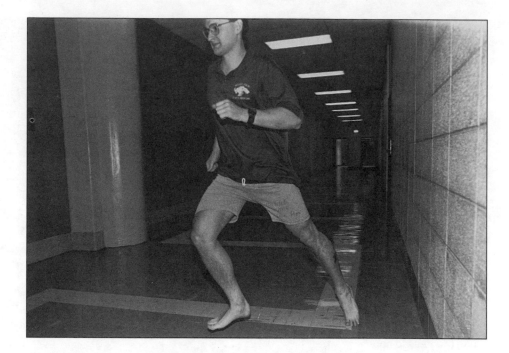

Figure 17.12
Explosive sprinting must be part of ankle rehabilitation. Begin with straight-ahead 5-yd sprints with gradual starting and stopping, progress to quick starts and stops, and then try cuts and turns.

distinct starts and stops (Figure 17.12). Also progress to sprinting in a lazy-S or figure-eight pattern, then in a sharp-Z pattern. Sprints should be performed simultaneously with hopping and jumping.

9. Hopping and sprinting without ice anesthesia
Here the patient gradually increases the duration of hopping, jumping, and sprinting beyond the period of anesthesia until he or she can perform these activities without the aid of the ice anesthesia.

10. Team drills
Have the recovering athlete begin at half speed and progresses to three-quarter speed and finally full speed (Figure 17.13). Pay particular attention during team drills and practice to how the athlete performs. All activities must be performed with proper mechanics. Any pain, hesitancy, or irregular movement indicates the athlete is not ready for the complexity of the activity. Have the athlete back off and perform at a lower level for a while. The ankle should be taped (Figure 17.14) for both team drills and team practice. (During earlier phases of cryokinetic exercising, the ankle need not—in fact, should not—be taped. The earlier exercises are performed indoors on a smooth surface where there is little chance of reinjury [none that I'm aware of after over 20 years of using and teaching the technique]. Not only is taping unnecessary, but it will also interfere with treatment. If you tape prior to numbing the ankle, the tape will reduce the effects of the ice. If you tape the ankle after numbing it, you will waste valuable exercising time. You only have 2 to 3 minutes of numbness to work with.)

A technique I have found useful during rehabilitation is to have the recovering athlete wear an "off-color" jersey (red unless his school colors are red) during team drills and reduced-intensity practice. This reminds coaches and other athletes that the injured athlete should be treated carefully. Excessive aggression either by a teammate or by the recovering athlete in response to an overly demanding coach might cause reinjury.

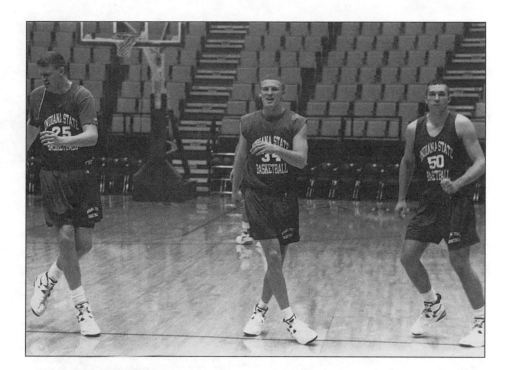

Figure 17.13 Athletes performing an individual agility drill at half speed. Gradually increase the tempo of the activity until they perform at full speed.

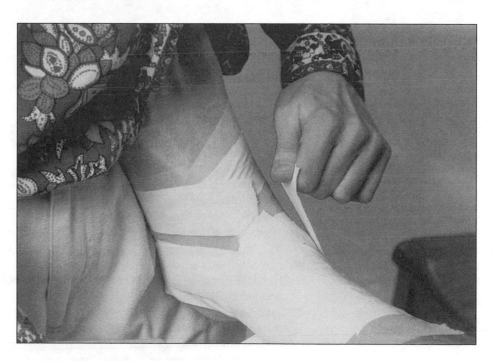

Figure 17.14 Tape the ankle for team drills and practice. Exercises performed in the training room generally need not be done with the ankle taped.

11. Team practice (Figure 17.15).
    Have the recovering athlete begin at reduced speed and intensity the first day and progress to full speed and intensity as quickly as possible.

Alternatives

If cold applications fail to provide enough pain relief for exercise, transcutaneous electrical nerve stimulation (TENS), or contrast baths may work. See chapters 9 and 11 for the theoretical basis for these alternatives.

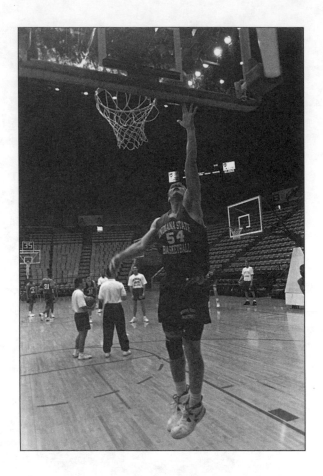

Figure 17.15
Perform team drills at half speed, and then gradually progress to full speed.

Key Points for Using Cryokinetics

- Cryokinetics is a combination of cold applications and active exercise.
- Cryokinetics results in much speedier rehabilitation than other forms of treatment.
- The cold applications provide a relative anesthesia so that active exercise can begin much more quickly than normal.
- Pain-free exercise is the key to cryokinetics (B23, C46).
- Cryokinetics has a built-in safety valve: Pain during numbness indicates that the exercise is too vigorous and the level of activity must be decreased.
- Judge the length of cold application by the patient's sensation rather than the time, but apply only for a maximum of 20 minutes during initial numbing and 5 minutes for renumbing.
- The initial numbing during the first treatment session is usually difficult for the patient. Explain to the patient that the intense pain is only temporary and that it will not occur during subsequent cold applications.
- Exercise while the body part remains numb, about 3 minutes.
- All exercise should be active (performed by the patient), progressive (increasing in both intensity and complexity), and free of pain.
- Perform exercise of progressively increasing intensity according to the patient's tolerance, as long as all exercise is performed smoothly and without pain.

- Constantly encourage the patient to progress from one level of activity to the next as quickly as possible, as long as the exercise can be performed without pain and in a normal, rhythmic, coordinated fashion.
- The key to cryokinetics is neither the time spent performing an activity nor the number of repetitions, but rather the ability to perform exercises of increasing difficulty properly and without pain.
- Don't allow the patient to limp.
- Have the patient perform weight training exercises once daily, after one of the cryokinetic sessions.
- For all phases of cryokinetic exercising up to team drills, the body part should not be taped.
- Have the athlete wear an "off-color" jersey while he or she is performing team drills and practicing at reduced intensity.

18

Relieving Acute Muscle Spasm: Cryostretch

Cryostretch combines three techniques for reducing muscle spasm: cold application, static stretching, and the hold-relax technique of proprioceptive neuromuscular facilitation (PNF) (B22, J40). Its purpose is to decrease muscle spasm, thereby allowing increased flexibility.

Cryostretch is similar to cryokinetics (chapter 17) in that exercise is performed while the body part is numbed, but it is different in the number of exercise sets and in the exercise itself. During cryostretch exercises, the affected muscle is alternately statically stretched and isometrically contracted.

Cryostretch begins with cold application—usually ice massage, ice pack, or large cold pack. Following numbness and interspersed with renumbing are three exercise bouts. Each bout lasts about 2-1/2 minutes and consists of two 65-second sets of exercise, with 20 seconds of relaxation between the two sets. The exercise sets consist of static stretching alternating with three repetitions of isometric (hold-relax) contractions.

The cryostretch technique is used whenever there is a need to reduce low-grade muscle spasm. Most muscle injuries (strains and contusions) result in some degree of spasm or tightness. Also, many mild muscle "pulls" are actually muscles in spasm rather than torn muscle fibers (E82, J61). In either case, the first step in rehabilitation is to reduce the spasm and reestablish pain-free range of motion (H51).

CRYOSTRETCH

Summary of Rationale for Cryostretching

See chapters 4 and 10–12 for a more complete theoretical basis for cryostretch.

EFFECTS

- Ice diminishes pain and muscle spasm.
- Static stretching overcomes the stretch reflex, decreasing muscle spasm.
- Relaxation is often greater after a near-maximal muscular contraction than it was before the contraction.

ADVANTAGES

- The combination of the three components into one procedure is more effective than any of the parts independently.
- Ice is relatively inexpensive; exercise is free.

DISADVANTAGES

- Ice is painful to some people.
- Melting ice can be messy.

INDICATIONS

- Any muscle with residual muscle spasm
- First-degree muscle strain
- A muscle that is stiff from prolonged disuse (immobilized)

CONTRAINDICATIONS

- Do not perform any exercise or activity that causes pain.
- Do not use ice on a person who is hypersensitive to cold.

PRECAUTIONS

- Pain must be used as a guideline. The patient should not attempt to consciously or willfully overcome pain.
- There may be an increase in pain 4 to 8 hours after treatment.
- Muscle may tear or pull if the static exercise begins too quickly or suddenly. There must be a gradual build-up to a maximal contraction.

Equipment Needed

- Ice cubes, ice packs, or cold packs
- Towel

Preapplication Procedures

PSYCHOLOGICAL PREPARATION

The initial numbing during the first treatment session is rarely as difficult for the patient as is immersion during cryokinetics, but there may be some pain before the body part numbs. Prepare the patient for this possibility.

Enlist the patient as a partner in the treatment. This is much easier in cryostretching than in cryokinetics, because the static stretching is usually the only activity that causes pain during cryostretch, and you directly control the intensity of the stretch.

Make sure the patient understands that recovery will be hindered if she or he ignores pain during stretching; you want to go to the limit, but not beyond.

Application Procedures

1. Numb the body part.
   a. Apply ice to the injured muscle or muscles:
      - Ice massage (with 6- 8-oz [80- 240-milliliter] ice cubes)
      - Ice bag (crushed ice in plastic bag)
      - Cold pack (commercial gel pack)

   b. Continue applying ice until the body part is numb (10–20 minutes; but remember that the goal is numbness, not 10–20 minutes of application). Some people cannot judge when they are numb, so stop application after 20 minutes if the patient has not yet reported numbness.

2. Have the patient engage in neuromuscular training.
   Before the first exercise bout, either before or immediately after the ice application, help the patient get the feel of contracting the proper muscle group. Without this neuromuscular training session, many patients will contract both the agonistic and antagonistic muscle groups when asked to contract the muscle in spasm later in the treatment session.

   Begin the training session by moving the patient's body part so that the affected muscle is lengthened. Then ask the patient to return the body part to the anatomical (starting) position, which requires contracting the affected muscle. For example, if the injury is to the hamstring muscle group, the patient lies supine on a table, and you lift the leg into the air. Move the leg to about 70% to 80% of its present range of motion—do not forcibly stretch it. Ask the patient to pull the heel back down to the table while keeping the leg straight (Figure 18.1), while you offer only minimal resistance. Repeat this motion three to four times against increasing resistance. Make sure that the affected muscle is the prime mover (i.e., that it performs most of the activity) and that all activity is within a

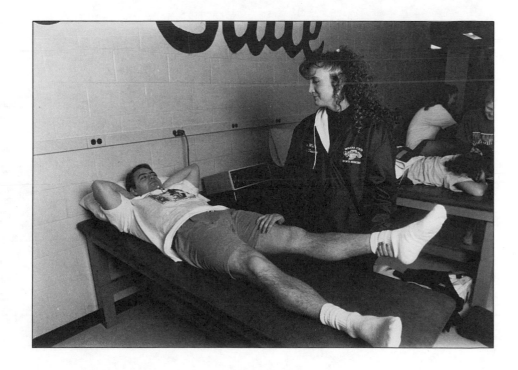

Figure 18.1 An athletic trainer teaching an athlete to contract only the specific involved muscle(s) prior to beginning cryostretch exercises. She lifts the limb into the air to within 20 to 30 degrees of the tightness. The athlete then actively returns the leg to the table, as shown. Repeat the exercise 3 to 4 times with the athletic trainer providing increased resistance each time.

comfortable range of motion. Correct the athlete if he or she attempts to move using muscles other than the target group.

3. Have the patient engage in cryostretching
   a. Begin by stretching the patient's affected muscle until pain or tightness is felt (Figure 18.2). Back off just a little (1°–3°) until the pain disappears.
   b. Hold the limb in that position for 20 seconds. During this time give the following instructions to the athlete: "In a moment, I want you to contract your muscle in the same way that you practiced earlier. This time, however, I will be holding it, so you may not be able to move your leg [or arm, etc.]. Do not contract the muscle quickly, or you may cause further injury. Start the contraction slowly and build up to a maximal contraction. When I tell you to stop, decrease your contraction slowly—not suddenly. Any questions? OK, begin" (Figure 18.3).
   c. The patient begins contracting the muscle. Encourage him or her to contract harder throughout the contraction.
   d. After 5 seconds, state, "Slowly, stop" as the signal to stop contracting the muscle.
   e. The muscle generally will be more relaxed following the isometric contraction than it was prior to it. So "take up the slack" by moving the patient's body part until the patient feels tightness or pain (Figure 18.4).
   f. Hold the patient in this second static stretch for 10 seconds.
   g. Repeat the isometric contraction, take up the slack, and perform the 10-second static stretch twice more.
   h. Rest the body part in the anatomical position for 20 seconds (Figure 18.5).
   i. Repeat the 65-second set of exercises as described in Steps a–h.
4. Perform a second and third sequence of renumbing and exercise by repeating Steps 1 and 3 twice more. Additional neuromuscular training (Step 2) is not necessary.

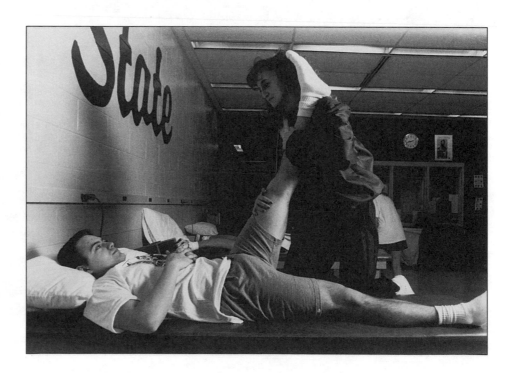

Figure 18.2 After the muscle is adequately cooled, stretch it until it feels tight, but not painful. Hold in this position for 20 seconds.

Figure 18.3 After the initial 20-second stretch, instruct the athlete to contract the muscles as hard as he can. The success of this stretch depends on keeping the muscle in its maximal stretched position during the isometric stretch. If the ratio of athletic trainer's arm strength to the injured muscle is to the athletic trainer's advantage, the athletic trainer can resist this contraction with his or her arms while standing on the floor. But if the involved muscle(s) are stronger than the athletic trainer, the athletic trainer may need to use his or her entire body to resist the contraction, as shown here.

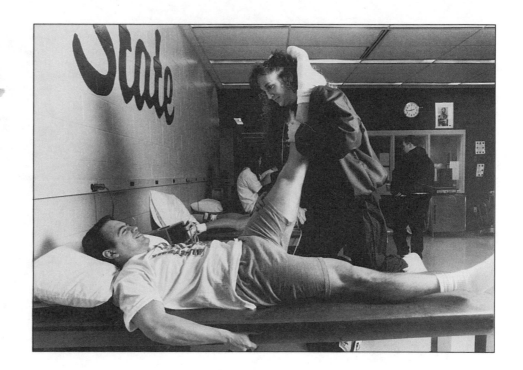

Figure 18.4 Take up the slack. Following the contraction, the muscle is often more relaxed than before the contraction, so the muscle can be stretched a few degrees further than the previous stretch. Hold the second (and each subsequent) stretch for 10 seconds.

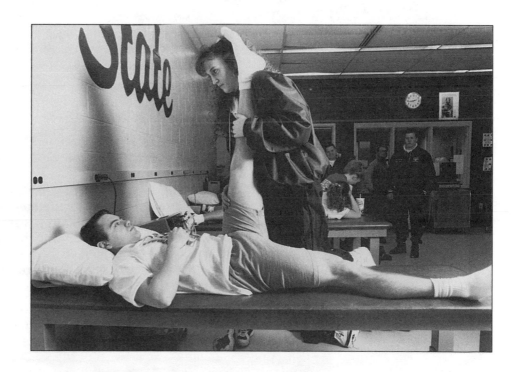

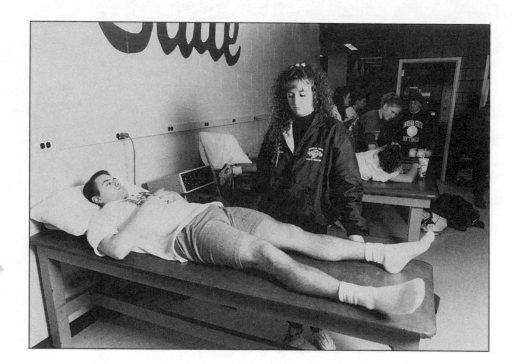

Figure 18.5
Following three sets of stretching and isometric contractions, return the limb to its anatomic position to rest for 20 seconds. Then repeat the entire exercise sequence.

Complete Cryostretch Treatment

- A complete cryostretch session consists of 10 to 20 minutes of ice application for initial numbness and three exercise bouts with numbness in between.
- Each exercise bout consists of two sets of passive-stretch/isometric contractions of approximately 65 seconds each with a 20-second rest in between.
- Always stretch as much as possible but within the limits of pain.
- Perform the entire treatment two or three times per day, with at least 3 hours between treatments.

COMBINED CRYOSTRETCH AND CRYOKINETICS

Once the muscle spasm begins to abate (often within 2–3 days), have the patient begin a protocol that combines cryostretch and cryokinetics. Each treatment session consists of an initial bout of cryostretch exercises, two or three bouts of cryokinetic exercises, and another bout of cryostretch exercises. Cold applications for numbness (or renumbing) precede each exercise bout. Begin cryokinetic exercises with manually resisted muscle contractions through a full range of motion and proceed through graded running, muscle strengthening, and team drills as explained in chapter 17. Make sure that all 10 elements of rehabilitation (chapter 4) are redeveloped. Follow these guidelines for combined cryostretch/cryokinetic exercises:

- During the second set of the first stretching bout, after the initial 20-second stretch, have the patient perform 6 to 10 repetitions of full range-of-motion contractions against manual resistance (Figure 18.6).
- Encourage the patient to work as hard as possible during the muscle contraction, especially at the end of the range of motion. Constantly encourage stronger contractions.

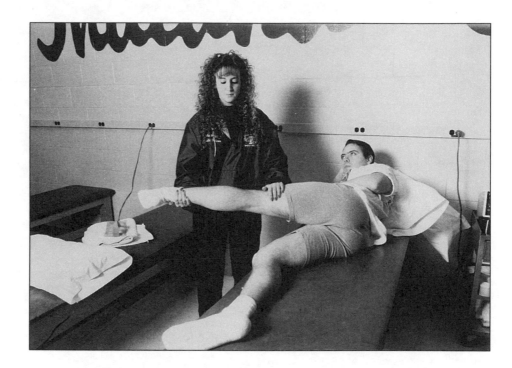

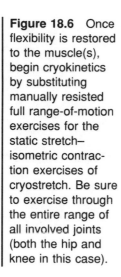

Figure 18.6 Once flexibility is restored to the muscle(s), begin cryokinetics by substituting manually resisted full range-of-motion exercises for the static stretch–isometric contraction exercises of cryostretch. Be sure to exercise through the entire range of all involved joints (both the hip and knee in this case).

- Perform only one set during each of the second and third exercise bouts. It should be the same as the second set of the first bout, that is, a 20-second passive stretch followed by 6 to 10 repetitions of manual-resistance full range-of-motion contractions.
- Once the strength begins to return (in 2–4 days), switch the patient to some type of isotonic weight lifting (using the daily adjustable progressive resistance exercise [DAPRE] technique) (J36, J38).
- Failure to either properly strengthen the muscle or resume full activity in a progressive, gradual way (as in the latter stages of cryokinetics) often results in reinjury to the muscle.

Key Points for Using Cryostretch

- Perform a brief neuromuscular training session prior to the first treatment to help the patient to get the feel of the proper muscular contraction.
- Each cryostretch treatment consists of three exercise bouts with renumbing between.
- Each cryostretch exercise bout consists of two sets of exercise of 65 seconds each with a 20-second rest between them.
- Each 65-second exercise set consists of static stretching interspersed with three isometric contractions of about 5 seconds each.
- Do not allow the patient to quickly begin or quickly stop the isometric contractions. Both transactions must be gradual.
- Always stretch as much as possible, but within the limits of pain.
- Once the muscle spasm releases and near full range of motion is possible, switch to a combined cryostretch and cryokinetics protocol. Perform two sets of cryostretch exercises with renumbing and three sets of cryokinetics between them.
- Continue through all 10 phases of rehabilitation until full sport activity is possible.

19

Postsurgical Cryotherapy

The three techniques that have been used most often for postsurgical cryotherapy are presented in this chapter: the AirCast Cryo Cuff, Dura*Kold packs, and the circulating cold-water machine. These units are described in chapter 15.

Although there is an increasing body of research supporting the use of postsurgical cryotherapy (see chapter 8), there is little research concerning optimal use of these devices. Please note, therefore, that the following application protocols are taken from manufacturers' suggestions.

AIRCAST CRYO CUFF

Cryo Cuff sleeves (see Figure 15.10, p. 205) are usually applied in the operating room over the surgical dressing, filled with chilled water, and worn constantly until the athlete leaves the hospital. "Refresh" the cuff every hour by draining the water back into the jug, rechilling it, and refilling the cuff by raising the jug into the air. This protocol results in skin interface temperatures ranging from 10° to 15°C (50° to 60°F).

Make sure the nursing staff regularly rechills the cuff on schedule. One way of doing so is to inform the patient of the importance of doing so, so he or she can remind busy nurses.

Send the Cryo Cuff unit home with the patient with instructions to continue using it as often as feasible until all symptoms are gone—that is, until he or she returns to normal activity.

DURA*KOLD PACKS

Dura*Kold packs are usually applied over a surgical dressing of gauze pads, surgical cotton pads, and an elastic bandage and secured with its elastic straps and Velcro. Leave the pack in place for 1-1/2 to 2 hours, remove and rechill for 1-1/2 to 2 hours, and then reapply to the surgical site. Continue alternating the pack between the freezer and the patient for 24 to 72 hours.

The advantage of Dura•Kold packs is their price and portability. They can be applied in the operating room and used throughout recovery. They can be chilled by the patient in any freezer unit. Their disadvantage is the lack of compression, which seems to be vital during postsurgical applications. This can be overcome with an elastic wrap applied over the pack.

CIRCULATING COLD-WATER MACHINES

The Polar Care cooler (see p. 206) and the Icy Hot machineare used in essentially the same manner. Apply the pads under or over the surgical dressing (under the dressing is more beneficial [E20]) in the operating room and use the device constantly while the patient is hospitalized. Their temperatures are high enough that constant application is possible.

Patients should also be given a cryotherapy product to use following discharge from the hospital. The Polar Care cooler is inexpensive and portable enough to be a home unit, but the Icy Hot machine is not. Either Dura*Kold or Cryo Cuff should be prescribed for home use.

20

Cryotherapeutic Techniques for Relieving Pain

Decreased pain is one of the primary objectives of numerous cryotherapeutic techniques. For most of these, decreasing pain is a means to an end—to allow additional therapeutic intervention. For instance, during cryokinetics cold is applied to decrease pain so that active exercise is possible. The cold applications without exercise are of no therapeutic value and may even hinder rehabilitation. On the other hand, the exercise intensity is severely restricted without prior cold-induced pain reduction.

In at least one instance—immediate care—decreased pain has nothing to do with the primary objective of the technique; it is simply an added benefit. During immediate-care procedures, cold is used to decrease metabolism and, thereby, secondary hypoxic injury. The decreased pain has no effect on decreasing metabolism, but it does add to the overall comfort of the patient.

For some types of pain, cryotherapeutic pain relief can be used as an end in itself. This chapter presents techniques for relieving four types of pain:

- Relieving menstrual cramps
- Treating headaches
- Painless injections and venipuncture
- Myofascial trigger point therapy

RELIEVING MENSTRUAL CRAMPS

Ice massage (J6) and acupressure may be used (J61) to relieve painful menstrual cramps in female athletes. Both techniques involve massaging an area 1 inch to the right of the L3 vertebral process. Massaging with ice may result in quicker relief and can be applied to a more generalized area (J6).

243

Application Procedures

1. Have patient lie prone.
2. Lift shirt so as to expose the lower back area.
3. Locate the L3 vertebral process (level of iliac crests; Figure 20.1).
4. Palpate area 1 inch to right of the L3 vertebra. Feel for a small nodule or area of extreme tenderness or sensitivity.
5. Massage tender area with finger (Figure 20.2) or ice cube (Figure 20.3) for 60 to 90 seconds. If pain or cramps subside, discontinue treatment; if not, continue treatment for up to 10 minutes.
6. Repeat treatment if pain or cramps return.

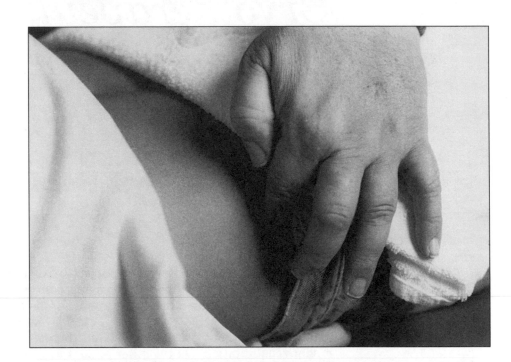

Figure 20.1 Locate the L3 vertebral process by drawing an imaginary line between the left and right iliac crests. Then palpate for a nodule about 1 inch to the right of the spinal column.

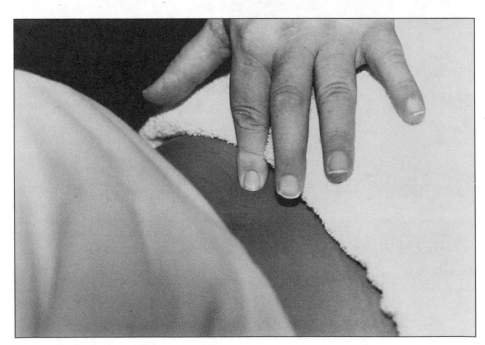

Figure 20.2 Massage the nodule with a finger for 60 to 90 sec to relieve severe menstrual cramps.

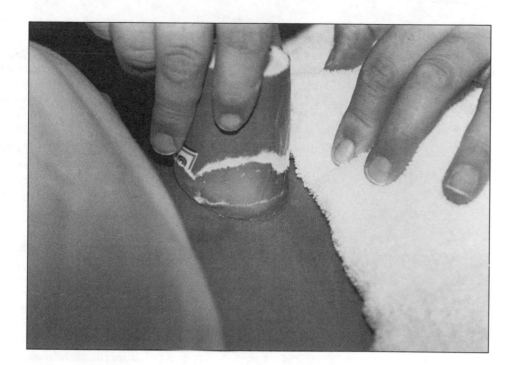

Figure 20.3 Ice massage to the low back for menstrual cramp relief.

TREATING HEADACHES

Two cryotherapeutic applications have been suggested for pain relief:

- Application of cold packs directly to the temples (B26, E84)
- Ice massage to the hoku acupressure point (LI-4) of the hand until the web space becomes numb or for 7 minutes (E67; Figure 20.4)

PAINLESS INJECTIONS AND VENIPUNCTURE

Pain caused by injections, intradermal testing with allergens, finger or ear pricks for blood counts, and venipuncture can be eliminated by cooling the

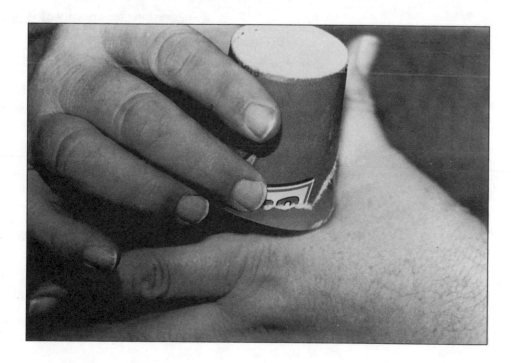

Figure 20.4 Ice massage to hoku (an acupressure point located in the web of the hand) for relief of headaches and toothaches.

skin below 10°C. Spray the skin for 3 to 5 seconds with a vapo-coolant (ethyl chloride or fluoromethane) to produce the desired analgesia. Be prepared to give the injection immediately; the analgesia only lasts 2 to 3 seconds.

Some people are adversely affected by the sudden shock of the spray, which can be worse than the pain of the needle. For such people, use a cotton ball saturated with the vapo-coolant for the application. The entire process takes 5 to 10 seconds, is not painful, and will result in 2 to 3 seconds of analgesia.

Application of a small amount of glycerol trinitrate to the skin a few minutes before and 30 to 60 seconds of ice massage immediately before venipuncture provides a simple and painless method of assisting venipuncture (J80). The glycerol trinitrate, a vasodilator, prevents the vasoconstriction that normally occurs with ice massage.

MYOFASCIAL TRIGGER POINT THERAPY

A myofascial trigger point is a localized palpable spot of deep hypersensitivity from which noxious impulses bombard the central nervous system to give rise to referred pain (E102). Stimulating the trigger point by palpation, ultrasound, or electrical muscle stimulation (J60) will set off referred pain and result in the "jump sign" (flinching motion), thus locating the trigger point. All trigger points in an area should be located and marked with a felt tip pen (J60). Each trigger point is then treated individually.

Noncryotherapeutic techniques for treating trigger points include injection with procaine (E99) and treatment with ultrasound or muscle stimulation (J60). Treatment with cryotherapy involves spraying with a vapo-coolant and stretching the involved tissue. Be careful not to chill underlying muscles (E24, E73, E99). Stretching the involved muscle following spraying is mandatory (E49, E73, E101, E103).

Application Procedures

One published set of suggestions for treatment is as follows (E101):

1. Guard against fire hazards.
2. Raise patient's head above the level to be sprayed and/or protect the head with a piece of fiberboard.
3. Hold the container 60 centimeters (2 feet) away from the trigger point.
4. Begin spraying at the trigger area, carrying over to the reference zone (area of referred pain).
5. Apply the stream at an acute angle.
6. Spray in one direction with a slow sweeping motion.
7. Repeat sweeps in rhythm of a few seconds on and off.
8. Lengthen interval between sweeps if aching develops.
9. Do not frost skin.
10. Stretch muscle by gentle movement.
11. Continue until pain disappears and tenderness at trigger area is lessened.
12. Stop if there is no relief after 5 minutes.

21

Miscellaneous Cryotherapeutic Techniques

An interesting grab bag of cryotherapeutic techniques exist that I present in this chapter, though not all of them are used for treating acute musculoskeletal conditions. Each technique in this miscellany utilizes local hypothermia in conjunction with

- medicated ice for abrasions,
- stretching connective tissue,
- cooling athletes during exercise in a hot environment,
- minimizing cold sores,
- minimizing blisters, and
- preventing hair loss during doxorubicin chemotherapy.

MEDICATED ICE FOR ABRASIONS

Athletes often suffer skin abrasions. Abrasions can become complicated injuries if they are not handled properly. Proper management includes the standard first aid of ice, compression, and elevation to limit pain, swelling, and secondary hypoxic injury. But you must also be concerned about bacterial contamination (H39).

Neither of the two most popular treatments for abrasions are comprehensive. One treats the injury like a sprain or strain with ice, compression, and elevation, ignoring the possibility of infection. The other treats the open wound by cleaning it and applying an antiseptic and sterile wound dressing (G34), but this treatment ignores the possibility of secondary hypoxic injury and swelling. The following technique (H39) combines the two treatments by using medicated ice cups (Figure 21.1). The antiseptic in the ice discourages bacterial propagation. The indications, contraindications, and precautions for any medication should be provided on the label.

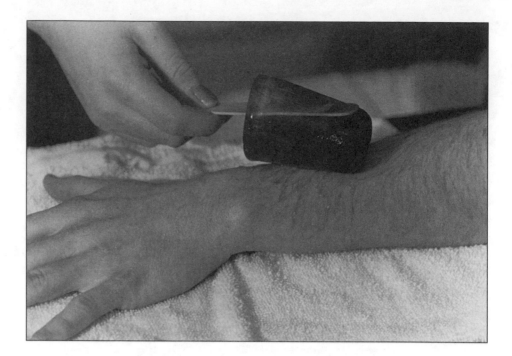

Figure 21.1 Ice massage with a medicated ice cup decreases pain as well as cleans and disinfects abrasions.

Ice acts as an analgesic. Using ice that contains lidocaine produces an even greater analgesic effect, which is necessary when brushing or picking dirt and debris out of an open wound. The decrease in pain from the ice and lidocaine also leads to a slowing of the pain-spasm-pain cycle, which helps enhance muscle function around the injury. It is easy to avoid wound infection when the injury is treated early and properly.

Equipment Needed

- 2-oz (60-milliliter) disposable cup
- Plastic stir sticks
- 2% lidocaine
- 10% povidone-iodine
- Distilled or boiled water

Preapplication Procedures

PREPARING MEDICATED ICE CUBES

1. Mix 1.5 oz (45 milliliters) of povidone-iodine solution with 0.5 oz (15 milliliters) of lidocaine solution.
2. Place the mixture in the cup.
3. Secure a stir stick vertically in the center of the cup with adhesive tape (see Figure 15.8, p. 203).
4. Freeze overnight.
5. Clearly label and isolate the medicated ice cups from other ice cups in the freezer so that they are not accidently used for general ice massage. (This would not cause problems, but it would be a waste of resources.)

Application Procedures

1. Seek the advice and approval of a physician before administering medicated ice.
2. Remove the ice cube from the cup.
3. Hold the stir stick and roll the ice back and forth along the lacerated skin for about 10 minutes.
4. As the ice melts, the medicines will flow into the damaged region and produce analgesic and antiseptic effects.
5. Debride the area (remove foreign materials using sterile gauze or tweezers).
6. Treat and protect the injured area as you would any open wound, emphasizing sterility.
7. Apply an ice pack for 20 to 30 minutes each hour until bedtime and apply compression continuously (except when applying or taking off the ice pack) for the first 24 to 72 hours after the injury.

STRETCHING CONNECTIVE TISSUE

The following technique (J66) was designed for treating connective tissue structures that are abnormally tight due to surgical shortening, transplantation, scarring, or immobilization contracture. Both heat and cold packs are applied during static stretching (Figure 21.2).

Equipment Needed

- 4 to 6 hot packs
- 2 cold packs
- 3 to 15 lbs (1.4 to 7 kilograms) of weights
- 8 to 10 feet (2.5 to 3 meters) of rope or cord
- Leverage system

Application Procedures

1. Heat the joint and tissue with hot packs for 35 to 75 minutes. Use two packs at a time to surround the joint, and change the packs every 15 to 20 minutes to obtain the maximum tolerable degree of heating. If the connective tissue is deep under other tissue, ultrasound or diathermy may be necessary to heat the tissue adequately.
2. Passively stretch the patient's tissue after 15 minutes of heating. Use a cable and pulley system to apply a moderate but tolerable force (3 to 15 pounds [1.4 to 7 kilograms]; Figure 21.3). Release the

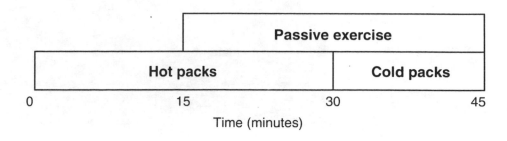

Figure 21.2
Diagram of the connective tissue stretching technique.

force every 5 to 10 minutes for about 30 seconds to allow the patient to move the body part and thus relieve any discomfort caused by the stretching.

3. Following 20 to 60 minutes of stretching with heat, remove the Hydrocollator packs.
4. Apply cold packs. (See Figure 21.4.)
5. Stretch the patient's tissue for an additional 15 minutes with the cold packs attached.
6. Have the patient repeat the protocol daily if possible, but at least three times per week.

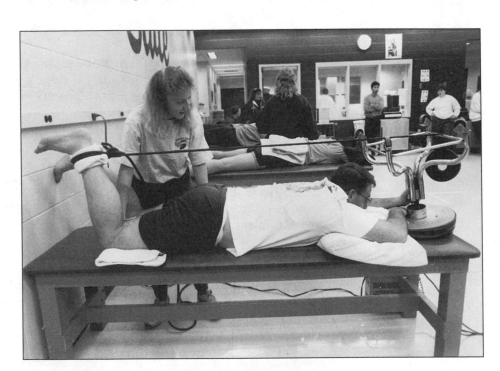

Figure 21.3 To stretch contracted connective tissue, apply gentle, constant tension to the joint. Here, a rope with a 5-lb weight is attached to the opposite end and is tied around the ankle and extended over an upside-down chair (fulcrum) so that the weight dangles.

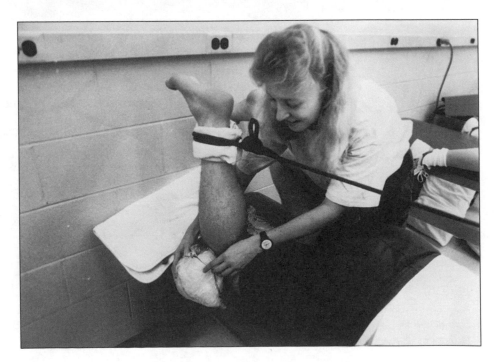

Figure 21.4 After 15 min of stretching with a hot pack on the knee, replace the hot pack with a cold pack and continue to stretch for an additional 15 min.

7. Total relaxation is necessary during the stretching. This requires a conscious effort by the patient and must be encouraged by the athletic trainer or therapist. Biofeedback devices have been helpful at times (J66).

COOLING ATHLETES DURING EXERCISE IN A HOT ENVIRONMENT

A variety of devices have been used to cool athletes during competition in the extreme heat, such as football in August in the southern United States. Removing heat from the body refreshes the athlete and helps him or her to participate longer (C69, J21, J42, J58, J63). Several cooling devices and techniques are listed here:

- Drape a towel soaked in ice water over the head (Figure 21.5).
- Place a fan on the sidelines and encourage athletes to remove their helmets, jerseys, and shoulder pads and stand in front of the fan.
- Wear an oversized vest made of nylon and lined with sheets of Dura*Kold plastic ice cubes (see chapter 15); this is actually a large Dura*Kold pack sewn by the manufacturer in the shape of a vest. It can be worn directly on the skin or over a T-shirt (Figure 21.6).
- Wear a cold pack around the neck or on top of the head. Some cold packs are constructed as neck collars and headbands to facilitate these applications.

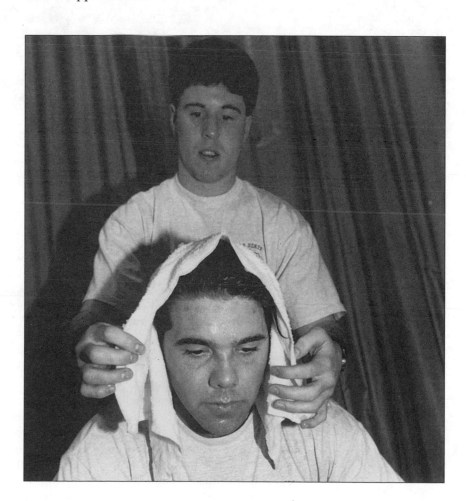

Figure 21.5 On very hot days, cool athletes with a cold towel draped over their head. Soak the towel in a slush bucket, wring it only lightly, and apply it directly to the scalp.

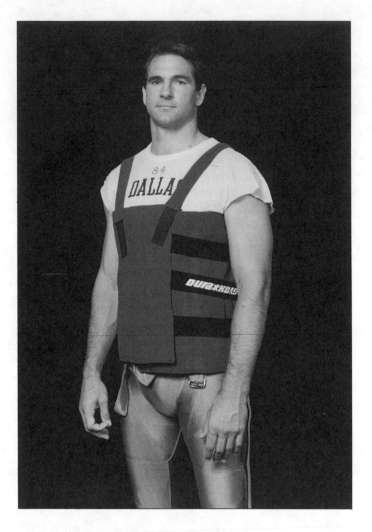

Figure 21.6 Dura*-Kold vests are popular with football teams in the South and industrial workers in hot factories. The vests are chilled in a freezer, stored in an insulated cooler, and then applied under the shoulder pads when the athlete needs to cool down.

- Use a "cool cape," an oversized, hooded vinyl rain coat attached to an air conditioner on wheels with 4-inch (10-centimeter) flexible plastic tubing (e.g., clothes dryer hose) (J64). Athletes stand or sit with the cool cape over them.

MINIMIZING COLD SORES

In one study (J15), cold sores were treated with ice packs for 90 to 120 minutes. In all 14 patients treated within 24 hours of onset of the prondrome, vesicles were reabsorbed without breaking or becoming purulent (runny), and healing was complete in 1 to 2 days. The 4 patients treated 36 hours or more following onset, however, developed full-fledged cold sores.

Application Procedures

1. As soon as you feel a cold sore coming on, wrap an ice cube with a wash cloth so that one fourth of the ice cube is exposed, or put it in a plastic bag. (The bag and wash cloth are to collect water as the ice cube melts, thus preventing dripping water.)
2. Hold the covered end of ice cube and apply the exposed end to the cold sore. Hold in place for 90 to 120 minutes (Figure 21.7), replacing the ice cube as needed.

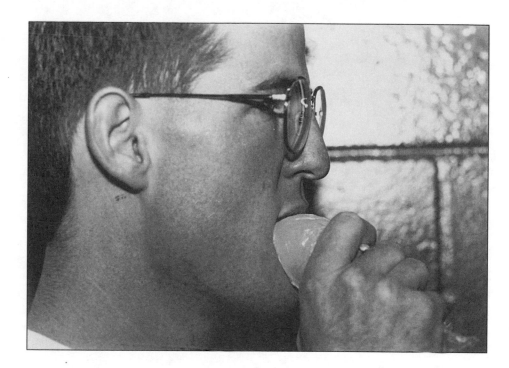

Figure 21.7 Ice cube in a plastic bag, when applied to a cold sore or fever blister on the lips as it begins to form, will prevent the blister from fully developing and hasten resolution of the problem.

MINIMIZING BLISTERS

Blisters, like cold sores, can be prevented by cold applications if applied quickly enough, but cold will do nothing for blisters once they are formed. The key is to catch the problem in the "hot spot" stage, just before the layers of skin separate and begin filling with fluid. A hot spot appears as a circle of bright red tissue at the point of irritation; it is called a hot spot because it feels warm or as if it is burning.

Athletes should be informed of hot spots and encouraged to be aware of them, especially during the initial days of their sport season. They should be allowed to stop practice so that they can immerse the hot spot in a slush bucket for 5 to 10 minutes. Such a policy will save much time lost from blisters.

PREVENTION OF HAIR LOSS DURING DOXORUBICIN CHEMOTHERAPY

Doxorubicin is one of the most active cytotoxic agents used in cancer chemotherapy, especially for advanced breast cancer (J4, J76). This treatment leads to severe hair loss, however. A number of investigators have found that hair loss is often prevented by local hypothermia (J4, J14, J22, J76). One (J4) treated 28 patients with a skullcap made of cold-gel packs. Twelve suffered no substantial scalp hair loss, even though 11 lost pubic and axillary hair. Ten others suffered some scalp hair loss, but not enough to require a wig. The remaining 6 suffered severe or total hair loss (all of these had biochemical abnormalities of liver function associated with hepatic metastasis).

References

To facilitate further reading and research in cryotherapy, I've attempted to organize this reference list according to the major thrust of the article. Obviously, there is overlap. Some articles could fit into multiple categories. But, it seemed the benefits of this type of organization outweighed the problems. Each section is assigned a letter and the articles within that section are alphabetized and numbered. So each reference is a combination of a letter and a number. The categories are:

A   Reviews and general articles.
B   Rehabilitation technique and theory. The main emphasis of the article is on technique, but some theory is discussed.
C   Circulatory and temperature responses.
D   Neurological effects.
E   Pain.
F   Spasm.
G   Metabolism and inflammation.
H   Immediate care and postsurgical cryotherapy.
I   Complications, contraindications and precautions.
J   Miscellaneous (mostly noncryotherapy).

A second aid to reading and research was to cross-reference each entry with the page(s) on which it is referenced. The last item of each entry is a number (or numbers) in parentheses. These numbers refer to the pages on which that entry is referenced. Thus if you are interested in a particular author and how I've quoted that author's work, you can find the author's name in the bibliography and then turn directly to the text pages where his or her work is quoted.

A third aid is an author index, which contains an alphabetical listing of the first three authors of each reference and the reference number of that entry.

REVIEWS COVERING MULTIPLE EFFECTS

A1.   American Academy of Orthopaedic Surgeons. Athletic Training and Sports Medicine. Park Ridge, IL: American Academy of Sports Medicine; 1991:96-123. (9, 150)

A2.   Bancroft H. Circulation in skeletal muscle. In : Hamilton WF, ed. Handbook of Physiology. Washington, DC: American Physiological Society; 1963; 2:1353-1384. (9, 20)

A3.   Bierman W. Therapeutic use of cold. JAMA. 1955; 157:1189-1192. (9, 17, 18)

A4.   Bryant T. A Manual for the Practice of Surgery. 3rd ed. Philadelphia, PA: Henry C Lea's Son; 1881:121, 961. (9, 15)

A5.   Burton AC, Edholm OG. Man in a Cold Environment. New York, NY: Hafner Publishing Co; 1969:129-147, 223-240. (9, 114)

A6. Carlson LD. Physiology of exposure to cold. Physiol Phys. December 1964; 2:1-7. (9, 20, 127, 128)

A7. Craig TT. Fundamentals of Athletic Training. 2nd ed. Chicago, Ill: American Medical Association; 1979:56. (9)

A8. Downey JA. Physiological effects of heat and cold. J Am Phys Ther Assoc. 1964; 44:713-717. (9, 20)

A9. Downey JA, Darling RC, Miller JM. The effects of heat, cold, and exercise on the peripheral circulation. Arch Phys Med Rehabil. 1968; 49:308-314. (9, 20, 112, 114)

A10. Dyment PG. Initial management of minor acute soft-tissue injuries. Pediatr Ann. 1988; 17:99-100, 102-106. (9)

A11. Everall M. Cold therapy. Nurs Times. 1976; 70:144-145. (9, 94, 99, 173)

A12. Fisher E, Solomon S. Physiological responses to heat and cold. In: Licht S, ed. Therapeutic Heat and Cold. 2nd ed. Baltimore, MD: Waverly Press; 1965:126-169. (9, 65, 122)

A13. Fox RH. Local cooling in man. Br Med Bull. 1961; 17:15-18. (9, 123, 165, 175, 176)

A14. Glick EN, Lucas M. Ice therapy. Ann Phys Med. 1969; 10:70-75. (9, 124, 163)

A15. Haines J. A study into a report on cold therapy. Physiotherapy. 1970; 56:501-502. (9, 17, 163, 164)

A16. Haines J. A survey of recent developments in cold therapy. Physiotherapy. 1967; 53:222-229. (9, 173)

A17. Kellett J. Acute soft tissue injuries: a review of the literature. Med Sci Sports Exerc. 1986; 18:489-500. (9, 15)

A18. Knight KL. Cold as a modifier of sports-induced inflammation. In: Leadbetter WB, Buckwalter JA, Gordon SL, eds. Sports-Induced Inflammation. Chicago, IL: American Academy of Orthopaedic Surgeons; 1990:463-477. (4, 9, 89, 173)

A19. Knight KL. Cryotherapy in sports medicine. In: Schriber K, Burke EJ, eds. Relevant Topics in Athletic Training. Ithaca, NY: Mouvement Publications; 1979:52-59. (9, 94, 163, 164, 171)

A20. Kowal MA. Review of physiological effects of cryotherapy. J Orthop Sports Phys Ther. September/October 1983; 5:66-73. (9, 20)

A21. LeBlanc J. Man in the Cold. Springfield, IL: Charles C Thomas Publisher, 1975:64-67. (9, 158)

A22. Lee JM, Warren MP. Cold Therapy in Rehabilitation. London, England: Belt and Hymen; 1978:69-71. (9, 15, 179)

A23. Lehman JF, DeLateur BJ. Diathermy and superficial heat, laser, and cold therapy. In: Kottke FJ, Lehman JF, eds. Krusen's Handbook of Physical Medicine and Rehabilitation. Philadelphia, PA: WB Saunders Co; 1990:283-367. (9)

A24. Lehman JF, DeLateur BJ. Cryotherapy. In: Lehman JF, ed. Therapeutic Heat and Cold. 3rd ed. Baltimore, MD: Williams & Wilkins; 1982:563-602. (9, 11, 135, 147, 164, 176)

A25. Lehman JF, Warren CG, Scham SM. Therapeutic heat and cold. Clin Orthop. 1974; 99:207-245. (9, 15, 71, 121)

A26. Licht S. History of therapeutic heat and cold. In: Lehman JF, ed. Therapeutic Heat and Cold. 3rd ed. Baltimore, MD: Williams & Wilkins; 1982:1-34. (9, 15)

A27. Licht S. Local cryotherapy. In Licht S, ed. Therapeutic Heat and Cold. 2nd ed. Baltimore, MD: Waverly Press; 1965:538-564. (9, 15, 172, 176, 183)

A28. Lorenze EJ, Caroutonis G, DeRosa AJ. Effect on coronary circulation of cold packs to hemiplegic shoulders. Arch Phys Med. 1960; 41:394-399. (9, 163)

A29. McLean DA. The use of cold and superficial heat in the treatment of soft tissue injuries. Br J Sports Med. March 1989; 23:53-54. (9, 89)

A30. McMaster WC. Cryotherapy. Physician Sportsmed. November 1982; 10:112-119. (9, 90, 134, 163)

A31. McMaster WC. A literary review on ice therapy in injuries. Am J Sports Med. 1977; 5:124-126. (9, 96, 163, 164)

A32. Meeusen R, Lievens P. The use of cryotherapy in sports injuries. Sports Med. 1986; 3:398-414. (9)

A33. Michlovitz S, Segal LR. Physical agents and electrotherapy techniques in hand rehabilitation. In: Stanley BG, Tribuzi SM, eds. Concepts in Hand Rehabilitation. Philadelphia, PA: FA Davis Co; 1992:216-237. (9)

A35. Murphy AJ. The physiological effects of cold application. Phys Ther Rev. 1960; 40:112-115. (9, 111)

A36. Nanneman D. Thermal modalities: heat and cold. Am Assoc Occup Health Nurs J. 1991; 39:70-75. (9)

A37. Oakes BW. Acute soft tissue injuries: nature and management. Aust Fam Physician. July 1981; 10(suppl):3-16. (9, 17)

A38. Olson JE, Stravino VD. A review of cryotherapy. Phys Ther. 1972; 53:840-853. (9, 147)

A39. Raptou AD. Cryotherapy: a brief review. South Med J. 1968; 61: 625-627. (9, 163, 173)

A40. Rawlinson K. Modern Athletic Training. New York, NY: Prentice-Hall Inc; 1961:48-49. (9, 163)

A41. Sherman S. Which treatment to recommend: hot or cold? Am Pharm. August 1980; 20:46-49. (9, 15, 89)

A42. Starkey C. Therapeutic Modalities for Athletic Trainers. Philadelphia, PA: FA Davis Co; 1993:6-17. (9, 16, 128)

A43. Thompson GE. Physiological effects of cold exposure. Int Rev Physiol, Environ Physiol II. 1977; 15:29-69. (9, 163, 164)

A44. Till D. Cold therapy. Physiotherapy. 1969; 55:461-466. (9, 89)

A45. Weise D, Smith C. Cold or heat: what will be your choice? First Aider. Winter 1993; 63:1, 12-13. (9)

A46. Wise D. Application of cold in treating soft tissue injury. Coaching Sci Update. 1979-1980:53. (9, 17, 94, 96, 111)

A47. Wise DD. Ice and the athlete. Physiother Can. 1973; 25:213-217. (9, 107, 108, 111)

REHABILITATION TECHNIQUE AND THEORY

B1. Abraham D. The hot and cold facts of injury treatment. Coaching Women's Basketball. July/August 1989; 2:28-30. (125)

B2. Anonsen RE. Evaluating injuries, protective devices, and cryokinetics in ice hockey. J Natl Athl Train Assoc. 1970; 5:16-19. (17)

B3. Behnke RS. Cold therapy. Athl Train. 1974; 9:178-179. (3, 10, 17, 85, 96, 111, 121, 123)

B4. Bennett D. Water at 67° to 69° Fahrenheit to control hemorrhage and swelling encountered in athletic injuries. J Natl Athl Train Assoc. 1961; 1f:12-14. (15, 109)

B5. Bergfeld J, Halpern B. Sports Medicine: Functional Management of Ankle Injuries. Kansas City, MO: The American Academy of Family Physicians; 1991:1-16. (92)

B6. Carbajal FJ, Nelson DO. The effect of cold pack application on the recovery from pitching a baseball. Athl J. February 1967; 47:8-11, 85-86. (166)

B7.   Cawley PW, France EP. Biomechanics of the lateral ligaments of the ankle: an evaluation of the effects of axial load and single plane motions on ligament strain patterns. Foot Ankle. October 1991; 12:92-99. (91, 167, 177)

B8.   DePodesta M. Cryotherapy in rehabilitation. Can Athl Train Assoc J. December 1979; 6:15-16. (94, 96, 111, 123)

B9.   Gieck J. Heat and cold: the mod modality. Schol Coach. June 1970; 29:25. (122)

B10.   Grant AE. Massage with ice (cryokinetics) in the treatment of painful conditions of the musculoskeletal system. Arch Phys Med Rehabil. 1964; 44:233-238. (3, 15-17, 121-123, 172)

B11.   Gray S. Cold, compression and elevation. Network News. September/October 1990; 16:14-15. (111, 121)

B12.   Gucker T. The use of heat and cold in orthopedics. In: Licht S., ed. Therapeutic Heat and Cold. New Haven, Conn: E Licht; 1965:398-406. (123)

B13.   Halvorson GA. Therapeutic heat and cold for athletic injuries. Phys Sportsmed. May 1990; 18:87-94.

B14.   Handling KA. Rehabilitating athletic injuries with cryotherapy. JOPERD. Jun 1982; 53:338-340. (10, 82)

B15.   Harvey J, Glick J. Stanish W, Teitz C. Tennis elbow: what's the best treatment? Phys Sportsmed. June 1990; 18:62-74. (11)

B16.   Hayden CA. Cryokinetics in an early treatment program. J Am Phys Ther Assoc. 1964; 44:990-993. (15, 17, 122, 172)

B17.   Hill PD. Effects of heat and cold on the perineum after episiotomy/laceration. J Obstet Gynecol Neonatal Nurs. 1989; 18:124-129. (101)

B18.   Hocutt JE. Cryotherapy. Am Fam Physician. March 1981; 23:141-144. (82, 96, 111, 123, 165, 207)

B19.   Johnson S, ed. A new treatment of musculoskeletal pain and injury. Reebok Instructor News. 1991; 4(4):4-5. (18)

B20.   Juvenal JP. Cryokinetics, a new concept in the treatment of injuries. Schol Coach. May 1966; 35:40-42. (10, 15, 17, 122)

B21.   Kalenak A, Medlar CE, Fleagle SB, Hockber WJ. Athletic injuries: heat vs. cold. Am Fam Physician. May 1975; 12:131-134. (15, 17, 109, 111, 112, 123, 124)

B22.   Knight KL. Cryostretch for muscle injuries. Physician Sportsmed. April 1980; 8:129. (50, 233)

B23.   Knight KL. Ankle rehabilitation with cryotherapy. Physician Sportsmed. November 1979; 7:133. (217, 230)

B24.   Laing DR, Dalley DR, Kirk JA. Ice therapy in soft tissue injuries. N Z Med J. 1973; 78:155-158. (15, 96, 123, 163, 179)

B25.   Lamboni P, Harris B. The use of ice, airsplints and high voltage pulsed galvanic stimulation in effusion reduction. Athl Train. 1983; 18:23. (91)

B26.   Lance JW. The controlled application of cold and heat by a new device (migra-lief apparatus) in the treatment of headache. Headache. 1988; 28:458-461. (245)

B27.   Meeroff JC. Cryotherapy for minor athletic injuries. Hosp Pract. 1985; 20:97-100. (179)

B28.   Michlovitz S, Smith W, Watkins M. Ice and high voltage pulsed stimulation in treatment of acute lateral ankle sprains. J Orthop Sports Phys Ther. 1988; 9:301-304. (91)

B29.   Moore RJ, Nicolette RL, Behnke RS. The therapeutic use of cold (cryotherapy) in the care of athletic injuries. J Natl Athl Train Assoc. 1967; 2:6. (15, 17, 123, 124)

B30. O'Connor FG, Sobel JR, Nirscl RP. Five-step treatment for overuse injuries. Physician Sportsmed. October 1992; 128-130, 135-142. (11)

B31. Ork H. Uses of cold. In: Kuprian W, ed. Physical Therapy for Sports. Philadelphia, Pa: WB Saunders Co; 1982; 62-68. (15, 96, 207)

B32. Peppard A, Riegler H. Ankle reconditioning with TNS. Physician Sportsmed. June 1980; 8:105-106. (125, 190)

B33. Puffer JC, Zachazewski JE. Management of overuse injuries. Am Fam Physician. September 1988; 38: 225-231. (11)

B34. Quillen WS, Rouillier LH. Initial management of acute ankle sprains with rapid pulsed pneumatic compression and cold. J Orthop Sports Phys Ther. 1982; 4:39-43. (91)

B35. Raether PR. The cold treatment, putting injuries on ice can be more complicated than it sounds. Runner. October 1983; 6:14. (109, 163, 164, 207)

B36. Rettig AC, Kraft DE. Treat ankle sprains fast: it pays. Your Patient Fitness. July/August 1991; 4:6-9. (47)

B37. Rivenburg DW. Physical modalities in the treatment of tendon injuries. Clin Sports Med. 1992; 11:645-659. (125)

B38. Rucinski TJ, Hooker DN, Prentice WE, Shields EW, Cote-Murray DJ. The effects of intermittent compression on edema in postacute ankle sprains. J Orthop Sports Phys Ther. 1991; 14:65-69. (91)

B39. Russell M, Breitbarth N. Innovative ice packs: food for thought. Urol Nurs. December 1990; 10:26. (114)

B40. Sawyer M, Zbieranek CK. The treatment of soft tissue after spinal injury. Clin Sports Med. 1986; 5:387-405. (246)

B41. Sloan JP, Hain R, Pownall R. Clinical benefits of early cold therapy in accident and emergency following ankle sprain. Arch Emerg Med. 1989; 6:1-6. (86)

B42. Stoddard G. Cold treatment of ankle sprains. Schol Coach. September 1969; 39:50-52. (17)

B43. Stokes M, Young A. Muscle weakness due to reflex inhibition: future research in different areas of rehabilitation. In: Proceedings of the 10th World Confederation for Physical Therapy, II. Sydney, Australia: Australian Physiotherapy Association; 1987:1056-1059. (50)

B44. Tepperman PS, Devlin M. Therapeutic heat and cold. Postgrad Med. 1983; 73:69-76. (15, 85)

B45. Tovel J. Ice immersion toe cap. Athl Train. 1980; 15:33. (220)

B46. Voight ML. Reduction of post traumatic ankle edema with high voltage pulsed galvanic stimulation. Athl Train. 1984; 19:278-279, 311. (91)

B47. Wedlick LT. The use of heat and cold in the treatment of sports injuries. Med J Aust. 1967; 54:1050-1051. (15, 17, 94, 207)

CIRCULATORY AND TEMPERATURE RESPONSES

C1. Abraham WM. Heat vs. cold therapy for the treatment of muscle injuries. Athl Train. 1974; 9:177. (17, 112, 123)

C2. Abramson DI. Circulation in the Extremities. New York, NY: Academic Press; 1957:268-291. (123)

C3. Aizawa Y, Shibata A, Tajiri M, Hirasawa Y. Reflex vasoconstriction to a cold stimulus for non-invasive evaluation of neurovascular function in man. Jpn Heart J. 1979; 20:301-305. (111, 119)

C4. Baker RJ, Bell GW. The effect of therapeutic modalities on blood flow in the human calf. J Orthop Sports Phys Ther. January 1991; 13:23-27. (117)

C5. Bancroft H, Edholm OG. The effect of temperature on blood flow and deep temperature in the human forearm. J Physiol. 1943; 102:5-20. (65, 111, 119, 123)

C6. Behnke RS. Cryotherapy and vasodilation. Athl Train. 1973; 8:106, 133-137. (17, 108, 109, 111, 112, 114, 123)

C7. Belitsky RB, Odam SJ, Hubley-Kozey C. Evaluation of the effectiveness of wet ice, dry ice, and Cryogen packs in reducing skin temperature. Phys Ther. 1987; 67:1080-1084. (67, 94)

C8. Bierman W, Friedlander M. The penetrative effect of cold. Arch Phys Ther. 1940; 21:585-592. (68, 70, 114)

C9. Bing HI, Carlsten A, Christiansen SV. The effect on muscular temperature produced by cooling normal and ultraviolet radiated skin. Acta Med Scand. 1945; 121:577-591. (65, 68, 70, 74, 176)

C10. Blair DA, Glover WE, Roddie IC. Vasomotor fibers to skin in the upper arm, calf, and thigh. J Physiol. 1960; 153:232-238. (74)

C11. Bocobo C, Fast A, Kingery W, Kaplan M. The effect of ice on intra-articular temperature in the knee of the dog. Am J Phys Med Rehabil. 1991; 70:181-185. (71)

C12. Bonney GLW, Hughes RA, Janus O. Blood flow through the normal human knee segment. Clin Sci. 1952; 11:167-181. (111)

C13. Borken N, Bierman W. Temperature changes produced by spraying with ethyl chloride. Arch Phys Med. 1955; 36:288-290. (68, 70, 71, 73)

C14. Boyer JT, Fraser JRE, Doyle AE. The haemodynamic effect of cold immersion. Clin Sci. 1960; 19:539.

C15. Cetas TC. Thermometry. In: Lehman JF, ed. Therapeutic Heat and Cold. 3rd ed. Baltimore, MD: Williams & Wilkins; 1982:35-69. (61)

C16. Chu DA, Lutt CJ. The rationale of ice therapy. J Natl Athl Train Assoc. 1969; 4:8-9. (17, 96, 107, 109, 111, 112, 124, 173)

C17. Cipriano LF, Goldman RF. Thermal responses of unclothed men exposed to both cold temperatures and high temperatures. J Appl Physiol. 1975; 39:796-800. (74)

C18. Clarke RSJ, Hellon RF, Lind AR. Vascular reactions of the human forearm to cold. Clin Sci. 1958; 17:165-179. (115, 116, 123, 175-177)

C19. Cobbold AF, Lewis OJ. Blood flow to the knee joint of the dog: effect of heating, cooling, and adrenaline. J Physiol. 1956; 13:379-383. (71)

C20. DonTigney RL. Effects of cold. Phys Ther. 1980; 60:219-220. Letter. (72, 73)

C21. Duff F, Greenfield ADM, Shepherd JT, Thompson ID, Whelan RF. The response to vasodilator substances of the blood vessels in fingers immersed in cold water. J Physiol. 1953; 121:46-54. (111, 119, 123)

C22. Edwards AG. Increasing circulation with cold. J Natl Athl Train Assoc. 1971; 6:15-16. (17, 107, 109, 111, 112, 121, 123)

C23. Edwards M, Burton AC. Correlation of heat output and blood flow in the finger, especially in cold-induced vasodilation. J Appl Physiol. 1960; 15:201-208. (112, 123)

C24. Ekholm J, Skoglund S. Intra-articular knee joint temperature variations in response to cooling and heating of the skin in the cat. Acta Physiol Scand. 1960; 50:175-185. (71, 73)

C25. Folkow B, Fox RH, Kro BJ, Odelran H, Thoren O. Studies on the reactions of the cutaneous vessels to cold exposure. Acta Physiol Scand. 1963; 58:342-354. (111, 119, 123)

C26. Fox RH, Wyatt HT. Cold-induced vasodilation in various areas of the body surface of man. J Physiol. 1962; 162:289-297. (112, 123)

C27. Goldschmidt S, Light AB. A cyanosis, unrelated to oxygen unsaturation, produced by increased peripheral venous pressure. Am J Physiol. 1925; 73:146-172. (122)

C28. Greenfield ADM. The circulation through the skin. In: Hamilton WF, ed. Circulation, Handbook of Physiology. Washington, DC: American Physiological Society; 1963; 2:1325-1351. (122)

C29. Greenfield ADM. The response to cold in the range 0-10°C. In: Wolsteholme GEW, Freeman JS, eds. Peripheral Circulation in Man. Boston, MA: Little Brown & Co; 1954:105-114. (123)

C30. Greenfield ADM, Shepherd JT. A quantitative study of the response to cold of the circulation through the fingers of normal subjects. Clin Sci. 1950; 9:323-334. (111, 112, 119, 123, 156)

C31. Grot RA. Interpretation of thermographic data for the identification of building heat loss. In: Madding RP, ed. Proceedings of the Society of Photo-Optical Instrumentation Engineers. Bellingham, WA: The Society of Photo-Optical Instrumentation Engineers; 1981:24-29. (62)

C32. Haimovici N. Three years experience in direct intra-articular temperature measurement. Prog Clin Biol Res. 1982; 107:453-461. (71)

C33. Ho SSW, Coel MN, Kagawa R, Richardson AB. The effect of ice on blood flow and bone metabolism in knees. Am J Sports Med 1994; 22:537-540. (117)

C34. Hobbs KT. Results of intramuscular temperature changes at various levels after the application of ice. Sport Health: Official Gazette Aust Sports Med. 1983; 1:15. (68)

C35. Horvath SM, Hollander JL. Intra-articular temperature as a measure of joint reaction. J Clin Invest. 1949; 28:469-473. (71, 145)

C36. Johannes SM, Knight KL. Temperature response during the warming phase of cryokinetics. Presented at the Indiana Interagency Research Seminar; April 1979; West Lafayette, IN. (68, 121, 155, 158, 220)

C37. Johnson DJ, Moore S, Moore J, Oliver RA. Effect of cold submersion on intramuscular temperature of the gastrocnemius muscle. Phys Ther. 1979; 59:1238-1242. (71-74)

C38. Jurkovich GJ, Pitt RM, Curreri PW, Granger DN. Hypothermia prevents increased capillary permeability following ischemia-reperfusion injury. J Surg Res. 1988; 44:514-521. (35)

C39. Keatinge WR. The effects of subcutaneous fat and of previous exposure to cold on the body temperature, peripheral blood flow and metabolic rate of men in cold water. J Physiol. 1960; 153:166-178. (71)

C40. Kern H, Fessl L, Trnavsky G, Hertz H. Kryotherapie: das verhalten der gelenkstemperatur unter eisapplikation: grundlage für die praktishe anwendung. Wien Klin Wochenschr. 1984; 22:832-837. (71, 72)

C41. Knight KL. Comparison of Blood Flow in Normal Subjects During Therapeutic Applications of Heat, Cold, and Exercise of Therapeutic Levels. Columbia: University of Missouri; 1977. Doctoral dissertation. (115, 119)

C42. Knight KL, Aquino J, Johannes SM, Urban CD. A re-examination of Lewis' cold-induced vasodilation in the finger and the ankle. Athl Train. 1980; 15:238-250. (4, 67, 72, 73, 113, 114, 158, 184)

C43. Knight KL, Bryan KS, Halvorsen JM. Circulatory changes in the forearm in 1, 5, 10, and 15°C water. Int J Sports Med. 1981; 4:281. Abstract. (19, 59, 71, 111, 115, 117, 119, 184)

C44. Knight KL, Carmody LW. Rewarming of the ankle and forearm following 30 minutes of ice water immersion. Presented at the 35th National Athletic Trainers Association Annual Meeting; June 1984; Nashville, TN. (67, 71, 73, 74, 113, 114, 184)

C45. Knight KL, Elam JF. Rewarming of the ankle, finger, and forearm after cryotherapy: further investigation of Lewis' cold-induced vasodilation. J Can Athl Ther Assoc. September 1981; 8:17-18. (16, 67, 71-74, 113, 114, 117, 158, 184)

C46.   Knight KL, Kluge, J, Varpolitti M, Hayes K. Knee skin temperature responses to applications of two types of cold packs over thick and thin surgical dressings. Med Sci Sports Exerc. 1990; 22:S100. Abstract. (67, 82, 101, 102, 111, 115, 122-124, 217, 230)

C47.   Knight KL, Londeree BR. Comparison of blood flow in normal subjects during therapeutic applications of heat, cold, and exercise. Med Sci Sports Exerc. 1980; 12:76-80. (10, 17, 19, 118)

C48.   Knight KL, Varpolitti M, Chase JA, Hayes K. Comparison of Dura*-kold compression ice wraps to crushed ice and refreezable flexible gel packs. Athl Train. 1990; 25:126. Abstract. (197, 199, 200)

C49.   Knight KL, Zwickler A. Skin temperature changes in male and female forearms during and after application of six different cold modalities. Presented at the National Athletic Trainers Association Annual Meeting and Clinical Symposium; June 1981; Fort Worth, TX. (16)

C50.   Lavelle BE, Snyder M. Differential conduction of cold through barriers. J Adv Nurs. 1985; 10:55-61. (94, 123)

C51.   Lennihan R, Mackereth MA. Ankle pressure in arterial occlusive disease involving the legs. Surg Clin North Am. 1973; 53:657-666. (62, 74, 108, 109, 111, 114, 117)

C52.   Lewis T. Observations upon the reactions of the vessels of the human skin to cold. Heart. 1930; 15:177-208. (108, 109)

C53.   Lowden BJ, Moore RJ. Determinants and nature of intramuscular temperature changes during cold therapy. Am J Phys Med. 1975;j 54:223-244. (71)

C54.   McMaster WC, Little S, Waugh TR. Laboratory evaluations of various cold therapy modalities. Am J Sports Med. 1978; 6:291-294. (71, 123, 197, 201)

C55.   Meehan JP. General body cooling and hand cooling. In: Fisher FR, ed. Protection and Functioning of the Hands in Cold Climates. Washington, DC: National Academy of Sciences National Research Council; 1957:45-62. (74)

C56.   Meeusen R, DeMeirleir K. Cryotherapy and microcirculation. Hung Rev Sports Med. 1991; 32:203-210. (117)

C57.   Merrick MA, Knight KL, Ingersoll CD, Potteiger JA. The effects of ice and compression wraps on intramuscular temperatures at various depths. J Athl Train. 1993; 29:236-245. (69)

C58.   Oosterveld FGJ, Rasker JJ, Jacobs JWG, Overmars HJA. The effect of local heat and cold therapy on the intraarticular and skin surface temperature of the knee. Arthritis Rheum. February 1992; 35:146-151. (71, 72)

C59.   Palmer JC, Knight KL. Ankle and thigh skin surface temperature changes with repeated ice pack application. J Athl Train. 1992; 27:138. (16, 60, 64, 67, 68, 73, 96)

C60.   Roos L, Knight KL. Blood flow and temperature changes in the forearm during and after application of three types of cold packs. Unpublished data on file in the Sports Injury Research Laboratory; 1981; Terre Haute, IN: Indiana State University. (73, 117, 184)

C61.   Schuster EG. Foot Blood Flow Changes During Treatment with Ice and/or Compression. University Park: Penn State University; 1988. Masters thesis. (117)

C62.   Seiyama A, Shiga T, Maeda N. Temperature effect on oxygenation and metabolism of perfused rat hindlimb muscle. Adv Exp Med Biol. 1990; 277:541-547. (78)

C63.   Sekins KM, Emery AF. Thermal science for physical medicine. In: Lehman JF, ed. Therapeutic Heat and Cold. 3rd ed. Baltimore, MD: Williams & Wilkins; 1982:70-132. (60)

C64. Senay LC Jr, Christensen M, Hertzman AB. Cutaneous vascular responses in finger and forearm during rising ambient temperatures. J Appl Physiol. 1960; 15:611-618. (74)

C65. Senay LC Jr, Prokop LD, Cronan L, Hertzman AB. Relation of local skin temperature and local sweating to cutaneous blood flow. J Appl Physiol. 1963; 18:781-785. (74)

C66. Shepherd JT. Physiology of the Circulation in Human Limbs in Health and Disease. Philadelphia, PA: WB Saunders Co; 1963; 101-163. (20, 68)

C67. Smith DR. The Comparative Effects of Heat, Cold, and Exercise on Local Blood Flow. Champaign-Urbana, IL: University of Illinois; 1971. Masters thesis. (73, 107)

C68. Taber C, Contryman K, Fahrenbruch J, LaCount K, Cornwall MW. Measurement of reactive vasodilation during cold gel pack applications to nontraumatized ankles. Phys Ther. 1992; 72:294-299. (115, 117)

C69. Van Beek E. Effects of reducing intramuscular temperature on delaying the onset of fatigue: an electomyographical analysis. Med Sci Sport. 1976; 8:75. (251)

C70. Wakin LG, Porter AN, Krusen FH. Influence of physical agents and of certain drugs on intra-articular temperature. Arch Phys Med Rehabil. 1951; 32:714-721. (71)

C71. Walton M, Roestenburg M, Hallwright S, Sutherland JC. Effects of ice packs on tissue temperatures at various depths before and after quadriceps hematoma: studies using sheep. J Orthop Sports Phys Ther. December 1986; 8:294-300. (73)

C72. Waylonis GW. The physiologic effects of ice massage. Arch Phys Med Rehabil. 1967; 48:37-42. (68-70, 114)

C73. Weston M, Taber C, Casgranda L, Cornwall M. Changes in local blood volume during cold gel pack application to traumatized ankles. J Orthop Sports Phys Ther. 1994; 19:197-199. (68, 117)

C74. Wolf SL. Contralateral upper extremity cooling from a specific stimulus. Phys Ther. 1971; 51:158-165. (71-74)

C75. Wolf SL, Basmajian JV. Intramuscular temperature changes due to localized cutaneous cold stimulation. Phys Ther. 1973; 33:1284-1288. (70)

C76. Zoller L. A comparative study of temperature changes in the ankle during applications of chemical cold packs and ice bags. Unpublished data on file in the Sports Injury Research Laboratory; 1980; Terre Haute: Indiana State University. (201)

NEUROLOGICAL EFFECTS

D1. Abramson DI, Chu LSW, Tuck S Jr, Lee SW, Richardson G, Levin M. Effect of tissue temperature and blood flow on motor nerve conduction velocity. JAMA. 1966; 198:1082-1088. (68, 111, 117-119, 135, 136)

D2. Abramson DI, Hlavova A, Rickert B, et al. Effects of ischemia on median and ulnar motor nerve conduction velocities at various temperatures. Arch Phys Med Rehabil. 1970; 51:463-470. (136)

D3. Bickford RG. The fibre dissociation produced by cooling human nerves. Clin Sci. 1939; 4:159-165. (129, 134)

D4. Blazevic A. Reaction of peripheral motor nerve to local cryomassage. Neurologija. 1983; 31:39-46.

D5. Boyd IA, Martin AR. Spontaneous subthreshold activity at mammalian neuromuscular junctions. J Physiol. 1956; 132:61-73. (138)

D6. Brust M, Toback S, Benton JG. Some effects of ultrasound and of temperature on contractions of isolated mammalian skeletal muscle. Arch Phys Med Rehabil. 1969; 50:677-694. (138)

D7.   Buchthal F, Rosenfalck A. Evoked action-potentials and conduction velocity in human sensory nerves. Brain Res. 1966; 3:1-122. (130, 131, 136)

D8.   Buller AJ, Kean CHC, Ranatunga KW, Smith JM. Quoted by: Ranatunga KW. Influence of temperature on isometric tension development in mouse fast and slow-twitch muscles. Exp Neurol. 1980;
70:211-218. (139, 140)

D9.   Chapman CE. The Effects of Muscle Cooling on the Stretch Reflex of
the Decerebrate Cat. London: University of Western Ontario; 1976.
Masters thesis. (134, 145)

D10. Chatfield PO. Hypothermia and its effects on the sensory nerves and
peripheral motor systems. Ann NY Acad Sci. 1959; 80:445-448. (138, 140)

D11. Clark DH. Effect of immersion in hot and cold water upon recovery
of muscular strength following fatiguing isometric exercise. Arch
Phys Med Rehabil. 1963; 44:365-368. (144)

D12. Clarke DH, Stelmach GE. Muscular fatigue and recovery curve parameters at various temperatures. Res Q. 1966; 37:468-479. (144)

D13. Clarke RSJ, Hellon RF, Lind AR. The duration of sustained contractions of the human forearm at different muscle temperatures. J
Physiol. 1958; 143:454-473. (141-145, 163, 177)

D14. Clendenin MA, Szumski AJ. Influence of cutaneous ice applications on
single motor units in humans. Phys Ther. 1971; 51:166-175. (17, 136, 177)

D15. Close R, Hoh JFY. Influence of temperature on isometric contractions
of rat skeletal muscles. Nature. 1968; 217:1179-1180. (138, 139)

D16. Coppin EG, Livingstone SD, Kuehn LA. Effects on handgrip strength
due to arm immersion at a 10°C water bath. Aviat Space Environ
Med. 1978; 49:1322-1326. (74, 141, 142, 176, 177)

D17. Cote DW. The Relationship of Temperature to Strength and Power
Production in Intact Human Skeletal Muscle. Tucson: University
of Arizona; 1979. Doctoral dissertation. (142, 177)

D18. DeJesus PV, Hausmanowa-Petrusewicz I, Barchi RL. The effect of
cold on nerve conduction of human slow and fast nerve fibers.
Neurology. 1973; 23:1182-1189. (130, 135)

D19. DeJong RH, Hersley WN, Wagman IH. Nerve conduction velocity during
hypothermia in man. Anesthesiology. 1966; 27:805-810. (135, 136, 138)

D20. Denny-Brown D, Adams RD, Brenner C, Doherty MM. The pathology
of injury to nerve induced by cold. J Neuropathol Exp Neurol. 1945;
4:305-323. (131)

D21. Dodt E. The behavior of thermoreceptors at low and high temperatures with special reference to Ebbecke's temperature phenomena.
Acta Physiol Scand. 1953; 27:295-314. (128)

D22. Dodt E, Zotterman Y. Mode of action of warm receptors. Acta Physiol
Scand. 1952; 26:345-357. (128)

D23. Doudoumopoulos AN, Chatfield PO. Effects of temperature on function
of mammalian (rat) muscle. Am J Physiol. 1959; 196;1197-1199. (140)

D24. Douglas WW, Malcolm JL. Effect of localized cooling on conduction
in cat nerve. J Physiol. 1955; 130:53-71. (130, 131, 144, 177)

D25. Dudley PH. The Effects of Cryotherapy and Static Stretching on
Residual Muscle Tension as Determined by Electromyography.
Huntsville, TX: Sam Houston State University; 1975. Masters the-
sis. (166, 167)

D26. Edelwejn Z. Trials of evaluation of conduction velocity in motor fibers
of different size under conditions of local hypothermia. Acta Physiol
Pol. 1964; 15:503-511. (136)

D27. Edwards RHT, Harris RC, Hultman E, Kaijer L, Koh D, Nordesjo LO.
Effect of temperature on muscle energy metabolism and endurance

during successive isometric contractions, sustained to fatigue, of the quadriceps muscle in man. J Physiol. 1972; 220:335-352. (145)

D28.   Eldred E, Lindsley DF, Buchwald JS. The effect of cooling on mammalian muscle spindles. Exp Neurol. 1960; 2:144-157. (130, 132-134, 145, 147)

D29.   Ferretti G, Ishii M, Moia C, Cerretelli P. Effects of temperature on the maximal instantaneous muscle power of humans. J Appl Physiol. 1992; 63:112-116. (140, 142, 143)

D30.   Foldes FF, Kuze S, Vizi ES, Deery A. The influence of temperature on neuromuscular performance. J Neurol Trans. 1978; 43:27-45. (137, 140)

D31.   Franz DN, Iggo A. Conduction Failure in myelinated and non-myelinated axons at low temperatures. J Physiol. 1968; 199:319-345. (131)

D32.   Gassel MM, Trojaborg W. Clinical and electrophysiological study of patterns of conduction times in distribution of sciatic nerve. J Neurol Neurosurg Psychiatry. 1964; 27:351-357. (135, 136)

D33.   Gasser HS. Nerve activity as modified by temperature changes. Am J Physiol. 1931; 97:254-270. (68, 131)

D34.   Grafstein B, Forman D, McEwen BS. Effects of temperature on axonal transport and turnover of protein in goldfish optic systems. Exp Neurol. 1972; 34:158-170.

D35.   Grob D. Spontaneous end-plate activity in normal subjects and patients with myasthenia gravis. Ann NY Acad Sci. 1971; 183:245-269. (138)

D36.   Gross GW. The effect of temperature on the rapid axoplasmic transport in C-fibers. Brain Res. 1973; 56:359-363. (135)

D37.   Gross JE. Depression of muscle fatigue curves by heat and cold. Res Q. 1958; 29:19-23. (144)

D38.   Halar EM, DeLisa JA, Brozovich FV. Nerve conduction velocity: relationship of skin, subcutaneous intramuscular temperatures. Arch Phys Med Rehabil. 1980; 61:199-203. (68, 130, 135, 136)

D39.   Halar EM, DeLisa JA, Soine TL. Nerve conduction studies in upper extremities: skin temperature corrections. Arch Phys Med Rehabil. 1983; 64:412-416. (130, 135, 136)

D40.   Hendrickson JD. Conduction Velocity of Motor Nerves in Normal Subjects and Patients With Neuromuscular Disorders. Minneapolis/St. Paul: University of Minnesota; 1966. Masters thesis. (130, 136)

D41.   Hensel H, Cutaneous thermoreceptors. In: Iggo A, ed. Handbook of Sensory Physiology. New York, NY: Springer, 1973; 11:79-110. (127, 128)

D42.   Hensel H. Neural processes in thermoregulation. Physiol Rev. 1973; 53:948-1017. (128, 154, 156)

D43.   Hensel H, Boman KKA. Afferent impulses in cutaneous sensory nerves in human subjects. J Neurophysiol. 1960; 23:564-578. (128)

D44.   Hensel H, Iggo A, Witt I. A quantitative study of sensitive cutaneous thermoreceptors with C afferent fibers. J Physiol. 1960; 153:113-126. (128)

D45.   Heslop JP, Howes EA. Temperature and inhibitor effects on fast axonal transport in a mulluscan nerve. J Neurochem. 1972; 19:1709-1716. (135)

D46.   Hill AV. The influence of temperature on the tension developed in an isometric twitch. Proc R Soc Lond. 1951; 138:349-354. (138)

D47.   Hoh JFY. Neural regulation of muscle activation. Exp Neurol. 1974; 45:241-256. (139)

D48.   Hunt CC. The effect of sympathetic stimulation on mammalian muscle spindles. J Physiol. 1960; 151:332-341. (147, 173)

D49.   Iggo A. Cutaneous thermoreceptors in primates and sub-primates. J Physiol. 1969; 200:403-430. (128, 129, 134, 136)

D50.   Johnson DJ, Leider FE. Influence of gold bath on maximum handgrip strength. Percept Mot Skills. 1977; 44:323-326. (141, 142, 177)

D51.   Johnson EW, Olsen KJ. Clinical value of motor nerve conduction velocity determination. JAMA. 1960; 172:2030-2035. (136)

D52.   Johnson KO, Phillips R. Tactile spatial resolution. J Neurophysiol 1981; 46:1177-1191.

D53.   Kato M. Conduction velocity of ulnar nerve and spinal reflex time measured by means of H-wave average adults and athletes. Tohoku J Exp Med. December 1960; 73:74-85. (135)

D54.   Kelly E, Fry WJ. Isometric twitch tension of frog skeletal muscle as a function of temperature. Science. 1958; 128:200-201. (140)

D55.   Koizumi K, Ushiyama J, Brooks CM. Effect of hypothermia on excitability of spinal neurons. J Neurophysiol. 1960; 23:421-431. (145)

D56.   Kraft GH. Effects of temperature and age on nerve conduction velocity in the guinea pig. Arch Phys Med Rehabil. 1972; 53:328-332. (135)

D57.   Krarup C. Temperature dependence of enhancement and diminution of tension evoked by staircase and by tetanus in rat muscle. J Physiol. 1981; 311:373-387. (138)

D58.   Lee JM, Warren MP, Mason SM. Effects of ice on nerve conduction velocity. Physiotherapy. 1978; 64:1-6. (130, 131, 136, 137)

D59.   Leyssius AT, Kalkman CJ, Bovill JG. Influence of moderate hypothermia on posterior tibial nerve somatosensory evoked potentials. Anesth Analg. 1986; 65:475-480.

D60.   Li CL. Effect of cooling on neuromuscular transmission in the rat. Am J Physiol. 1958; 194:200-206. (136-138)

D61.   Li CL, Gouras P. Effect of cooling on neuromuscular transmission in the frog. Am J Physiol. 1958; 192:464-470. (136-138)

D62.   Lind AR. Muscle fatigue and recovery from fatigue induced by sustained contraction. J Physiol. 1959; 147:162-177. (143)

D63.   Lippold OLJ, Nicholls JG, Redfearn JWT. A study of the afferent discharge produced by cooling a mammalian muscle spindle. J Physiol. 1960; 153:218-231. (136, 145)

D64.   Lowitzsch K. Hopf HC, Galland J. Changes of sensory conduction velocity and refractory periods with decreasing tissue temperature in man. J Neurol. 1977; 216(3):181-188. (130-132)

D65.   Ludin HP, Beyeler F. Temperature dependence of normal sensory nerve action potential. J Neurol. 1977; 216:173-180. (130-132)

D66.   Maclagan J, Zaimis E. The effect of muscle temperature on twitch and tetanus in the cat. J Physiol. 1957; 137:89P-90P. (139)

D67.   McGown HL. Effect of cold application on maximal isometric contraction. Phys Ther. 1967; 42:185-192. (141)

D68.   McLeod JG. Digital nerve conduction in the carpal tunnel syndrome after mechanical stimulation of the finger. J Neurol Neurosurg Psychiatry. 1966; 29:12-22. (130)

D69.   Mense S. Effects of temperature on the discharges of muscle spindles and tendon organs. Pfügers Arch. 1978; 374:159-166. (132-134)

D70.   Michalski WJ, Seguin JJ. The effects of muscle cooling and stretch on muscle secondary ending in the cat. J Physiol. 1975; 253:341-356. (132-134)

D71.   Michalski WJ, Seguin JJ. Effects of muscle cooling on spindle activity and monosynaptic reflexes. Pro Can Fed Biol Sci. 1971; 14:557. (133, 145)

D72.   Moberg E. The role of cutaneous afferents in position sense, kinesthesia, and motor function of the hand. Brain. 1983; 106:1-19. (134)

D73.   Newton MJ, Lehmkehl D. Muscle spindle response to body heating and localized muscle cooling: implications for relief of spasticity. J Am Phys Ther Assoc. 1965; 45:91-105. (132)

D74.   Oaklander AL, Spencer, PS. Cold blockade of axonal transport activates premitotic activity of Schwann cells and Wallerian degeneration. J. Neurochem 1988; 50:490-496. (135)

D75. Ochs S, Smith C. Low temperature slowing and cold-block of fast axoplasmic transport in mammalian nerves in vitro. J Neurobiol. 1975; 6:85-102. (135)

D76. Oliver RA, Johnson DJ. The effect of cold water baths on posttreatment leg strength. Physician Sportsmed. November 1976; 2:67-69. (142)

D77. Paintal AS. Conduction in mammalian nerve fibers. In: Desmedt JE, ed. New Developments in Electromyography and Clinical Neurology. Basel, Switzerland: Karger; 1973; 2:19-41. (131)

D78. Paintal A.S. A comparison of the nerve impulses of mammalian non-medullated nerve fibers with those of the smallest diameter medullated fibers. J Physiol. 1967; 193: 523-533. (131)

D79. Paintal AS. The influence of diameter of medullated nerve fibers of cats on the rising and falling phases of the spike and its recovery. J Physiol. 1966; 184:791-811. (130)

D80. Paintal AS. Block of conduction in mammalian myelinated nerve fibers by low temperatures. J Physiol. 1965; 180:1-19. (130, 134, 135)

D81. Paintal AS. Effects of temperature on conduction in single vagal end saphenous myelinated nerve fibers of the cat. J Physiol. 1965; 180:20-49. (130, 134, 135)

D82. Paintal AS. Vagal afferent fibers. Ergeb Physiol. 1963; 52:74-156. (131)

D83. Petajan JH, Daube JR. Effects of cooling the arm and hand. J Appl Physiol. 1965; 20:1271-1274. (67, 114)

D84. Petajan JH, Watts N. Effects of cooling on the triceps surae reflex. J Am Phys Med. 1962; 41:240-251. (65, 67, 70, 73, 145, 146, 165)

D85. Poloni AE, Sala E. Conduction velocity of ulnar and median nerves stimulated through twinneedle electrode. Electroencephalogr Clin Neurophysiol. 1962; 22 (suppl):17-19. (136)

D86. Provins KA, Morton R. Tactile discrimination and skin temperature. J Appl Physiol. 1960; 15:155-160. (130, 134)

D87. Rall JA. Effects of temperature on tension, tension-dependent heat, and activation heat in twitches of frog skeletal muscle. J Physiol. 1979; 291:265-275. (140)

D88. Ranatunga KW. Temperature-dependence of shortening velocity and rate of isometric tension development in rat skeletal muscle. J Physiol. 1982; 329:465-483. (140, 141)

D89. Ranatunga KW. Influence of temperature on the velocity of shortening and rate of tension development in mammalian (rat) skeletal muscle. J Physiol. 1981; 316:35P-36P. (140)

D90. Ranatunga KW. Influence of temperature on isometric tension development in mouse fast and slow-twitch skeletal muscles. Exp Neurol. 1980; 70:211-218. (138-140)

D91. Ranatunga KW. Changes produced by chronic denervation in the temperature dependent isometric contractile characteristics of rat fast and slow twitch skeletal muscles. J Physiol. 1977; 273:255-262. (139)

D92. Ranatunga KW, Wylie SR. Temperature-dependent transitions in isometric contractions of rat muscle. J Physiol. 1983; 339:87-95. (140)

D93. Ricker K, Hertel G. Increased voltage of the muscle action potential of normal subjects. J Neurol. 1977; 216:33-38. (138, 139)

D94. Stephenson DG, Williams DA. Calcium-activated force response in fast and slow-twitch skinned muscle fibers of the rat at different temperatures. J Physiol. 1981; 317:281-302. (140)

D95. Stevens JC. Temperature and the two-point threshold. Somatosens Mot Res. 1989; 6:275-284. (128, 129)

D96. Stevenson GC, Collins WF, Randt CT, Saurwein TD. Effects of induced hypothermia on subcortical evoked potentials in the cat. Am J Physiol. 1958; 194:423-426. (137)

D97. Thornton RJ, Blakeney C, Feldman SA. The effects of hypothermia on neuromuscular conduction. Br J Anaesth. 1976; 48:264. (137, 139)

D98. Tilney LG, Porter KR. Studies on the microtubules in heliozoa II: the effect of low temperature on these structures in the formation and maintenance of the axopodia. Cell Biol. 1967; 34:327-343. (135)

D99. Tleulin SZ, Kleinbock IY, Tsitsurin VI. Effect of peripheral heating and cooling on spinal reflex activity. Neirofiziologiia. 1973; 5:181-185. (146)

D100. Truong XT Wall BJ, Walker SM. Effects of temperature on isometric contraction of rat muscle. Am J Physiol. 1964; 207:393-396. (138, 140)

D101. Walker SM. The relation of stretch and of temperature to contraction of skeletal muscle. Am J Phys Med. 1960; 39:234-258. (136, 138)

D102. Weeks VD, Travell J. How to give painless injections. AMA Scientific Exhibits. 1957; 57:318-322. (130)

D103. Wolf SL, Letbetter WD, Basmajian JV. Effects of a specific cutaneous cold stimulus on single motor unit activity of medial gastrocnemius muscle in man. Am J Phys Med. 1976; 55:177-183. (68, 136, 177)

D104. Yarnitsky D, Ochoa JL. Warm and cold specific somatosensory systems; psychophysical thresholds, reaction times, and peripheral conduction velocities. Brain. 1991; 114:1819-1826. (127)

D105. Zotterman Y. Thermal sensations. In: Field J, ed. Handbook of Physiology. Washington, DC: American Physiological Society; 1959; 1:431-458. (128)

D106. Zotterman Y. Special senses: thermal receptors. Am Rev Physiol. 1953; 15:357-372. (128, 129)

PAIN

E1. Abramson DI, Tuck S Jr, Lee SW, et al. Vascular basis for pain due to cold. Arch Phys Med Rehabil. 1966; 47:300-305. (123, 156)

E2. Adams T, Smith RE. Effects of chronic cold exposure on finger temperature responses. J Appl Physiol. 1962; 17:317-322. (158-160)

E3. Adriaensen H, Gybels J, Handwerker HO, van Hees J. Response properties of thin myelinated (A-δ) fibers in human skin nerves. J Neurophysiol. 1983; 49:111-122. (128)

E4. Arendt-Nielsen L, Gotliebsen K. Segmental inhibition of laser-evoked brain potentials by ipsi- and contralaterally applied cold pressor pain. Eur J Appl Physiol. 1992; 64:56-61. (164)

E5. Ashby EC. Abdominal pain of spinal origin. Ann R Coll Surg Engl. 1977; 59:242-246. (47, 50, 173)

E6. Baker SL, Kirsch I. Cognitive mediators of pain and tolerance. J Pers Soc Psychol. 1991; 61:504-510. (158)

E7. Barnard JDW, Lloyd JW. Cryoanalgesia. Nurs Times. 1977; 73:897-899. (105, 165)

E8. Bhagat B. Effect of chronic cold stress on catacholamine levels in rat brain. Psychopharmacologia. 1969; 16:1-4. (151, 161)

E9. Bond MR. Pain: Its Nature, Analysis and Treatment. 1st ed. New York, NY: Churchill Livingstone; 1979:3-50. (150)

E10. Bonica JJ. The need for a taxonomy of pain. Pain. June 1979; 6:247. (150)

E11. Borg GAV. Psychophysical bases of perceived exertion. Med Sci Sports Exerc. 1982; 14:377-381. (150, 151, 153)

E12. Brooks K. Effects of cold on baragnosis. J Athl Train 1995; 30:S-36, Abstract. (134)

E13. Bugaj R. The cooling, analgesic, and rewarming effects of ice massage on localized skin. Phys Ther. 1975; 55:11-19. (67, 73, 155, 165)

E14.   Burgess JA, Sommers EE, Truelove EL, Dworkin SF. Short-term effect of two therapeutic methods on myofascial pain and dysfunction of the masticatory system. J Prosthet Dent. 1988; 60:606-610. (161, 167)

E15.   Byrne M, Troy A, Bradley LA, Marchisello PJ, Geisinger KF, Van der Heide L, Prieto EJ. Cross validation of the factor structure of MPQ. Pain. 1982; 13:193. (150)

E16.   Carman KW, Knight KL. Habituation to cold-pain during repeated cryokinetic sessions. J Athl Train. 1992; 27:223-230. (121, 153, 158-160)

E17.   Chapman CE. Can the use of physical modalities for pain control be rationalized by the research evidence? Can J Physiol Pharmacol. 1991; 69:704-712. (4, 149, 165)

E18.   Chatonnet J, Cabanac M. The perception of thermal comfort. Int J Biometeorol. 1965; 9:183-193. (60, 163)

E19.   Chery-Croze S. Relationship between noxious cold stimuli and the magnitude of pain sensation in man. Pain. 1983; 15:265-269. (154)

E20.   Creager CL, Knight KL. Temperature and pain changes resulting from post surgical (arthroscopy) application of cold packs. Athl Train. 1991; 26:168. (100-102, 125, 134, 166, 205)

E21.   Croze S, Duclaux R. Thermal pain in humans: influence of the rate of stimulation. Brain Res. 1978; 157:418-421. (157, 158)

E22.   Darian-Smith I, Johnson KO, Dykes R. 'Cold' fiber population innervating palmar and digital skin of the monkey: responses to cooling pulses. J Neurophysiol. 1973; 36:325-346. (128-168)

E23.   Denegar CR, Perrin DH. Effect of transcutaneous electrical nerve stimulation, cold, and a combination treatment on pain, decreased range of motion, and strength loss associated with delayed onset muscle soreness. J Athl Train. 1992; 27:200-206. (151, 152, 166-168, 172)

E24.   Ellis M. The relief of pain by cooling of the skin. Br Med J. 1961; i:240-252. (163, 246)

E25.   Ellis M. The treatment of pain by ethylchloride and other cooling sprays. Practitioner. 1961; 187:367-370. (163)

E26.   Enander A. Performance and sensory aspects of work in cold environments: a review. Ergonomics. 1984; 27:365-378. (177)

E27.   Evans T. The effects of cooling on agility. J Athl Train, 1994; 29:179 abstract. (134, 147, 176, 177)

E28.   Gammon GD, Starr I. Studies on the relief of pain by counter-irritation. J Clin Invest. 1941; 20:13-20. (164)

E29.   Gerard RW. The physiology of pain: abnormal states in causalgia and related phenomena. Anesthesiology. 1951; 12:1-13. (168)

E30.   Gerig BK. The effects of cryotherapy upon ankle proprioception. Athl Train. 1990; 25:119. (134)

E31.   Glynn CJ, Lloyd JW, Bernard JDW. Cryoanalgesia in the management of pain after thoracotomy. Thorax. May 1980; 5:325-327. (105, 165, 166)

E32.   Gracely RH. Pain measurement in man. In: Ng LKY, Bonica JJ, eds. Pain, Discomfort and Humanitarian Care. New York, NY: Elsevier/North Holland; 1980; 111-137. (150)

E33.   Gracely RH. Psychophysical assessment of human pain. In Bonica JJ, ed. Advances in Pain Research and Therapy. New York, NY: Raven Press; 1979; 3:805-824. (150)

E34.   Halkovich LR, Personius WJ, Clamann HP, Newton RA. Effect of fluorimethane spray on passive hip flexion. Phys Ther. 1981; 61:185-189. (168)

E35.   Havenith G, van de Linde EJG, Heus R. Pain, thermal sensation and cooling rates of hands while touching cold materials. Eur J Appl Physiol. 1992; 65:43-51. (134, 153-155, 157, 177, 183)

E36. Hellström B. Local Effects of Acclimatization to Cold in Man. Oslo, Norway: University Press; 1965. (74)

E37. Huskisson EC. Visual analogue scales. In: Melzack R, ed. Pain Measurement and Assessment. New York, NY: Raven Press; 1983; 33-40. (121, 151, 167)

E38. Ingersoll CD, Knight KL, Merrick MA. Sensory perception of the foot and ankle following therapeutic applications of heat and cold. J Athl Train. 1992; 27:231-234. (130, 134, 163)

E39. Ingersoll C, Mangus B. Sensations of cold reexamined: a study using the McGill pain questionnaire. Athl Train. 1991; 26:240-245. (153)

E40. Ingersoll CD, Mangus BC. Habituation to the perception of the qualities of cold-induced pain. J Athl Train. 1992; 27:218-222. (121, 153, 161-163)

E41. Isabell WK, Durrant E, Myrer W, Anderson S. The effects of ice massage, ice massage with exercise, and exercise on the prevention and treatment of delayed onset muscle soreness. J Athl Train. 1992; 27:208-217. (166, 167)

E42. Jaremko ME, Silbert L, Mann T. The differential ability of athletes and nonathletes to cope with two types of pain: a radical behavioral model. Psychol Record. 1981; 31:265-275. (149)

E43. Jensen MP, Karoly P, Braver S. The measurement of clinical pain intensity: a comparison of six methods. Pain. 1986; 27:117-126. (152)

E44. Joucken K, Michel L, Schoevaerdts JC, Mayne A, Randour P. Cryoanalgesia for post-thoracotomy pain relief. Acta Anaesthesiol Belg. 1987; 38:179-183. (165)

E45. Kanui TI. Thermal inhibition of nocicoceptor-driven spinal cord neurones in the cat: a possible neuronal basis for thermal analgesia. Brain Res. 1967; 402:160-163. (163, 164)

E46. Kato DJ. Effect of Static stretch and Ice Immersion on Pitching Performance after Induced Muscle Performance. Terre Haute: Indiana State University; 1985. Masters thesis. (166, 167, 177)

E47. Klepack RK, Dowling J, Hauge G. Sensitivity of the McGill Pain Questionnaire to intensity and quality of laboratory pain. Pain. 1981; 10:199.

E48. Knight KL, Ingersoll CD, Trowbridge CA, Connolly TA, Cordovia ML, Hyink LL, Welch SM. The effects of cooling the ankle, the triceps surae, or both on functional agility. J Athl Train. 1994; 29:165. Abstract. (134, 176, 177)

E49. Kraus H. Prevention and treatment of ski injuries. J Trauma. 1961; 1:457-463. (10, 121, 173, 174, 246)

E50. Kraus H. Evaluation and treatment of muscle functions in athletic injury. Am J Surg. 1959; 98:353-362. (163, 168, 177)

E51. Kraus H. Use of surface anesthesia in treatment of painful motion. JAMA. 1941; 116:2582-2583. (158, 159, 163, 168)

E52. Kraus H. Neue distorsionsbehandlung. Wein Klin Wochenschr. 1935; 48:1014. (168)

E53. Kreh A, Anton F, Gilly H, Handwerker HO. Vascular reactions correlated with pain due to cold. Exp Neurol. 1984; 85:533-546. (157)

E54. Kunkel EC. Phasic pains induced by cold. J Applied Physiol. 1949; 12:811-824. (153-156)

E55. Lake NC. An investigation in to the effects of cold upon the body. Lancet. 1917; 2:557-562. (183)

E56. LaMotte RH, Thalhammer JG. Response properties of high-threshold cutaneous cold receptors in the primate. Brain Res. 1982; 244:279-287. (128)

E57. Landen BR. Heat or cold for the relief of pain in musculoskeletal injuries. Phys Ther. 1967; 47:1126-1128. (17, 172)

E58.   LaReviere J, Osternig LR. The effect of ice on joint position sense. J Sports Rehabil 1994; 3:58-67. (134, 150)

E59.   LeBlanc J. Adaptive mechanisms in humans. Ann NY Acad Sci. 1966; 134:721-732. (51, 74)

E60.   LeBlanc J, Dulac S, Côté J, Girard B. Autonomic nervous system and adaptation to cold in man. J Appl Physiol. 1975; 39:181-186. (73, 74, 114, 160, 162)

E61.   LeBlanc J, Potvin P. Studies on habituation to cold pain. Can J Physiol Pharmacol. 1966; 44:287-293. (153, 158, 160, 161)

E62.   LePivert PJ. Basic considerations of the cryolesion. In: Albin RJ, ed. Handbook of Cryosurgery. New York, NY: Marcell Dekker Inc; 1980:15-68. (105, 152, 160, 165)

E63.   Livingstone SD. Changes in cold-induced vasodilation during arctic exercises. J Appl Physiol. 1976; 40:455-457. (74, 150, 191)

E64.   Lloyd JW, Barnard JDW, Glynn CJ. Cryoanalgesia: a new approach to pain relief. Lancet. 1976; 2:932-934. (105, 165)

E65.   MacKenzie RA, Burke D, Skuse NF, Lethlean AK. Fibre function and perception during cutaneous nerve block. J Neurol Neurosurg Psychiatry. 1975; 38:865-873. (128)

E66.   McCaffery M. Nursing approaches to nonpharmacological pain control. Int J Nurs Stud. 1990; 27:1-5. (101, 103, 165)

E67.   McCaffery M. Nursing Management of the Patient With Pain. Philadelphia, PA: JB Lippincott Co; 1979. (3, 149, 245)

E68.   Melzack R. The McGill Pain Questionnaire: major properties and scoring methods. Pain. 1975; 1:277. (153)

E69.   Melzack R, Gutte S, Gonshor A. Relief of dental pain by ice massage of the hand. Can Med Assoc J. 1980; 122:189. (166)

E70.   Melzack R, Jeans ME, Stratford JG, Monks RC. Ice massage and transcutaneous electrical stimulation: comparison of treatment for low-back pain. Pain. 1980; 9:209-217. (167)

E71.   Melzack R, Toorgerson WS. On the language of pain. Anesthesiology. 1971; 34:50. (55, 150)

E72.   Melzack R, Wall PD. Pain mechanisms, a new theory. Science. 1965; 150:971-979. (163, 164, 166, 174)

E73.   Mennell JM. The therapeutic use of col. J Am Orthop Assoc. 1975; 74:1146-1158. (163-165, 168, 246)

E74.   Miller MF, Barabasz AF, Barabasz M. Effects of active alert and relaxation hypnotic inductions on cold pressor pain. J Abnorm Psych. 1991; 100:223-226. (158)

E75.   Miller CR, Webers RL. The effects of ice massage on an individual's pain tolerance level to electrical stimulation. J Orthop Sports Phys Ther. 1990; 12:105-110. (167)

E76.   Moret V, Forster A, Laverriere MC, Lambert H, Gaillard RC, Bourgeois P, Haynal A, Gemperle M, Buscher E. Mechanism of analgesia induced by hypnosis and acupuncture: is there a difference? Pain. 1991; 45:135-140. (158)

E77.   Newton RA. Contemporary views on pain and the role played by thermal agents in managing pain symptoms. In: Michlovitz SL, ed. Thermal Agents in Rehabilitation. Philadelphia, PA: FA Davis Co; 1986:19-48. (50)

E78.   Nielson AJ. Spray and stretch for relief of myofascial pain. Phys Ther. 1978; 58:567-569. (168)

E79.   Nimchick PSR, Knight KL. Effects of wearing a toe cap or a sock on temperature and perceived pain during ice water immersion. Athl Train. 1983; 18:144-147. (114, 153, 168, 220)

E80.   Ohnhaus EE, Adler R. Methodological problems in the measurement of pain: a comparison between the verbal rating scale and the visual analogue scale. Pain. 1975; 1:379. (151)

E81.   Parsons CM, Goetzl FR. Effect of induced pain on pain threshold. Proc Soc Exp Biol Med. 1945; 60:327-329. (164)

E82.   Peppard A. Myotonic muscle distress: a rationale for therapy. Athl Train. 1973; 8:166-169. (50, 168, 174, 233)

E83.   Reading AE. A comparison of MPQ in chronic and acute pain. Pain. 1982; 13:185. (150)

E84.   Robbins LD. Cryotherapy for headache. Headache. 1989; 29:598-600. (245)

E85.   Roberts D, Pizzarelli G, Lepore V, Al-Khaja N, Belboul A, Dernevik L. Reduction of post-thoracotomy pain by cryotherapy of intercostal nerves. Scand J Cardiovasc Surg. 1988; 22:127-130. (128, 165)

E86.   Saumet JL, Chery-Croze S, Duclaux R. Response of cat skin mechanothermal nociceptors to cold stimulation. Brain Res Bull. 1985; 15:529-532. (128)

E87.   Scott J, Huskisson EC. Vertical and horizontal analogue scales. Ann Rheum Dis. 1979; 38:560. (151, 157)

E88.   Shiomi K. Relations of pain threshold and pain tolerance in cold water with scores on Maudsley personality inventory and manifest anxiety scale. Percept Mot Skills. 1978; 47:1155-1158. (153, 154, 158)

E89.   Shumate M, Worthington EL. Effectiveness of components of self-verbalization training for control of cold pressor pain. J Psychosom Res. 1987; 31:301-310. (153, 158)

E90.   Stangel L. The value of cryotherapy and thermotherapy in the relief of pain. Physiother Can. 1975; 27:135-139. (165)

E91.   Streator S. The role of sensory information on affective pain. J Athl Train. 1994; 29:166. Abstract. (121, 159)

E92.   Strempel H. Adaptive modification to cold II: long term experiments with 24 hour intervals. Eur J Appl Physiol. 1978; 38:17-24. (158-160)

E93.   Strempel H. Adaptive modification to cold. Eur J Appl Physiol. 1976; 36:19-25. (160)

E94.   Svacina L. Pain Control #10. Longmont, CO: Staodynamics Inc; 1977:1-3. (149, 150)

E95.   Talag T. Residual muscle soreness as influenced by concentric, eccentric and static contractions. Res Q. 1973; 44:458-469. (150, 151)

E96.   Thieme H. Knee joint position sense following therapeutic applications of heat and cold. Indiana University; 1993. Masters thesis. (134)

E97.   Thompson JM, McFarland GK, HIrsch JE, Tucker SM, Bowers AC. Comfort. Clin Nurs. St Louis, Mo: CV Mosby CO; 1986:1971-1983. (150)

E98.   Torebjork HE. Afferent C units responding to mechanical, thermal, and chemical stimuli in human non-glaborus skin. Acta Physiol Scand 1974; 92:374-390. (128, 134, 168)

E99.   Travell J. Ethyl chloride spray for painful muscle spasm. Arch Phys Med. 1952; 33:291-298. (163, 165, 168, 246)

E100. Travell J. Treatment of painful disorders of skeletal muscles. NY State J Med. 1948; 48:2050-2059. (163)

E101. Travell J, Rinzler SH. Influence of ethyl chloride spray on deep pain and ischemic contraction of skeletal muscle. Fed Proc. 1949; 8:339. (82, 164, 246)

E102. Travell J, Rinzler SH. The myofascial genesis of pain. Postgrad Med. 1952; 11:425-434. (173, 246)

E103. Travell J, Simons DG. Myofascial Pain and Dysfunction: The Trigger Point Manual. Baltimore, Md: Williams & Wilkins; 1983:714. (168, 246)

E104. Underwood FB, Kremser GL, Finstuen K, Greathouse DG. Increasing involuntary torque production by using TENS. J Orthop Sports Phys Ther. 1990; 12:101-104. (167)

E105. Weisenberg M. Psychological intervention for the control of pain. Behav Res Ther. 1987; 25:301-312. (149, 158)

E106. Wells HS. Temperature equalization for the relief of pain. Arch Phys Med Rehabil. 1947; 28:135-139. (153, 156)

E107. Wolf S, Hardy JD. Studies on pain: observations on pain due to local cooling and factors involved in the "Cold Pressor" effect. J Clin Invest. 1941; 20:521-533. (67, 154, 156, 157, 160)

E108. Worthington EL Jr. Effect of cognitive strategy content and length of instructions on cold pressor pain tolerance. Percept Mot Skills. 1982; 55:1175-1178. (153, 158, 159)

E109. Worthington EL, Feldman DA. Presentational style of therapeutic directive and response to cold pressor pain. Percept Mot Skills. 1981; 53:506. (158, 159)

E110. Yackzan L, Adams C, Francis KT. The effects of ice massage on delayed muscle soreness. Am J Sports Med. 1984; 12:159-164. (121, 166, 167)

E111. Yarnitsky D, Ochoa JL. Release of cold-induced burning pain by block of cold-specific afferent input. Brain. 1990; 113:893-902. (128)

E112. Zelman DC, Howland EW, Nichols SN, Cleeland CS. The effects of induced mood on laboratory pain. Pain. 1991; 46:105-111. (158)

SPASM

F1. Backlund L, Tiselius P. Objective measurement of joint stiffness in rheumatoid arthritis. Acta Rheum Scand. 1967; 13:275-288. (176)

F2. Bassett SW, Lake BM. Use of cold applications in the management of spasticity. Phys Ther Rev. 1958; 28:333-334. (172, 175)

F3. Boes MC. Reduction of spasticity by cold. J Am Phys Ther Assoc. 1962; 42:29-32. (172)

F4. Boynton BI, Garramone PM, Buca JT. Observations on the effects of cool baths for patients with multiple sclerosis. Phys Ther Rev. 1959; 39:297-307. (172)

F5. Chambers R. Clinical uses of cryotherapy. Phys Ther. 1969; 49:245-249. (111, 172)

F6. DonTigney RL, Shelton KW. Simultaneous use of heat and cold in treatment of muscle spasm. Arch Phys Med Rehabil. 1962; 43:148-150. (17, 172)

F7. Ferretti G, Ishii M, Moia C, Cerretelli P. Effects of temperature on the maximal instantaneous muscle power of humans. J Appl Physiol. 1992; 63:112-116. (177)

F8. Fox WF. Human performance in the cold. Hum Factors. 1967; 9:203-220. (176)

F9. Gaydos GF. Effects of local hand cooling on manual performance. J Appl Physiol. 1958; 12:376-380. (176)

F10. Giesbrecht GG, Bristow GK. Decrement in manual arm performance during whole body cooling. Aviation Space Evniron Med. 1992; 63:1077-1081. (175-177)

F11. Hamilton GF. Mobilization of the proximal interphalangeal joint. Phys Ther. 1967; 47:1111-1114. (172)

F12. Hartviksen K. Ice therapy in spasticity. Acta Neurol Scand. 1962; 38(suppl 3):79-84. (70, 73, 172)

F13.   Hunter J, Kerr EH, Whillans MG. The relationship between joint stiffness upon exposure to cold and the characteristics of synovial fluid. *Can J Med Sci.* 1952; 30:367-377. (176, 177)

F14.   Hunter J, Willians MG. A study of the effects of cold on joint temperature and mobility. *Can J Med Sci.* 1951; 29:255-262. (175-177)

F15.   Johns RJ, Wright V. Relative importance of various tissues in joint stiffness. *J Appl Physiol.* 1962; 17:824-828. (176)

F16.   Kelley M. Effectiveness of a cryotherapy technique on spasticity. *Phys Ther.* 1969; 49:349-353. (17, 172)

F17.   Knott M. Some suggestions for reducing spasticity in neurological conditions. *Sjukgymnastem.* 1969; 27:7-8. (15, 16, 172)

F18.   Knott M, Barafoldi ED. Treatment of whiplash injuries. *Phys Ther Rev.* 1961; 41:573-577. (15, 16, 172, 177, 220)

F19.   Knutsson E. Physical therapy techniques in the control of spasticity. *Scand J Rehabil Med.* 1973; 5:167-169. (4, 171, 173)

F20.   Knutsson E. On effects of local cooling upon motor functions in spastic paresis. *Prog Phys Ther.* 1970; 1:124-131. (172)

F21.   Knutsson E. Topical cryotherapy in spasticity. *Scand J Rehabil Med.* 1970; 2:159-163. (172, 173)

F22.   Knutsson E, Lindblom U, Martensson A. Differences in effects in gamma and alpha spasticity induced by the gaba derivative baclofen (lioresal). *Brain.* 1973; 96:29-46. (171, 173)

F23.   Knutsson E, Mattsson E. Effects of local cooling on monosynaptic reflexes in man. *Scand J. Rehabil Med.* 1969; 1:126-132. (173)

F24.   Knutsson E, Odeen I, Franzen H. The effects of therapeutic exercise under local hypothermia in patients with spastic pareses. *Sjukgymnastem.* 1969; 27:137-139. (173)

F25.   Lane LE. Localized hypothermia for relief of pain in musculoskeletal injuries. *Phys Ther.* 1971; 51:182-183. (17, 172)

F26.   LeBlanc JS. Impairment of manual dexterity in the cold. *J Appl Physiol.* 1956; 9:62-64. (176)

F27.   Lehman JF, Masock AJ, Wareen CG, Koblanski JN. Effect of therapeutic temperatures on tendon extensibility. *Arch Phys Med Rehabil.* 1970; 51:481-487. (175)

F28.   Levine MG, Kabat H, Knott M, Voss DE. Relaxation of spasticity by physiological techniques. *Arch Phys Med Rehabil.* 1954; 35:214-223. (15, 16, 172)

F29.   Mackworth NH. Finger numbness in vary cold winds. *J Appl Physiol.* 1953; 5:533-543. (167, 177)

F30.   Mead S, Knott M. Topical cryotherapy: use for relief of pain and spasticity. *Calif Med.* 1966; 105:179-181. (15, 16, 172)

F31.   Mead S, Knott M. Ice therapy in joint restriction, spasticity, and certain types of pain. *Gen Pract.* 1961; 30:16-18. (15, 16, 172)

F32.   Mecomber SA, Hermarr RM. Effects of local hypothermia on reflex and voluntary activity. *Phys Ther.* 1971; 51:271-282. (172, 175-177)

F33.   Miglietta O. Action of cold on spasticity. *Am J Phys Med.* 1973; 52:198-205. (139, 172)

F34.   Miglietta OE. Electromyographic characteristics of clonus and influence of cold. *Arch Phys Med.* 1964; 45:508-512. (172)

F35.   Miglietta OE. Evaluation of cold in spasticity. *Am J Phys Med.* 1962; 41:148-151. (146, 173)

F36.   Price R, Lehman JF. Influence of muscle cooling on the viscoelastic response of the human ankle to sinusoidal displacements. *Arch Phys Med Rehabil.* 1990; 71:745-748. (175)

F37. Provens KA, Clarke RSJ. The effect of cold on manual performance. *J Occup Med.* 1960; 2:169-176. (175, 176)

F38. Rockafeller LE. The use of cold packs for increasing joint range of motion: a study. *Phys Ther Rev.* 1958; 38:564-566. (172)

F39. Ruiz DH, Myrer JW, Durrant E, Fellingham GW. Cryotherapy and sequential exercise bouts following cryotherapy on concentric and eccentric strength in the quadriceps. *J Athl Train.* 1993; 28:320-323. (147, 177)

F40. Schiefer RE, Kok R, Lewis MI, Meese GB. Finger skin temperature and manual dexterity-some inter group differences. *Appl Ergon.* 1984; 15:135-141. (177)

F41. Sechrist WC, Stull GA. Effects and mild activity, heat applications, and cold applications on range of joint movement. *Am Corr Ther J.* 1969; 23:120-123. (177)

F42. Showman J, Wedlick LT. The use of cold instead of heat for the relief of muscle spasm. *Med J Aust.* 1963; 50:612-614. (17, 145)

F43. Teichner WH. Manual dexterity in the cold. *J Appl Physiol.* 1957; 11:333-338. (177)

F44. Urbscheit N, Bishop B. Effects of cooling on the ankle jerk and H-response in hemiplegic patients. *Phys Ther.* 1970; 50:1041-1049.

F45. Urbscheit N, Johnston R, Bishop B. Effects of cooling on the ankle jerk and H-response in hemiplegic patients. *Phys Ther.* 1971; 51:983-987. (173)

F46. Viel E. Treatment of spasticity by exposure to cold. *Phys Ther Rev.* 1959; 39:598-599. (172)

F47. Vincet MJ, Tipton MJ. The effects of cold immersion and hand protection on grip strength. *Aviat Space Environ Med.* 1988; 59:738-741. (176)

F48. Warren CG, Lehman JF, Koblanski JN. Heat and stretch procedures: an evaluation using rat tail tendon. *Arch Phys Med Rehabil.* 1976; 57:122-126. (173, 175)

F49. Warren CG, Lehman JF, Koblanski JN. Elongation of rat tail tendon: effect of load and temperature. *Arch Phys Med Rehabil.* 1971; 52:465-474. (175, 176)

F50. Wolf SL, Knutsson E. Effects of skin cooling on stretch reflex activity in triceps surae of the decerebate cat. *Exp Neurol.* 1975; 49:22-35. (172, 175)

F51. Wolf SL, Ledbetter WD. Effect of skin cooling on spontaneous EMG activity in triceps surae of the decerebrate cat. *Brain Res.* 1975; 91:151-155. (173)

F52. Wright V, Johns RJ. Physical factors concerned with the stiffness of normal and diseased joints. *Bull Johns Hopkins Hosp.* 1960; 106:215-231. (176)

METABOLISM AND INFLAMMATION

G1. Abakumova EA. Effect of hypothermia on inflammation. *Stomatologiia (Mosk).* 1978; 57:19-21. English abstract. (9, 81, 82)

G2. Abbott TR. Oxygen uptake following deep hypothermia. *Anaesthesia.* 1977; 32:524-532. (79)

G3. Abramson DI, Kahn A, Tuck S, Turman GA, Rejal H, Fleischer CJ. Relationship between a range of tissue temperature and local oxygen consumption in the resting forearm. *Lab Clin Med.* 1957; 50:789. (78)

G4. Albin MS, White RJ, Acosta-Rua G, Yason D. Study of functional recovery produced by delayed localized cooling after spinal cord injury in primates. *J Neurosurg.* 1968; 29:113-120. (80)

G5. Albin MS, White RJ, Locke GS, Massopust LC, Kretchmer HE. Localized spinal cord hypothermia. *Anesth Analg.* 1967; 46:8-15. (80)

G6.   Angell WW, Rikkers L, Doug E, Shumway NE. Organ viability with hypothermia. *J. Thorac Cardiovasc Surg.* 1969; 58:619-624. (79)

G7.   Augustynowicz SD, Sochacka ZD, Szmurlo WF, Stryjecki JK, Pawtel B. Low Temperature technique in preservation of organs and tissues. *Acta Med Pol.* 1978; 19:127-132. (79)

G8.   Bingham R. The therapeutic effect of cold in bone and joint infection: part I. *Am J Orthop Surg.* 1968; 10:158-165. (82, 100)

G9.   Bingham R. The therapeutic effect of cold in bone and joint infection: conclusion. *Am J. Orthop Surg.* 1968; 10:186-189. (82)

G10. Blair E. *Clinical Hypothermia.* New York, NY: McGraw-Hill Book Co; 1964:22-30. (77, 78)

G11. Blalock A. A comparison of the effects of the local application of heat and of cold in the prevention and treatment of experimental traumatic shock. *Surgery.* 1942; 11:356-359. (79)

G12. Bloch M. Cold water for burns and scalds. *Lancet.* 1968; 1:695. (80)

G13. Bloch M. Hypothermia in the treatment of burn injury: a critical evaluation. *Br J. Plast Surg.* 1966; 57:347-360. (80)

G14. Blomgren I, Eriksson E, Bagge U. The effect of different cooling temperatures and immersion fluids on post-burn oedema and survival of the partially scalded hairy mouse ear. *Burns.* 1985; 11:161-165. (80)

G15. Boykin JV, Crute SL. Mechanisms of burn shock protection after severe scald injury by cold-water treatment. *J. Trauma.* 1982; 22:859-866. (80, 81)

G16. Bricolo A, Ore GD, DaPian R, Faccioli F. Local cooling in spinal cord injury. *Surg Neurol.* August 1976; 6:101-106. (80)

G17. Brinker MR, Timberlake GA, Goff JM, Rice JC, Kerstein MD. Below-knee physiologic cryoanesthesia in the critically ill patient. *J Vasc Surg.* 1988; 7:433-438. (104)

G18. Brooks B, Duncan GW. The influence of temperature on wounds. *Ann Surg.* 1941; 114:1069-1075. (81)

G19. Buch B, Papert AI, Shear M. Microscopic changes in rate tongue following experimental cryosurgery. *J Oral Pathol.* 1979; 8:94-102. (8)

G20. Casley-Smith JR. An electron microscopic study of injured and abnormally permeable lymphatics. *Ann NY Acad Sci.* 1964; 116:803-828. (10)

G21. Civalero LA, Moreno JR, Senning A. Temperature conditions and oxygen consumption during deep hypothermia. *Acta Chir Scand.* 1962; 123:179-188. (78)

G22. Clancy WG Jr. Tendinitis and plantar fasciitis in runners. In: D'Ambrosia R, Drez D Jr, eds. *Prevention and Treatment of Running Injuries.* Thorofare, NJ: Charles B Slack; 1982:77-87. (27)

G23. Cohn LH, Collins JJ. Local cardiac hypothermia for myocardial protection. *Ann Thorac Surg.* 1974; 17:135-145. (78)

G24. Coté DJ, Prentice WE, Hooker DN, Shields EW. Comparison of three treatment procedures for minimizing ankle sprain swelling. *Phys Ther.* 1988; 68:1072-1076. (91)

G25. Delorme EJ. Experimental cooling of the blood stream. *Lancet.* 1952; 263:914-915. (77)

G26. Demling RH, Mazess RB, Wolberg W. The effect of immediate and delayed cold immersion on burn edema formation and resorption. *J Trauma.* 1979; 19:59-60. (80)

G27. Dillard DH. Cogenital heart disease: definitive surgery during infancy. *Surg Rounds.* January 1981; 4:24-31. (79)

G28.   Dorwart BB, Hansel JR, Schumacher HR. Effects of heat, cold and mechanical agitation on crystal-induced arthritis in the dog. *Arthritis Rheum.* 1973; 16:540-556. (71, 81, 122)

G29.   Drucker WR. Rationale for hypothermia in therapy of hypovolemia. In: Mills LC, Moyer JH, eds. *Shock and Hypotension.* New York, NY: Grune & Stratton; 1965:670-677. (78)

G30.   Duncan GW, Blalock A. Shock produced by crush injury. *Arch Surg.* 1942; 45:183-194. (79)

G31.   Enneking WF. *Principles of Musculoskeletal Pathology.* Gainesville, FL: Storter Printing Co; 1970:351. (30)

G32.   Enright LP, Staroscik RN, Reis RL. Left ventricular function after occlusion of the ascending aorta. *J Thorac Cardiovasc Surg.* 1970; 60:737-745. (78)

G33.   Epstein MF, Crawford JD. Cooling in the emergency treatment of burns. *Pediatrics.* 1973; 52:430-432. (80)

G34.   Fashouer TF, LoBello CM. Artificial turf abrasions. *Physician Sportsmed.* November 1983; 11:65. (247)

G35.   Ferrer JM, Grikelare GF, Armstrong D. Some effects of cooling on scald burns in the rat. *Surg Forum.* 1962; 13:486-487. (80)

G36.   Freeman NE. Influence of temperature on the development of gangrene in peripheral vascular disease. *Arch Surg.* 1940; 40:326-333. (78)

G37.   Gott VL, Bartlett M, Long DM, Lillehie CW, Johnson JA. Myocardial energy substances in the dog heart during potasisum and hypothermic arrest. *J Appl Physiol.* 1962; 17:815-818. (78)

G38.   Griepp RB, Stinson EB, Shumway NE. Profound local hypothermia for myocardial protection during open-heart surgery. *J Thorac Cardiovasc Surg.* 1973; 66:731-741. (79)

G39.   Hagerdal M, Harp J, Nilsson L, Siesjo BK. The effect of induced hypothermia upon oxygen consumption in the rat brain. *J Neurochem.* 1975; 24:311-322. (79, 80)

G40.   Hansebout RR, Lamont RN, Kamath MV. The effects of local cooling on canine spinal cord blood flow. *Can J Neurol Sci.* 1985; 12:83-87. (80)

G41.   Hansebout RR, Tanner JA, Romero-Sierra C. Current status of spinal cord cooling in the treatment of acute spinal cord injury. *Spine.* 1984; 9:508-511. (80)

G42.   Harris ED, McCroskery PA. The influence of temperature in fibril's stability on degradation of cartilage collagen by rheumatoid syovial collagenase. *N Engl J Med.* 1974; 290:1-6. (81, 82)

G43.   Hegnauer AH, D'Amato HE. Oxygen consumption and cardiac output in the hypothermic dog. *Am J Physiol.* 1954; 178:138-142. (78)

G44.   Ikemoto Y, Kobayashi H, Usui M, Ishii S. Changes in serum myoglobin levels caused by tourniquet ischemia under ormothermic and hypothermic conditions. *Clin Orthop.* 1988; 234:296-302. (78)

G45.   Iung OS, Wade FV. The treatment of burns with ice water, phisohex, and partial hypothermia. *Ind Med Surg.* 1963; 32:365-370. (78)

G46.   Jennings RB, Ganote CE, Reimer KA. Ischemic tissue injury. *Am J Pathol.* 1975; 81:179-198. (80)

G47.   Jennings RB, Hawkins HK, Lowe JE, Hill ML, Klotman S, Reimer KA. Relatioship between high energy phosphage and letal injury in myocardial ischemia in the dog. *Am J Pathol.* 1978; 92:187-214. (80)

G48.   Kelly MJ, Wheatley R, Smith JHF, Thomas WEG. Cooling prevents ischaemic testicular damage after spermatic cord clamping in rats. *Int J. Androl.* 1987; 10:721-726. (78)

G49.   King TC, Price PB. Surface colling following extensive burns. *JAMA.* 1963; 83:677-678. (80)

G50.   Knight KL. Effects of hypothermia on inflammation and swelling. *Athl Train.* 1976; 11:7-10. (9, 15, 31, 85, 88, 124)

G51.   Kohnlein HE, Larnpere G. Experiments and clinical observations on cold water treatment of fresh burns. *Chir Plast (Berl).* 1972; 1:216-221. (80)

G52.   Kvitsinskaya EA, Krivulis DB, Sorokin YA. Effect of hypothermia on metabolism in the liver during preservation. *Bull Exp Biol Med.* 1978; 86:179-182. (79, 82)

G53.   Lamberti JJ, Cohn LH, Laks H, Braunwald NS, Collins JJ Jr, Castaneda AR. Local cardiac hypothermia for myocardial protection during correction of congenital heart disease. *Ann Thorac Surg.* 1975; 20:446-454. (79, 90)

G54.   Langohr JL, Rosenfield L, Owen CR, Cope O. Effect of therapeutic cold on the circulation of blood and lymph in thermal burns. *Arch Surg.* 1949; 59:1031-1044. (80)

G55.   Lungren C, Muren A, Zederfeldt B. Effect of cold-vasoconstriction on wound healing in the rabbit. *Acta Chir Scand.* 1959; 118:14. (9, 82)

G56.   MacDonald DJF. Current practice of hypothermia in British cardiac surgery. *Br J Anaesth.* 1975; 47:1011-1016. (79)

G57.   Manson AD, Williams HB, Woolhouse FM. Correlation of edema formation, hemoconcentration, and mortality in experimental burns treated with hypothermia. *Surg Forum.* 1964; 15:469-471. (80)

G58.   Marcove RC. cryosurgery in the treatment of giant cell tumors of bone. *Clin Orthop.* 1978; 134:275-289. (8)

G59.   Michenfelder JD, Theye RA. Hypothermia: effect on canine brain and whole-body metabolism. *Anesthesiology.* 1968; 29:1107-1112. (78)

G60.   Mirkovitch V, Robinson JWL, Comba A, Fischer A, Winistorfer B, Vouron J. Influence of short-term hypothermia upon the normal of ischaemic dog kidney. *Cryobiology.* 1976; 13:168-176. (80)

G61.   Movat HZ. The acute inflammatory reaction. In: Movat HZ, ed. *Inflammation, Immunity, and Hypersensitivity.* 2nd ed. New York, NY: Harper & Row; 1978:2-161. (30, 90)

G62.   Najafi H. Comment following: Griepp RB, Stinson EB, Shumway NE. Profound local hypothermia for myocardial protection during open-heart surgery. *J Thorac Cardiovasc Surg.* 1973; 66:732-741. (31, 79)

G63.   Nordstrom CH, Rehncrona S. Reduction of cerebral blood flow and oxygen consumption with a combination of barbituate anesthesia and induced hypothermia in the rat. *Acta Anesthesiol Scand.* 1978; 22:7-12. (78)

G64.   Nugent GR. Prolonged hypothermia. *Am J Nurs.* 1960; 60:967-970. (77)

G65.   Ofeigsson OJ, Mitchell R, Patrick RS. Observations on the cold water treatment of cutaneous burns. *J Pathol.* 1972; 108:145-150. (79)

G66.   Orr KD, Fainer DC. Cold injuries in Korea during winter of 1950-51. *Medicine.* 1952; 31:77. (80)

G67.   Osterholm J. The pathophysiological response to spinal cord injury: the current status of related research. *J Neurosurg.* 1972; 40:5-33. (180)

G68.   Osterman AL, Heppenstall RB, Sapega AA, Katz M, Chance B, Sokolow D. Muscle ischemia and hypothermia: a bioenergetic study using [31]phosphorus nuclear magnetic resonance spectrosocpy. *J Trauma.* 1984; 24:811-817. (78)

G69.   Popovic V, Popovic P. *Hypothermia in Biology and Medicine.* New York, NY: Grune & Stratton Inc; 1974:79-115, 215. (77-79)

G70.   Poy NG, Williams HB, Woolhouse FM. The alteration of mortality rates in burned rates using early excision, homografting, and hypothermia, alone and in combination. *Plast Reconstr Surg.* 1965; 35:198-206. (80)

G71. Pushkar NS, Sandorminsky BP. Cold treatment of burns. *Burns.* 1982; 9:101-110. (80)

G72. Race D, Cooper E, Rosenbaum M. Hemorrhagic shock: the effect of prolonged low flow on the regional distribution of blood and its modification by hypothermia. *Ann Surg.* 1968; 167:454-466. (78)

G73. Rao KS, Schultz RW, Feinberg H, Levitsky S. Metabolic evidence that regional hypothermia induced by cold saline protects the heart during ischemic arrest. *J Surg Res.* 1976; 20:421-425. (78)

G74. Repolgle R, Cutiletta AF, Arcilla RA, Lin CY. Ischemic cardiac arrest: left ventricular contractility and cyclic AMP in the human heart. Presented at the Eighth European Society for Experimental Surgery; May 2, 1973; Oslo, Norway. (78)

G75. Rippe B, Grega GJ. Effects of 150 prenaline and cooling on histamine induced changes of capillary permeability in the rat hindquarter vascular bed. *Acta Phisiol Scand.* 1978; 103:252-262. (81, 90)

G76. Robbins SL, Cotron RS. *Poathologic Basis of Disease.* 2nd ed. Philadelphia, PA: WB Saunders Co; 1979:22-90. (30, 31, 36, 80)

G77. Ryan GB, Majno G. *Inflammation.* Kalamazoo, MI: The Upjohn Co; 1977:1-80. (26, 28, 31, 38)

G78. Ryan TJ. The blood vessels of the skin. *J Invest Dermatol.* 1976; 67:110-118. (31, 78)

G79. Salsbury RE, McKeel DW, Mason AD. Ischemic necrosis of the intrinsic muscle of the hand after thermal injuries. *J Bone Joint Surg.* 1974; 56A:1701. (80)

G80. Sapega AA, Heppenstall RB, Sokolow DP, et al. The bioenergetics of preservation of limbs before replantation. *J Bone Joint Surg.* 1988; 70A:1500-1513. (78)

G81. Sapsford RN, Blackstone EH, Kirklin JW, et al. Coronary perfusion versus cold ischemic arrest during aortic valve surgery. *Circulation.* 1974; 49:1190-1199. (79)

G82. Schmidt KL, Ott VR, Rocher G, Schaller H. Heat, cold and inflammation: a review. *Z Rheumatol.* 1979; 38:391-404. (81)

G83. Seiyama A, Shiga T, Maeda N. Temperature effect on oxygenation and metabolism of perfused rat hindlimb muscle. *Adv Exp Med Biol.* 1990; 277:541-547. (78)

G84. Simmons RL, Foker JE, Lower RR, Najarian JS. Transplantation. In: Schwartz SI, Lilleh RC, Shires GT, Spencer FC, Stoher EH, eds. *Principles of Surgery.* 2nd ed. St. Louis, MO: McGraw Hill Book Co; 1974; 1:349-442. (79)

G85. Southard JH, Lindell SL, Belzer FO. Energy metabolism and renal ischemia. *Ren Fail.* 1992; 14:251-255. (79)

G86. Stewart GJ, Ritchie WGM, Lynch PR. Venous endothelial damage produced by massive sticking and emigration of leukocytes. *Am J Pathol.* 1974; 74:507-532. (31)

G87. Svanes K. Studies in hypothermia, I: the influence of deep hypothermia on the formation of cellular exudate in acute inflammation in mice. *Acta Anaesthesiol Scand.* 1964; 8:143-156. (81)

G88. Svanes K. Studies in hypothermia, II: the influence of deep hypothermia on the formation of fluid exudate in acute inflammation in mice. *Acta Anaesthesiol Scand.* 1964; 8:157-166. (81)

G89. Swan H, Patton BC. The current status of hypothermia in cardiovascular surgery. *Prog Cardiovasc Dis.* 1961; 4:228-258. (79)

G90. Uihlein A, Terry HR, Martin JT. Induced hypothermia in neurologic surgery. *Modern Medicine.* October 1960; 28:134-136. (79)

G91.   Vogt MT, Farber E. On the molecular pathology of the ischemic renal cell death: reversible and irreversible cellular and mitochondrial metabolic alterations. *Am J Pathol.* 1968; 53:1-26. (80)

G92.   Wiedeman MP, Brigham MP. The effects of cooling on the microvasculature after thermal injury. *Microvasc Surg.* 1971; 3:154-161. (80)

G93.   Wilson CE, Sasse CW, Musselman MW, McWhorter CA. Cold water treatment of burns. *J Trauma.* 1963; 3:477-482. (80)

G94.   Wright JG, Kerr JC, Valeri CR, Hobson RW. Regional hypothermia protects against ischemia-reperfusion injury in isolated canine gracilis muscle. *J Trauma.* 1988; 28:1026-1031. (78)

G95.   Zachariassen KE. Hypothermia and cellular physiology. *Arctic Med Res.* 1991; 50:13-17. (182)

IMMEDIATE CARE AND POSTSURGICAL CRYOTHERAPY

H1.   Allen FM. Reduced temperature in surgery, I: surgery of limbs. *Am J Surg.* 1941; 52:225-237. (104, 166, 181)

H2.   Appenzeller H, Ross CT. Utah: can a student trainer be held to the same standard of care of a physician or surgeon? *Sports Courts.* Summer 1984; 5:11-13. (180)

H3.   Aukland K, Nicolaysen G. Interstitial fluid volume: local regulatory mechanisms. *Physiol Rev.* 1981; 61:556-643. (34)

H4.   Barnes L. Cryotherapy: putting injury on ice. *Physician Sportsmed.* June 1979; 7:130-136. (15, 217)

H5.   Basur RL, Shephard E, Mouzas GL. A cooling method in the treatment of ankle sprains. *Practitioner.* 1976; 216:708-711. (86)

H6.   Bert JM, Strak JG, Maschka K, Chock C. The effect of cold therapy on morbidity subsequent to arthroscopic lateral retinacular release. *Orthop Rev.* 1991; 20:755-758. (100)

H7.   Blomgren I, Bagge U, Johansson BR. Effects of cooling after scald injury to a dorsal skin fold of mouse. *Scand J Plast Reconstr Surg.* 1985; 19:1-9. (80)

H8.   Blomgren I, Eriksson E, Bagge U. Effect of cold water immersion on edema formation in the scalded mouse ear. *Burns.* 1982; 9:17-20. (80)

H9.   Boland AL: Rehabilitation of the injured athlete. In: Strauss RH, ed. *Sports Medicine and Physiology.* Philadelphia, PA: WB Saunders Co; 1979:226-234. (3, 85, 94, 96)

H10.   Cohn BT, Draeger RI, Jackson DW. The effects of cold therapy in the postoperative management of pain in patients undergoing anterior cruciate ligament reconstruction. *Am J Sports Med.* 1989; 17:344-349. (100, 101, 166)

H11.   Condit RE, Kalenak A. Letter and reply: wound repair. *Am Fam Pract.* April 1976; 13:28, 30. (10)

H12.   Cramer Products. *Athletic Training in the Seventies.* Gardner, KS: Cramer Products Inc; 1970:29. (94)

H13.   Crossman LW, Ruggiero WF, Hurley V, Allen FM. Reduced temperature in surgery, II: amputation for peripheral vascular disease. *Arch Surg.* 1942; 44:139-156. (104, 166)

H14.   Downer A. Cryotherapy for animals. *Mod Vet Pract.* 1978; 59:659-662. (94)

H15.   Droegemeuller W. Cold sitz baths for relief of perineal pain. *Clin Obstet Gynecol.* 1980; 23:1039-1043. (101)

H16.   Farry PJ, Prentice NG, Hunter AC, Wakelin CA. Ice treatment of injured ligaments: an experimental model. *N Z Med J.* 1980; 91:12-14. (103)

H17. Fashouer TF, LoBello CM. Aftificial turf arasions. *Physician Sportsmed.* November 1983; 11:64.

H18. Garrett WE. Muscle strain injuries: clinical and basic aspects. *Med Sci Sports Exerc.* 1990; 22:436-443. (92)

H19. George F. Editorial comment. In: Anderson JL, George F, Krakauer LJ, Shephard RJ, Torg JS, eds. *1983 year Book of Sports Medicine.* Chicago, IL: Year Book Medical Publishers, Inc; 1983:365-386. (87)

H20. Gibbel MI, Atkins RA, Burns A. The use of dry ice refrigeration when delaying an inevitable amputaiton. *Am J Surg.* 1960; 99:326-329. (104)

H21. Guyton AC. Integrative hemodynamics. In: Sodeman WA Jr, Sodeman WA, eds. *Pathologic Physiology.* 5th ed. Philadelphia, PA: WB Saunders Co; 1977:149-176. (20, 33, 34, 36)

H22. Hafen BQ, Karren KJ. *First Aid and Emergency Care Workbook.* 3rd ed. Englewood, CO: Morton Publishing Co; 1984; 178, 262. (94)

H23. Hargens AR. Fluid shifts in vascular and extravascular spaces during and after simulated weightlessness. *Med Sci Sports Exerc.* 1983; 15:421-427. (89, 92)

H24. Hecht PJ, Bachmann S, Booth RE, Rothman RH. Effects of thermal therapy on rehabilitation after total knee arthroplasty. *Clin Orthop.* 1983; 178:198-201. (100, 101)

H25. Hirata I. *The Doctor and the Athlete.* Philadelphia, PA: JB Lippincott Co; 1974; 76,328. (94, 96, 122)

H26. Hocutt JE, Jaffe R, Rylander CR, Bebbe JK. Cryotherapy in ankle spairs. *Am J Sports Med.* 1982; 10:316-319. (87, 101)

H27. Holloway GA, Daly CH, Kennedy D, Chirmoskey J. Effects of external pressure loading on human skin blood flow measured by ^{133}Xe clearance. *J Appl Physiol.* 1976; 40:597-600. (89)

H28. Hovig T, Dodds WJ, Rowsell HC, Mustard JF. The transformation of hemostatic platelet plugs in normal and factor IX deficient dogs. *Am J Pathol.* 1968; 53:355-374. (32, 88, 89)

H29. Jedzinsky J, Marck J, Ochonsky P. Effects of local cold and heat therapy on traumatic oedema of the rat hind paw I. effects of cooling on the course of traumatic oedema. *Acta Univ Palacki Olomuc Fac Med.* 1973; 66:185-201. (103)

H30. Johnson MG. Potential role of the lymphatic vessel in regulating inflammatory events. *Surv Synthesis Pathol Res.* 1983; 1:111-119. (10, 33)

H31. Johnson S, ed. The RICE principles *Reebok Instructor News.* 1991; 4(4):4. (85)

H32. Jorgensen L, Borchgrevink CF. The platelet plug in normal persons, I: the histological appearance of the plug 15-20 minutes and 24 hours after the bleeding and its role in the capillary haemostasis. *Acta Pathol Microbiol Scand.* 1963; 57:40-56. (28)

H33. Kaempffe FA. Skin surface temperature reduction after cryotherapy to a casted extremity. *J Orthop Sports Phys Ther.* 1989; 10:448-450. (102)

H34. Klafs CE, Arnheim DD. *Modern Principles of Athletic Training.* St. Louis, MO: CV Mosby Co; 1977:84,244. (15, 16, 89, 93, 94, 221)

H35. Larson CB, Gould M. *Orthopedic Nursing.* 9th ed. St. Louis, MO: CV Mosby Co; 1978:445-446. (109)

H36. Lee JM, Warren MP. *Cold Therapy in Rehabilitation.* London, England: Belt & Hymen; 1978:69-81. (10, 82, 179, 187, 190)

H37. Levick JR, Michel CC. The effects of position and skin temperature on the capillary pressures of the fingers and toes. *J Physiol.* 1978; 274:97-109. (92)

H38. Levy S, Marmar E. Cold compression after TKA can reduce blood loss and pain. Presented at the American Orthopedic Society for Sports Medicine; February 18, 1993; San Francisco, Calif. Reprinted in *Orthop Today*, June 1993:17. (100, 101, 166)

H39. MacLeod J. Treating abrasions with medicated ice. *Physician Sportsmed*. August 1985; 13:155. (247)

H40. Mancuso DL, Knight KL. Effects of prior physical activity on skin surface temperature response of the ankle during and after a 30-minute ice pack application. *J Athl Train*. 1992; 27:242-249. (16, 68)

H41. Matsen FA, Questad K, Matsen AL. The effect of local cooling on postfracture swelling. *Clin Orthop*. 1975; 109:201-206. (103)

H42. Mattacola CG, Perrin DH. Effects of cold water application on isokinetic strength of the plantar flexors. *J Athl Train*. 1992; 27:136. (177)

H43. McDonald WD, Guthrie JD. Cryotherapy in the postoperative setting. *J Foot Surg*. 1985; 24:438-441. (103)

H44. McFarland RG. Normal and abnormal blood coagulation: a review. *J Clin Pathol*. 1948; 1:113-143. (32, 88, 89)

H45. McLean JI. A refrigerator, so useful in the training room. Coach Athl. 1967; Jan:12; 22-24. (94)

H46. McMaster WC, Liddle S. Cryotherapy influence on posttraumatic limb edema. *Clin Orthop*. 1980; 150:283-287. (16, 68, 103)

H47. Mirkin G. Hot and cold: when to apply each to a running injury. *Runner*. Aug 1980; 22-23. (86, 94, 102, 185)

H48. Mlynarczyk JM. Temperature changes during and after ice pack application of 10, 20, 30, 45, and 60 minutes. Terre Haute: Indiana State University; 1984. Masters thesis. (16, 67, 94, 96)

H49. Mustard JF, Packham MA. The reaction of the blood to injury. In: Movat HZ, ed. *Inflammation, Immunity, and Hypersensitivity*. 2nd ed. New York. NY: Harper & Row; 1978:557-665. (28)

H50. Mutschler TA, D'Antonio JA, Ferguson GM, Morsch R, Spinola A. Cold therapy reduces blood loss after primary TKA; but pain and swelling are unaffected. Presented at the American Orthopedic Society for Sports Medicine; February 18, 1993; San Francisco, Calif. Reprinted in *Orthop Today*. June 1993:16. (100, 101)

H51. Oakes BW. Hamstring muscle injuires. *Aust Fam Physician*. 1984; 13:587-591. (233)

H52. Ogden W, Biser J, Akers K, Lyttle C. Constant cold therapy for total joint replacements. Presented to the Piedmont Orthopaedic Society; May 1990. (100, 103)

H53. Omer GE, Brobeck AG. An evaluation of ice application with postoperative dressings. *Clin Orthop*. 1971; 81:117-121. (101)

H54. Papenheimer JR, Soto-Rivera A. Effective osmotic pressure of the plasma proteins and other quantities associated with the capillary circulation in the hindlimbs of cats and dogs. *Am J Physiol*. 1948; 152:471-491. (33, 97)

H55. Paletta FX, Shehadi SI, Mudd JG. Hypothermia and tourniquet ischemia. *Plast Reconstr Surg*. 1962; 29:531-538. (104)

H56. Post JB, Knight KL. Ankle skin temperature changes with a repeated ice pack application. *J Athl Train*. 1992; 27:136. (16, 67, 73, 96)

H57. Ramler D, Roberts J. A comparison of cold and warm sitz baths for relief of postpartum perineal pain. *J Obstet Gynecol Neonatal Nurs*. 1986; 15:471-474. (101)

H58. Rembe EC. Use of cryotherapy on the postsurgical theumatoid hand. *Phys Ther*. 1970; 50:19-23. (103)

H59. Ryan AJ. Technological advances in sports medicine and in the reduction in sports injuries. *Exerc Sport Sci Rev.* 1973; 1:285-312. (3, 15, 85)

H60. Sabiston KB, Prentice WE, Hooker DH, Shields EW. The effects of intermittent compression and cold on reducing edema in postacute ankle sprains. *J Athl Train.* 1992; 27:140. (68, 91)

H61. Schaubel HJ. The local use of ice after orthopedic procedures. *Am J Surg.* 1946; 72:711-714. (99-101, 166)

H62. Scheffler NM, Sheitel PL, Lipton MN. Use of Cryo/Cuff for the control of postoperative pain and edmea. *J Foot Surg.* 1992; 31:141-148. (100, 101)

H63. Schwartz SI, Lillehei RC, Shires GT, Spencer FC, Storer EH. In: Schwartz SI, ed. *Principles of Surgery.* 2nd ed. New York, NY: McGraw-Hill Book Co; 1974:290.

H64. Schwartz SI, Troup SB. Hemostasis, surgical bleeding, and transfusion. In: Schwartz SI, ed. *Principles of Surgery.* 2nd ed. New York, NY: McGraw Hill Book Co; 1974:97-132. (16, 28, 89)

H65. Shafer K. *Medical-Surgical Nursing.* 7th ed. St. Louis, MO: CV Mosby Co; 1980:231-232, 704-880. (104)

H66. Slagle GW. ICE: this initial 3-step treatment can mean a quicker recovery. *The First Aider.* 1979; 48(7):7. (94)

H67. Slocum DB. Treatment of football injuries. *Athl Train.* 1972; 7:77-89. (89)

H68. Smith MP. Reduction of postoperative pain. *Northwest Med.* 1964; 63:698-701. (99)

H69. Snedeker J, Recine V, MacCartee C. Cryotherapy and the athletic injury. *Athl Journal.* 1974. (15, 94)

H70. Starkey JA. Treatment of ankle sprains by simultaneous use of intermittent compression and ice packs. *Am J Sports Med.* 1976; 4:142-144. (10, 17)

H71. Stevens DM, D'Angelo JV. Frostbite due to improper use of frozen gel pack. *N Engl J Med.* 1978; 299:1415. (95, 199)

H72. Thorndike A. Frequency and nature of sports injuries. *Am J Surg.* 1959; 98:316-324.

H73. Urban CD, Knight KL. Insulating effects of elastic wraps used in ice, compression, and elevation. Presented at the Indiana Intergency Research Seminar; April 1979; West Lafayctte, IN. (16, 94, 95)

H74. Varpalotai M, Knight KL. Pressures exerted by elastic wraps applied by beginning and advanced student athletic trainers to the ankle and the thigh with and without an ice pack. *Athl Train.* 1991; 26:246-250. (16, 67, 95, 96)

H75. Wallace L, Knortz K, Esterson P. Immediate care of ankle injuires. *J Orthop Sports Phys Ther.* 1979; 1:46-50. (94)

H76. Watt AJ, ed. *Early Care of the Injured Patient.* Philadelphia, PA: WB Saunders Co; 1982:413. (15)

H77. Weatherall DJ, Bunch C, Sharp AA. The blood and blood-forming organs. In: Smith LH Jr, Thier SO, eds. *Pathophysiology: the Biological Principles of Disease.* Philadelphia, PA: WB Saunders Co; 1981:326-479. (28)

H78. Weisman G. Introduction. In: Weissman G, ed. *Mediators of Inflammation.* New York, NY: Plenum Press; 1974:1-9. (90)

H79. Wilkerson GB. Management of the acute inflammatory response following joint trauma. *Sports Med Update.* Fall 1992; 7:12-15,28. (91, 103)

H80. Wilkerson GB. Treatment of the inversion ankle sprain through synchronous application of focal compression and cold. *Athl Train.* 1991; 26:220-237. (103)

H81.   Wilkerson GB. Treatment of ankle sprains with external compression and early mobilization. *Physician Sportsmed.* June 1985; 13:83. (47, 103)

H82.   Wilkerson LA. Ankle injuires in athletes. *Pri Care.* 1992; 19:377, 386-392. (53)

H83.   Zuidema GD, Rutherford RB, Ballinger WF. *The Management of Trauma.* 3rd ed. Philadelphia, PA: WB Saunders Co; 1979:849. (15)

H84.   Ikemoto Y, Kobayshi H, Usui M, Ishii S. Changes in serum myoglobin levels caused by tourniquet ischemia under normothermic and hypothermic conditions. *Clin Orthop Rel Res.* 1988; 234:296-302. (104)

COMPLICATIONS, CONTRAINDICATIONS, AND PRECAUTIONS

I1.   Barber JM, Dillman PA, *Emergency Patient Care.* Reston, VA: Reston Publishing Co; 1981:550-553. (180-182)

I2.   Bassett FH, Kirkpatrick JS, Englehardt DL, Malone TR. Cold-induced nerve injury. *Am J Sports Med.* 1992; 20:516-518. (185, 188)

I3.   Browse NL. Raynaud's phenomenon and blood viscosity. *Br J Surg.* 1981; 68:520. (191)

I4.   Bushby PA, Hoff ES, Hankes GH. Microscopic tissue alterations following cryosurgery of canine skin. *J Am Vet Med Assoc.* 1978; 173:177-181. (182, 183)

I5.   Coffman JD, Davies WT. Vasospastic diseases: a review. *Prog Cardiovasc Dis.* 1975; 18:123-146. (191)

I6.   Collins K, Storey M, Peterson K. Peroneal nerve palsy after cryotherapy. *Physician Sportsmed.* May 1986; 14:105-108. (185, 188)

I7.   Covington DB, Bassett FH. When cryotherapy injuires: the danger of peripheral nerve damage. *Physician Sportsmed.* March 1993; 21:78-93. (16, 94, 185, 188)

I8.   De Loecker R, Penninckx F. Biochemical and functional aspects of recovery of mammalian systems from deep sub-zero temperatures. *Symp Soc Exp Biol.* 1987; 41:407-427. (23, 188)

I9.   Denny-Brown D, Brenner C. paralysis of nerve induced by direct pressure and by tourniquet. *Arch Neurol Physiol.* 1944; 51:1-26. (183, 185)

I10.   Drez D, Faust DC, Evans IP. Cryotherapy and nerve palsy. *Am J Sports Med.* 1981; 9:256-257. (96, 185, 188)

I11.   Edholm OG, Fox RH, Lewis HE, MacPherson HE. Cold injury. *J Physiol.* 1957; 139:14P-15P. (184)

I12.   Elliot FA. *Clinical Neurology.* 2nd ed. Philadelphia, PA: WB Saunders Co; 1961. (187)

I13.   Escher S, Tucker A. Preventing, diagnosing, and treating cold urticaria. *Physician Sportsmed.* December 1992; 20:73-84. (190)

I14.   Franks F, Mathias SF, hatley RHM. Water, temperature and life. *Philos Trans R Soc Long.* 1990; 326:517-533. (182)

I15.   Fuhrman FA. Experimental frostbite: oxygen consumption and anaerobic glycolysis of rat tissues after freezing and colling in vitro. *J Appl Physiol.* 1957; 10:244-230. (183)

I16.   Gage AA. What temperature is lethal for cells? *J Dermatol Surg Oncol.* 1979; 5:459-460. (182, 183)

I17.   Geller M. Cold-induced cholinergic urticaria: case report. *Ann Allergy.* 1989; 63:29-30. (190)

I18.   Goldberg EE, Pittman DR. Cold sensitivity syndrome. *Ann Intern Med.* 1959; 50:505-511. (188, 190)

I19.   Granberg PO. Freezing cold injury. *Arctic Med Res.* 1991; 50(suppl 6):76-79. (182, 183)

I20.   Green GA, Zachazewski JE, Jordan SE. Peroneal nerve palsy induced by cryotherapy. *Physician Sportsmed.* September 1989; 17:63-70. (183, 185)

I21.   Harvey CK. An overview of cold injuries. *J Am Podiatr Med Assoc.* 1992; 82:436-438. (184, 185, 188, 190)

I22.   Hirvonen J. Vital reactions to frostbite of the ear and paw skin in guinea pigs exposed to the cold. *Z Rechtsmed.* 1990; 103:249-256. (182)

I23.   Juhlin L, Shelley WB. Role of most cell and basophil in cold urticaria with associated systemic reactions. *JAMA.* 1961; 177:371-377. (188)

I24.   Keahey TM, Indrisano J, Kaliner MA. A case study on the induction of clinical tolerance in cold urticaria. *J Allergy Clin Immunol.* 1988; 82:256-261. (188, 190)

I25.   Keatinge WR, Cannon P. Freezing point of human skin. *Lancet.* 1960; 1:11-14. (181)

I26.   Kegerreis S. The construction and implementation of functional progressions as a component of athletic rehabilitation. *J Orthop Sports Phys Ther.* 1983; 5:14-19. (46)

I27.   Kreyberg L. Local freezing. *Proc R Soc.* 1957; 147:546-547. (183)

I28.   Kulka JP. Cold injury of the skin. *Arch Environ Health.* 1965; 11:484-497. (183)

I29.   Kulka JP. Microcirculatory impairment as a factor in inflammatory tissue damage. *Ann NY Acad Sci.* 1964; 116:1018-1044. (183)

I30.   Lewis T, Love WS. Vascular reactions of the skin to injury. Part III. Some effects of freezing, of cooling, and of warming. *Heart.* 1926; 13:27-60. (122, 183)

I31.   Lyons R. Bicycle ergometer for injured athletes. *Physician Sportsmed.* August 1974; 2:65. (54)

I32.   Malone Tr, Englehardt DL, Kirkpatrick JS, Bassett FH III. Nerve injury in athletes caused by cryotherapy. *J Athl Train.* 1992; 27:235-237. (85, 185, 188)

I33.   Maltby NH, Ind PW, Causon RC, Fuller RW, Taylor GW. Leukotriene E$_4$ release in cold urticaria. *Clin Exp Allergy.* 1989; 19:33-36. (188)

I34.   Meryman HT. Mechanism of freezing injury in clinical frostbite. In: Viereck EG, ed. *Proceedings, Symposia on Arctic Biology and Medicine, IV: Frostbite.* Washington, DC: Office of Technical Services, US Dept of Commerce; 1964:1-11. (182, 188)

I35.   Meryman HT. Tissue freezing and local cold injury. *Physiol Rev.* 1957; 37:233-251. (114, 180-182)

I36.   Molnar GW, Hughes AL, Wilson O, Goldman RF. Effect of skin wetting on finger cooling and freezing. *J Appl Physiol.* 1973; 35:205-207. (182)

I37.   Molnar GW, Wilson O, Goldman RF. Analysis of events leading to frostbite. *Int J Biometeor.* 1972; 16:247-258. (157, 183)

I38.   Morton R, Porovins KA. Finger numbness after acute local exposure to cold. *J Appl Physiol.* 1960; 15:149-154. (177)

I39.   Mundth ED. Studies on the pathogenesis of cold injury, microcirculatory changes in tissue injured by freezing. In: Vilreck EG, ed. *Proceedings, Symposia on Artic Biology and Medicine, IV: Frostbite.* Washington, DC: Office of Technical Services, US Dept of Commerce; 1964:51-72. (182)

I40.   Neittaanmaki H. Cold Urticaria. *J Am Acad Dermatol.* 1985; 13:636-644. (188)

141. Nelson SL, Lassen NA. Measurement of digital blood pressure after local cooling. *J Appl Physiol.* 1977; 43:907-910. (191)

142. Nukada H, Pollock M, Allpress S. Experimental cold injury to peripheral nerve. *Brain.* 1981; 104:779-811. (187)

143. Ormerod AD, Kobza-Black A, Dawes J, Murdoch RD, Koro O, Barr RM, Greaves MW. Prostaglandin D2 and histamine release in cold urticaria unaccompanied by evidence of platelet activation. *J Allergy Clin Immunol.* 1988; 82:586-589. (188)

144. Ormerod AD, Kobza-Black A, Milford-Ward A, Greaves MW. Combined cold urticaria: clinical characterization and laboratory findings. *Br J Dermatol.* 1988; 118:621-627. (190)

145. Page EH, Shear NH. Temperature-dependent skin disorders. *J Am Acad Dermatol.* 1988; 18:1003-1019. (180, 182, 184, 185, 190, 191)

146. Parker JT, Small NC, Davis PG. Cold-induced nerve palsy. *Athl Train.* 1983; 18:76. (185, 188)

147. Pegg DE. Mechanisms of freezing damage. *Symp Soc Exp Biol.* 1987; 41:363-378. (182)

148. Pegg DE, Diaper MP. On the mechanism of injury to slowly frozen erythrocytes. *Biophys J.* 1988; 54:471-488. (182)

149. Perry TM, Miller FN. *Pathology: A Dynamic Introduction to Medicine and Surgery.* 2nd ed. Boston, MA: Little Brown & Co; 1971:219. (182)

150. Post PW, Daniels F Jr, Binford RT Jr. Cold injury and the evolution of "white" skin. *Hum biol.* 1975; 47:65-80. (183)

151. Proulx RP. Southern California frostbite. *J Am Coll Emerg Phys.* 1976; 5:618. (96, 180, 184)

152. Reade PC. Cryosurgery in dental practice. *Int Dent J.* 1979; 29:1-11. (182)

153. Rotella RJ, Campbell MS. Systematic desensitization: psychological rehabilitation of injured athletes. *Athl Train.* 1983; 18:140-142. (55)

154. Saner HE, Wurbel H, Gurtner HP, Mahler F. Increased peripheral vasoconstrictor reaction upon local cold in patients with coronary heart disease. *Int J Microcirc Clin Exp.* 1989; 8:127-134. (191)

155. Schoning P. Frozen cadaver: antemortem versus postmortem. *Am J Forensic Med Pathol.* March 1992; 13:18-20. (183)

156. Shelley WB, Caro WA. Cold erythemia. *JAMA.* 1962; 180:639-642. (188)

157. Sigler RW, Evans R III, Horakava Z, Ottesen E, Kaplan AP. The role of cyproheptadine in treatment of cold urticaria. *J Allergy Clin Immunol.* 1980; 65:309. (190)

158. Spittell JA. Raynaud's phenomenon and allied vasospastic conditions. In: Jergens JL, Spittell JA, Fairbairn JF, eds. *Allen-Barker-Hines Peripherial Vascular Diseases.* 5th ed. Philadelphia, PA: WB Saunders Co; 1980:555-583. (188, 191)

159. Spittell JA. Vascular syndromes related to environmental temperature. In: Jergens JL, Spittell JA, Fairbairn J, eds. *Allen-Barker-Hines Peripheral Vascular Diseases.* 5th ed. Philadelphia, PA: WB Saunders Co; 1980:585-605. (182)

160. Sunderland S. *Nerve and Nerve Injuries.* New York, NY: Churchill Livingstone; 1978:186-188. (131, 187)

161. Wagner WO. Urticaria: a challenge in diagnosis and treatment. *Postgrad Med.* 1988; 83:321-325. (70, 188, 190)

162. Washburn B. Frostbite: what it is, how to prevent it, emergency treatment. *N Engl J Med.* 1962; 266:974-989. (180, 181)

163. Whitaker DK. Cryosurgery of the oral mucosa: a study of the mechanism of tissue damage. *Dent Pract.* 1972; 22:2. (182)

I64. Wilson O, Goldman RF. Role of air temperature and wind in the time necessary for a finger to freeze. *J Appl Physiol.* 1970; 29: 658-664. (157, 180, 181, 183)

MISCELLANEOUS (MOSTLY NONCRYOTHERAPY)

J1. Abramson DI, Kahn A, Tuck S, Turman GA, Rejal S, Fleischer CJ. Relationship between a range of tissue temperature and local oxygen uptake in the human forearm, I: changes observed under resting conditions. *J Clin Invest.* 1958; 37:1031-1038. (123)

J2. Abramson DI, Mitchell RE, Tuck S, Bell Y, Zayas AM. Changes in blood flow, oxygen uptake, and tissue temperature produced by the topical application of wet heat. *Arch Phys Med Rehabil.* 1961; 42:305-318. (123)

J3. Allwood MJ, Burry HS. The effects of local temperature on blood flow in the human foot. *J Physiol.* 1954; 124:345-357. (117)

J4. Anderson JE, Hunt JM, Smith IE. Prevention of doxorubicin-induced alopecia by scalp cooling in patients with advanced breast cancer. *Br Med J.* 1981; 282:423-424. (254)

J5. Anshel MH, Wrisberg CA. Reducing warm-up decrement in the performance of the tennis serve. *J Sport Exerc Psychol.* 1993; 15:290-303.

J6. Arnold L. Treating menstrual cramps. *First Aider.* Oct 1983; 43:10. (134)

J7. Bancroft H, Dornhorst AC. The blood flow through the human calf during rhythmic exercise. *J Physiol.* 1949; 190:402-411. (123)

J8. Bevan R. *The Athletic Trainer's Handbook.* Englewood Cliffs, NJ: Prentice Hall; 1956:63-75. (15)

J9. Bilik SE. *The Trainer's Bible.* 8th ed. New York, NY: TJ Reed & Co; 1946:257-263. (15)

J10. Black JE. Blood flow requirements of the human calf after walking and running. *Clin Sci.* 1959; 18:89-93. (123)

J11. Costil DL. Muscle rehabilitation after knee surgery. *Physician Sportsmed.* May 1977; 5:71-84. (50)

J12. Danzier S. Ice-packs for cold-sores. *Lancet.* 1978; 1:103. (252)

J13. Dayton OW. *Athletic Training and Conditioning.* New York, NY: Ronald Press; 1960:121-127. (15, 45)

J14. Dean JC, Salmon SE, Griffin KS. Prevention of doxorubicin-induced hair loss wth scalp hypothermia. *N Engl J Med.* 1979; 301:1427-1429. (254)

J15. Dehn E, Torp RP. Treatment of joint injuries by immediate mobilization. *Clin Orthop.* 1971; 77:218-231. (8, 10, 17, 47, 50, 92, 173)

J16. DeLee JC. Tissue remodeling and response to therapeutic exercises. In: Leadbetter WB, Buckwalter JA, Gordon SL, eds. *Sports-Induced Inflammation.* Chicago, Ill: American Academy of Orthopaedic Surgeons; 1990:547-554. (37, 40)

J17. Delorme TL. 1948; (46)

J18. DePalma MT, DePalma B: The use of instruction and the behavioral approach to facilitate injury rehabilitation *Athl Train.* 1989; 24: 217-219. (17, 45, 47)

J19. deVries HA. *Physiology of Exercise.* 4th ed, Dubuque, IA: WC Brown Publishers; 1986:297-301. (62, 68)

J20. Duffley HM, Knight KL. Ankle compression variability using the elastic wrap, elastic wrap with a horseshoe, edema II boot, and air-stirrup brace. *Athl Train.* 1989; 24:320-323. (92)

J21.   Duke PM, Reinach SG. A study to determine the effects of ice on fatigued muscle in long distance runners. *Proceedings of the 10th World Confederation for Physical Therapy, II*. Sydney: Australian Physiotherapy Association; 1987:1056-1059. (251)

J22.   Edelstyn GA, MacDonald M, MacRae KD. Doxorubicin-induced hair loss and possible modification by scalp cooling. *Lancet*. 1977; 11:253-254. Letter. (254)

J23.   Enwemeka CS. Inflammation, cellularity, and fibrillogenesis in regenerating tendon: implications for tendon rehabilitation. *Phys Ther*. 1989; 69:816-825. (38, 41, 49)

J24.   Fantone JC. Basic concepts in inflammation. In: Leadbetter WB, Buckwalter JA, Gordon SL, eds. *Sports-Induced Inflammation*. Chicago, IL: American Academy of Orthopaedic Surgeons; 1990:25-53. (21, 22, 27, 36)

J25.   Ferkel RD, Karzel RP, Pizzo WD, Friedman MJ, Fischer SP. Arthroscopic treatment of anterolateral impingement of the ankle. *Am J Sports Med*. 1991; 19:440-446. (91)

J26.   Fisher BD, Baracos VE, Shnitka TK, Mendryk SW, Reid DC. Ultrastructural events following acute muscle trauma. *Med Sci Sports Exerc*. 1900; 22:185-193. (22, 37)

J27.   Goslen JB. Wound healing for the dermatologic surgeon. *J Dermatol Surg Oncol*. 1988; 14:959-972. (37)

J28.   Greenburg RS. The effects of hot packs and exercise on local blood flow. *Phys Ther*. 1972; 52:273-278. (123)

J29.   Guyton AC. *Textbook of Medical Physiology*. 5th ed. Philadelphia, PA: WB Saunders Go; 1976:404-407. (22, 23, 34, 92)

J30.   Hudson A, Nelson R. *University Physics*. Chicago, IL: Harcourt Brace Jovanovich; 1982:420-424. (64)

J31.   Humphreys PW, Lind AR. The blood flow through active and inactive muscles of the forearm during sustained handgrip contractions. *J Physiol*. 1963; 166:120-135. (123)

J32.   Hunt TK. Disorders of wound healing. *World J Surg*. 1980; 4:271-277. (37)

J33.   Jarvinen M. Healing of a crush injury in rat striated muscle, IV: effect of early mobilization and immobilization on the tensile properties of gastrocnemius muscle. *Acta Chir Scand*. 1976; 142:47-56. (47)

J34.   Jarvinen M. Healing of a crush injury in rat striated muscle, III: a microangiographical study of the effect of early mobiliztion and immobilization on capillary in growth. *Acta Pathol Microbiol Immunol Scand*. 1976; A84:85-94, (8, 47)

J35.   Jarvinen M. Healing of a crush injury in rat striated muscle, II: a histological study of the effect of early mobilization and immobilization on the repair process. *Acta Pathol Microbiol Immunol Scand*. 1975; A83:269-282. (8, 47)

J36.   Knight KL. Guidelines for rehabilitation of sports injuries. In: Harvey JS, ed. *Clinics in Sports Medicine: Rehabilitation of the Injured Athlete*. Philadelphia, PA: WB Saunders Co; 1985; 4:405-416. (145, 50, 239)

J37.   Knight KL. Quadriceps strengthening with the DAPRE technique: case studies with neurological implications. *Med Sci Sports Exerc*. 1985; 17:646-650. (43, 50, 222)

J38.   Knight KL. Knee rehabilitation using a daily adjustable progressive resistance exercise technqiue. *Am J Sports Med*. 1979; 7:336-337. (50-52, 222, 239)

J39.   Knight KL. Total injury rehabilitation. *Physician Sportsmed*. August 1979; 7:111. (45, 47)

J40. Knott M, Voss DE. *Proprioceptive Neuromuscular Facilihtion, Patterns and Techniques.* 2nd ed. New York, NY: Harper & Row; 1968:99. (50, 233)

J41. Konradsen L, Holmer P, Sondergaard L. Early mobilizing treatment for grade III ankle ligament injuries. *Foot Ankle.* 1991; 12:69-73. (47)

J42. Kruk B, Kaciuba-Uscilko H, Nazar K, Greenleaf JE, Kozlowski S. Hypothalamic, rectal, and muscle temperatures in exercising dogs: effect of cooling. *J Appl Physiol.* 1985; 58:1444-1448. (251)

J43. Kvist H, Jarvinen M. Sorvari T. Effect of mobilization and immobilization on the healing of contusion injury in muscle: a preliminary report of a histological study in rats. *Scand J Rehabil Med.* 1974; 6:137-140. (47)

J44. Leadbetter WB. An introduciton to sports-induced soft-tissue inflammation. In Leadbetter WB, Buckwalter JA, Gordon SL, eds. *Sports-Induced Inflammation.* Chicago, IL: American Academy of Orthopaedic Surgeons; 1990:3-23. (8, 9, 22, 27, 36)

J45. Lehman JF, DeLateur BJ. Therapeutic heat. In: Lehman JF, ed. *Therapeutic Heat and Cold.* 3rd ed. Baltimore, MD: Williams & Wilkins; 1982: 404-562. (10, 175)

J46. Lephart SM, Perrin DH, Fu FH, Minger K. Functional performance tests for the anterior cruciate ligament insufficient athlete. *Athl Train.* 1991; 26:44-50. (134)

J47. Levin S. Ealry mobilization speeds recovery. *Physician Sportsmed.* August 1993; 21:70-74. (47)

J48. Martinez-Hernandez A, Amenta PS. Basic concepts in wound healing In: Leadbetter WB, Buckwalter JA, Gordon SL, eds. *Sports-Induced Inflammation.* Chicago, Ill: American Academy of Orthopaedic Surgeons; 1990:55-101. (128)

J49. Mayor MB, Biglow JR. Making a rockerboard for ankle rehabilitation. *Physician Sportsmed.* October 1991; 19:75-78. (36)

J50. McCluskey GM, Blackburn TH, Lewis T. A treatment for ankle sprains. *Am J Sports Med.* 1976; 4:158-161. (221, 222)

J51. McKeag DB. Overuse injuries: the concept in 1992. *Prim Care.* 1991; 18:851-865. (11)

J52. Milch DL. Rehabilitation exercise following inversion ankle sprains. *J Am Podiatr Med Assoc.* 1986; 76:577-580. (53)

J53. Morehead JJ. *Traumatotherapy: The Treatment of the Injured.* Philadelphia, PA: WB Saunders Co; 1931:17-18. (15)

J54. Morrissey MC. Reflex inhibition of thigh muscles in knee injury: causes and treatment. Sports Med. 1989; 7:263-276. (49)

J55. Nathan PW. The gate control theory of pain. *Brain.* 1976; 99:123-148. (124)

J56. National Safety Council. *First Aid and CPR.* Boston, MA: Jones and Bartlett Publishers; 1991. (94, 180)

J57. Niinikoski J. Effect of oxygen supply on wound healing and formation of experimental grandulation tissue. *Acta Physiol Scand.* 1969. Suppl. 334:1-72. (41)

J58. Olschewski H, Bruck K. Thermoregulatory, cardiovascular, and muscular factors related to exercise after precooling. *J Appl Physiol.* 1988; 64:803-811. (251)

J59. Omega International Corporation. *The Temperature Handbook.* Standford, CT: Omega International Corp; 1991; 27:29-228. (61)

J60. Peppard A. Trigger-point therapy for myofascial pain. *Physician Sportsmed.* June 1981; 9:161-162. (246)

J61. Prentice BE. Acupressure massage to relieve menstrual cramps. *Physician Sportsmed.* March 1981; 9:171. (233, 243)

J62.   Prizmetal M, Wilson C. The nature of the peripheral resistance in arterial hypertension with special reference to the vasomotor system. *J Clin Sci.* 1936; 15:63-83. (123)

J63.   Quirion A, Boisvert P, Brisson GR, DeCarufel D, Laurencelle L, Dulac S, Vogelaere P, Therminarias A. Physiological adjustments of facial cooling during exercise. *J Sports Med Phys Fitness.* 1990; 30:264-267. (251)

J64.   Rx for overheating. *Popular Sci.* February 1992; 96:19. (252)

J65.   Ryan JB, Hopkinson WJ, Wheeler JH, Arciero RA, Swain JH. Office management of the acute ankle sprain. *Clin Sports Med.* 1989; 8:477-495. (53)

J66.   Sapega AA, Quedenfeld TC, Moyer RA, Butler RA. Biological factors in range-of-motion exercise. *Physician Sportsmed.* December 1981; 9:57-65. (50, 175, 249, 251)

J67.   Schurman DJ, Goodman SB, Smith RL. Inflammation and tissue repair. In: Leadbetter WB, Buckwalter JA, Gordon SL, eds. *Sports-Induced Inflammation.* Chicago, IL: American Academy of Orthopaedic Surgeons; 1990:547-554. (36)

J68.   Serway RA, Faughn JS. *College Physics.* Philadelphia, PA: WB Saunders Col; 1989: 279-289. (64)

J69.   Silver IA. The measurement of oxygen tension in healing tissue. *Progr Resp Res.* 1969; 3:124-135. (38)

J70.   Stanish WD. Overuse injuries in athletes: a perspective. *Med Sci Sports Exerc.* 1983; 16:1-7. (11)

J71.   Strandness DE. Exercise testing in the evaluation of patients undergoing direct arterial surgery. *J Cardiovasc Surg.* 1970; 11:192-200. (123)

J72.   Sumner DS, Strandness DE. The relationship between calf blood flow and ankle pressure in patients with intermittent claudication. *Surgery.* 1969; 65:763-771. (123)

J73.   Thomas CL, ed. *Taber's Cyclopedic Medical Dictionary.* 16th ed. Philadelphia, Pa: FA Davis Co; 1989. (60, 150, 163, 172, 174, 180-182, 184, 188, 191)

J74.   Thorsson O, Hemdal B, Lilja B, Westlin N. The effect of external pressure on intramuscular blood flow at rest and after running. *Med Sci Sport Exerc.* 1987; 19:469-473. (187)

J75.   Thorsson O, Ahlgren L, Hemdal B, Lilja B, Westlin N. The effect of local cold application on intramuscular blood flow are rest and after running. *Med Sci Sport Exerc.* 1985; 17:710-713. (68, 117)

J76.   Timothy AR, Bates TD, Hoy AM. Influence of scalp hypothermia on doxorubicin related alopedia. *Lancet.* 1980; 1:663. Letter. (254)

J77.   Tonnesen KH. Blood flow through muscle during rhythmic contraction measured by 133 Xenon. *Scand J Clin Lab Invest.* 1964; 16: 646-654. (123)

J78.   Toomey SJ. Four-square ankle rehabilitation exercises. *Physician Sportsmed.* September 1986; 14:281. (185, 224)

J79.   Trott A. Mechanisms of surface soft tissue trauma. *Ann Emerg Med.* 1988; 17:1279-1283. (180, 184)

J80.   Williams S, Hecker JF, Effect of glyceryl trinitrate and ice on dilaton of hand veins. *Anaesthesia.* 1991; 46:14-16. (246)

J81.   Willis WD, Grossman RC. *Medical Neurobiology.* St Louis, MO: CV Mosby; 1973. (128)

J82.   Hargens AR (Ed): Tissue, Fluid, Pressure, and Composition. Baltimore: Williams & Wilkins, 1981, p. 31. (34)

J83.   Ehrlick HP, Grislis C, Hunt TK. Metabolic and circulatory contributions to oxygen gradients in wounds. Surgery. 1972:578-583. (40)

Author Index

Subject Index

Credits

Figure 3.4 is from *Aspects of Acute Inflammation* (p. 18), by A.G. MacLeod, 1969, Kalamazoo, MI: Upjohn Company. Copyright 1973 by Upjohn Company. Reprinted with permission.

Figure 3.6 is from *Aspects of Acute Inflammation* (p. 19), by A.G. MacLeod, 1969, Kalamazoo, MI: Upjohn Company. Copyright 1973 by Upjohn Company. Reprinted with permission.

Figure 3.9 is from *Aspects of Acute Inflammation* (p. 35), by A.G. MacLeod, 1969, Kalamazoo, MI: Upjohn Company. Copyright 1973 by Upjohn Company. Reprinted with permission.

Figure 3.23 is from "The Measurement of Oxygen Tension in Healing Tissue," by I.A. Silver, 1969, Progress in Respiration Research, 3, pp. 124-135. Copyright 1969 by S. Karger.

Figure 3.24 is from "Measurement of Wound Oxygen with Implanted Silastic Tube," by J. Niinikoski and T.K. Hunt, 1972, Surgery, 71, pp. 22-26. Copyright 1972 by Mosby-Year Book, Inc. Reprinted with permission.

Figure 5.6 is from "The Effects of Ice and Compression Wraps on Intramuscular Temperatures at Various Depths," by M.A. Merrick, K.L. Knight, C.D. Ingersoll, and J.A. Potteiger, 1993, *Journal of Athletic Training*, 28, pp. 236-245. Copyright 1993 by National Athletic Trainers' Association, Inc. Reprinted with permission.

Figure 5.7 is from "The Physiologic Effects of Ice Massage," by G.W. Waylonis, 1967, *Archives of Physical Medicine and Rehabilitation*, 48, pp. 37-42. Copyright 1967 by W.B. Saunders Co. Reprinted with permission.

Figure 5.8 is from "Ice Therapy in Spasticity," by K. Hartviksen, 1962, Acta Neurologica Scandinavica, Supplementum, 38(3). Copyright 1962 by Munksgaard. Reprinted with permission.

Figure 5.9 is from "Rewarming of the Ankle, Finger, and Forearm After Cryotherapy," by K. Knight and J.F. Elam, 1981, *Journal of the Canadian Athletic Therapy Association*, 8(3), pp. 17-18. Copyright 1981 by the Canadian Athletic Therapy Association. Reprinted with permission.

Figure 6.1 is from *Clinical Hypothermia*, by E. Blair, 1964, New York: McGraw Hill. Copyright 1964 by McGraw Hill.

Figure 6.2 is from "The Influence of Temperature in Fibril's Stability on Degradation of Cartilage Collagen by Rheumatoid Synovial Collagenase," by E.D. Harris, and P.A. McCroskery, 1974, *New England Journal of Medicine*, 290, pp. 1-6. Copyright 1974 by Massachusetts Medical Society. Reprinted with permission.

Figure 7.2 is from "Effects of Hypothermia on Inflammation and Swelling," by K.L. Knight, 1976, *Journal of Athletic Training*, 11, pp. 7-10. Copyright 1976 by National Athletic Trainers' Association, Inc. Reprinted with permission.

Figure 9.1 is from "Observations upon the Reactions of the Vessels of the Human Skin to Cold," by T. Lewis, 1930, *American Heart*, 15, pp. 177-208. Copyright 1930 by Mosby-Year Book, Inc.

Figure 9.6 is from "A Re-examination of Lewis' Cold-induced Vasodilation in the Finger and the Ankle," by K.L. Knight, J. Aquino, S.M. Johannes, and C.D. Urban, 1980, *Journal of Athletic Training*, 15, pp. 248-250. Copyright 1980 by National Athletic Trainers' Association, Inc. Reprinted with permission.

Figure 9.7 is from "Effects of Wearing a Toe Cap or a Sock on Temperature and Perceived Pain During Ice Water Immersion," by P.S.R. Nimchick, and K.L. Knight, 1983, *Journal of Athletic Training*, 18, pp. 144-147. Copyright 1983 by National Athletic Trainers' Association, Inc. Reprinted with permission.

Figure 9.8 is from "Measurement of Reactive Vasodilation During Cold Gel Pack Application to Nontraumatized Ankles," by C. Taber, K. Countryman, J. Fahrenbruch, K. LaCount, and M.W. Cornwall, 1992, *Physical Therapy Journal*, 72, pp. 294-299. Copyright 1992 by American Physical Therapy Association. Reprinted with permission.

Figure 9.9 is from "Vascular Reactions of the Human Forearm to Cold," by R.S.J. Clarke, R.F. Hellon, and A.R. Lind, 1958, *Clinical Science*, 17, pp. 165-179. Copyright 1958 by Portland Press Ltd.

Figure 9.12 is from "Effect of Tissue Temperature and Blood Flow on Motor Nerve Conduction Velocity," by D.I. Abramson, L.S.W. Chu, S. Tuck Jr., S.W. Lee, G. Richardson, and M. Levin, 1966, *Journal of the American Medical Association*, 198, pp. 1082-1088. Copyright 1966 by American Medical Association. Reprinted with permission.

Figure 10.1 is from "Cutaneous Thermoreceptors in Primates and Sub-primates," by A. Iggo, 1969, *Journal of Physiology*, 200, pp. 403-430. Copyright 1953 by The Physiological Society. Reprinted with permission.

Figure 10.2 is from "Special Senses: Thermal Receptors," by Y. Zotterman, 1953, *Annual Reviews in Physiology*, 15, pp. 357-372. Copyright 1953 by The American Physiological Society. Reprinted with permission.

Figure 10.3 is from "Changes of Sensory Conduction Velocity and Refractory Periods with Decreasing Tissue Temperature in Man," by K. Lowitzsch, H.C. Hopf, and J. Galland, 1977, *Journal of Neurology*, pp. 181-188. Copyright 1977 by Springer-Verlag New York. Reprinted with permission.

Figure 10.5 is from "Nerve Conduction Velocity: Relationship of Skin, Subcutaneous Intramuscular Termperatures," by E.M. Halar, J.A. DeLisa, and F. Brozovich, 1980, *Archives of Physical Medicine and Rehabilitation*, 61, pp. 199-203. Copyright 1980 by W.B. Saunders Co. Reprinted with permission.

Figure 10.6 is from "Effects of Ice on Nerve Conduction and Velocity," by J.M. Lee, M.P. Warren, and S.M. Mason, 1978, *Physiotherapy*, 64, pp. 1-6. Copyright 1978 by Physiotherapy: Journal of the Chartered Society of Physiotherapy. Reprinted with permission.

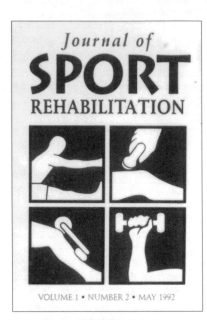
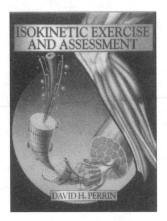
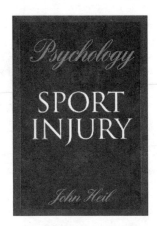